Diversity in Action

Steve H. Koh • Gabriela G. Mejia
Hilary M. Gould
Editors

Diversity in Action

Case Studies in Cultural Psychiatry

Springer

Editors
Steve H. Koh
Department of Psychiatry
University of California San Diego
San Diego, CA, USA

Gabriela G. Mejia
Department of Psychiatry
University of California San Diego
San Diego, CA, USA

Hilary M. Gould
Department of Psychiatry
University of California San Diego
San Diego, CA, USA

ISBN 978-3-030-85400-3 ISBN 978-3-030-85401-0 (eBook)
https://doi.org/10.1007/978-3-030-85401-0

This Springer imprint is published by the registered company Springer Nature Switzerland AG
The registered company address is: Gewerbestrasse 11, 6330 Cham, Switzerland

Contents

Contributors

Philip J. Candilis, MD, DFAPA Department of Psychiatry and Behavioral Sciences, George Washington University School of Medicine and Health Sciences, Washington, DC, USA

Saint Elizabeths Hospital, Washington, DC, USA

Nancy Catherine Colimon-Ardila, MD Nuevo Atardecer, Geriatric Center, Mexicali, BC, Mexico

Gregory Evangelatos, MD Department of Psychiatry, Kaweah Delta Medical Center, Visalia, CA, USA

Omar Ghosn, MD Department of Psychiatry, University of California San Diego, San Diego, CA, USA

Mollie Gordon, MD Menninger Department of Psychiatry and Behavioral Sciences, Baylor College of Medicine, Bellaire, TX, USA

Kimberly Gordon-Achebe, MD Department of Psychiatry & Behavioral Sciences, Tulane University School of Medicine, New Orleans, LA, USA

University of Maryland, New Orleans, LA, USA

Hilary M. Gould, PhD Department of Psychiatry, University of California San Diego, San Diego, CA, USA

Donald M. Hilty, MD, MBA Mental Health Service, Northern California Veterans Administration Health Care System, Mather, CA, USA

Department of Psychiatry & Behavioral Sciences, University of California Davis, Sacramento, CA, USA

Alan Hsu, MD Department of Psychiatry, VA San Diego Healthcare System/ University of California San Diego, San Diego, CA, USA

Steven Huege, MD, MSEd Department of Psychiatry, University of California San Diego, San Diego, CA, USA

Steve H. Koh, MD, MPH, MBA Department of Psychiatry, University of California San Diego, San Diego, CA, USA

Sanaz Kumar, MD Department of Psychiatry and Behavioral Sciences, George Washington University School of Medicine and Health Sciences, Washington, DC, USA

Rahul Lauhan, MD Department of Psychiatry, VA San Diego Healthcare System/ University of California San Diego, San Diego, CA, USA

Christine Le, MD Department of Psychiatry, Kaweah Delta Medical Center, Visalia, CA, USA

Jeanne Maglione, MD Department of Psychiatry, VA San Diego Healthcare System/University of California San Diego, San Diego, CA, USA

Gabriela G. Mejia, BS Department of Psychiatry, University of California San Diego, San Diego, CA, USA

Aaron Meyer, MD Department of Psychiatry, University of California San Diego, San Diego, CA, USA

Bernardo Ng, MD, FAPA Department of Psychiatry, University of California San Diego, San Diego, CA, USA

Sun Valley Behavioral Medical and Research Centers, Imperial, CA, USA

Nuevo Atardecer, Geriatric Center, Mexicali, BC, Mexico

Mexican Psychiatric Association, Mexico City, Mexico

David Nissan, MD Department of Psychiatry, Naval Medical Center San Diego, San Diego, CA, USA

Priti Ojha, MD Department of Psychiatry, University of California San Diego, San Diego, CA, USA

Joanna Ortega, MPH Department of Psychiatry and Behavioral Sciences, University of California Davis, Sacramento, CA, USA

Teresa Pan, PhD Department of Psychiatry, VA San Diego Healthcare System/ University of California San Diego, San Diego, CA, USA

Rachel Ann Paul, LCSW Department of Psychiatry, Rady Children's Hospital, San Diego, CA, USA

Rachel Robitz, MD Department of Psychiatry and Behavioral Sciences, University of California Davis, Sacramento, CA, USA

Daniel D. Sewell, MD Department of Psychiatry, University of California San Diego, San Diego, CA, USA

Juan Sosa, MD Department of Psychiatry, Kaweah Delta Medical Center, Visalia, CA, USA

Hannah Cherian Sweet, MD UCSD Division of Child & Adolescent Psychiatry, Rady Children's Hospital, San Diego, CA, USA

Jessica Thackaberry, MD Department of Psychiatry, University of California San Diego, San Diego, CA, USA

G. Andrew Valasquez, MD Department of Psychiatry, Kaweah Delta Medical Center, Visalia, CA, USA

Savannah L. Woodward, MD Department of Psychiatry, Naval Medical Center San Diego, San Diego, CA, USA

Introduction 1

Hilary M. Gould, Gabriela G. Mejia, and Steve H. Koh

As a medical specialty often referred to as an art, psychiatry requires creative approaches to assessing and treating patients with complicated histories across contexts. As each individual's mental health experience is different within one's cultural construct, it is important to weigh how mental illness presents in specific cultural settings [1]. The field of psychiatry has advanced significantly from utilizing a purely western perspective to interpret behavioral presentations to incorporating concepts of cultural competency and cultural humility [2].

Cultural psychiatry is a discipline formed out of medicine, anthropology, and social psychology. Relative to other disciplines, it is a young and developing field. The American Psychiatric Association initially focused on evaluating "cultural bound syndromes" and symptoms experienced by non-majority populations through a westernized and colonial lens [3]. This comparative approach focused on the "exotic other." Culture was defined as a specific unit characterized by a group's race, ethnicity, country of origin, and/or social status. As the field of cultural psychiatry evolved, training and education emphasized understanding the cultural context of specific mental illnesses and providing appropriate psychiatric care in ethnically diverse populations. Psychiatric diagnoses and symptoms therefore are not strictly biological and are influenced by experiences and environments, including transmission of generational norms and cultural manifestations of mental illness. Clinical treatments address wide-ranging issues, such as bereavement after loss, psychiatric sequelae of stigmatized subgroups, and the care of individuals with serious mental illness. More recently, there has been a shift toward reducing inequities and understanding the larger structural and systemic contributions affecting mental health prevalence and manifestation.

In a modern and globalized world, a broader idea of culture has developed. Beginning in the twentieth century, anthropologists expanded their studies of

H. M. Gould · G. G. Mejia · S. H. Koh (✉)
Department of Psychiatry, University of California San Diego, San Diego, CA, USA
e-mail: hgould@health.ucsd.edu; ggmejia@health.ucsd.edu; shkoh@health.ucsd.edu

S. H. Koh et al. (eds.), *Diversity in Action*,
https://doi.org/10.1007/978-3-030-85401-0_1

village communities to industrial enterprises. They used ethnographic principles to examine workforce, college campuses, labor unions, prisons, and other groups that shared a common cultural system. The study of these groups helped provide an understanding of unique dynamics and hierarchies, how organizational principles evolved over time, and the relationship between the institution and larger society. Inherent in this framework is a recognition that cultural worlds are "temporary, ever-changing constructions that emerge from interactions between individuals, communities, and larger ideologies and institutional practices" [4].

Furthermore, in clinical practice, it is critical to not focus exclusively on the dyadic cultural differences between the psychiatrist and the patient. The larger environment or cultural context in which the two individuals interact must be understood to provide optimal care. This larger context extends beyond the physical space (e.g., outpatient clinical practice versus hospital-based consult liaison practice) and is influenced by legal and institutional constructs (e.g., legal aspects involved in human trafficking or military culture). It is not sufficient to deliver psychiatric care without an understanding of the larger construct within which a patient exists. Therefore, throughout this book, a broad view of culture is used when presenting research, clinical case examples, and training recommendations across unique settings and patient populations. It is hoped that the reader will benefit from understanding the dynamic aspect of a culture which spans beyond racial and ethno-specifics of our patients and encompasses the larger context in which we find them.

Cultural Constructs in the DSM-5

The fifth edition of the *Diagnostic and Statistical Manual of Mental Disorders* [5] incorporates more elements of culturally competent care than any previous edition of the manual. The DSM-IV listed culture-bound syndromes (i.e., pattern of aberrant behaviors that are localized to a specific society or culture, such as *ataque de nervios*), while the current edition dedicates more thoughtful and updated context to cultural presentations. It includes a clinical interview tool (i.e., "Cultural Formulation Interview," CFI) and describes elements critical to culturally sensitive diagnoses and care (e.g., "Glossary of Cultural Concepts of Distress"). Recommendations include attending to cultural factors when contemplating specific diagnoses. For example, considering primary language when diagnosing specific learning disorders or intellectual disabilities, understanding religious beliefs and practices when psychotic symptoms are present, and appreciating trends unique to certain cultural groups regarding over or underemphasized cognitive or somatic complaints. Rather than the notion of the culture-bound syndrome from older editions of the DSM, three new concepts are presented in the DSM-5: (1) cultural syndrome, or symptoms found in specific cultural groups; (2) cultural idioms of distress, the shared way of communicating suffering; and (3) cultural explanations, the perceived cause(s) and etiology of symptoms [5].

The DSM-5 defines culture as "systems of knowledge, concepts, rules, and practices that are learned and transmitted across generations. Culture includes language, religion and spirituality, family structures, life-cycle stages, ceremonial rituals, and customs, as well as moral and legal systems" [5]. This definition primarily focuses on cultures specific to race/ethnicity and country of origin. The CFI includes 16 questions intended to highlight key elements of the patient's cultural identity (e.g., values, orientations, knowledge, practices, geographical origin, migration, language, religion, sexual orientation, race/ethnicity, developmental experiences), their social network's influence as sources of stress or support, cultural interpretations of presenting symptoms, and factors affecting help-seeking behavior [5]. Cultural considerations are deemed critical for evidence-based psychiatric care, including enhancing the therapeutic relationship, accurately diagnosing disorders, obtaining relevant clinical information (e.g., coping strategies), and improving efficacy of treatments.

Definition of Culture to Improve Clinical Care

In the modern world, culture has multiple meanings that affect understanding and applications in psychiatry [6]. Throughout this book, chapter authors define culture broadly and explore several aspects of social behavior and norms, including attitudes, beliefs, habits, rituals, behaviors, values, interactions, language, knowledge, and stories as depicted in Fig. 1.1. Inherent in its definition is

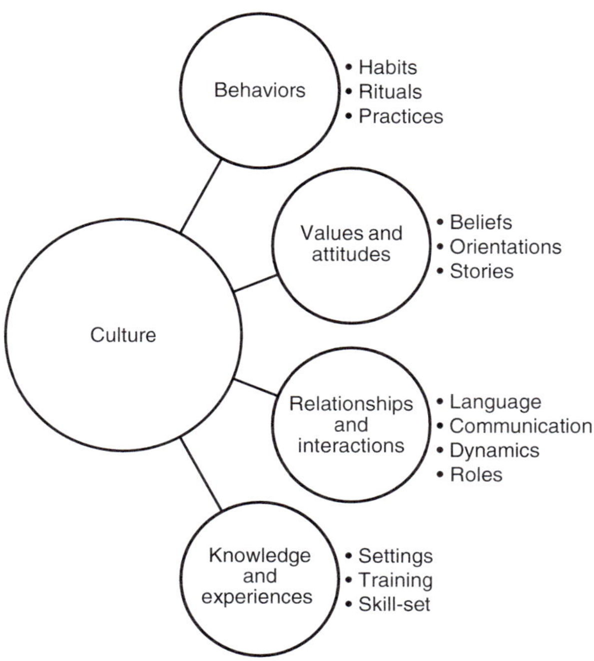

Fig. 1.1 Schematic of elements that define culture

recognition that culture has both external and internal representations [7]. External representations encompass institutions, traditions, and activities. In contrast, internal representations include interpretations, ascribed meaning, and importance set by the individual. Culture affects all aspects of mental health care delivery, including identification of a problem, acceptable treatment options, and access to services.

In addition to examining specific subgroups with shared backgrounds, chapter authors will aim to look at cultures across experiences and settings. For example, anthropologists have studied psychiatry training as assimilation into a shared cultural organization [8]. In a department of psychiatry, there is a unique culture of shared characteristics passed down from experts in the field, as well as faculty, prior trainees, and cohort members in the university and hospital settings. This "culture" of academic psychiatry encompasses language (e.g., psychiatric terminology), interests and values (e.g., improving patient outcomes), training backgrounds and skill sets (e.g., medical school and residency), beliefs (e.g., medical model and scientific method), habits and daily rituals (e.g., meetings and sessions), and so on. There are subgroups within the larger cultural group, such as residents, attendings, allied health professionals, and administrative support; those who work in inpatient, consult-liaison, outpatient, or research settings; and those in general clinics/tracks compared to specialized or disorder-specific clinics or research laboratories. While these subcultures exist, the group members may be further categorized by membership to other subgroups, identities, and cultures that they may share with their colleagues (e.g., race, class, sexual orientation, gender identity, age). Individuals are not limited to one cultural group and instead are often impacted by the intersection of several cultural identities coupled with their unique experiences and interpretations.

Cultural groups are constantly changing in response to both internal and external factors derived from shared experiences. For example, although generational transmission of cultural norms is inherent in the definition, other local and global changes of the era contribute to adaptations in cultural beliefs and practices. Even the authors of the DSM-5 echo this sentiment, "like culture and DSM itself, cultural concepts may change over time in response to both local and global influences" [5]. Using the department of psychiatry example, residents 10 years ago are likely quite different from present day residents due to a number of local (e.g., current leadership within the department) and large-scale external factors (e.g., less national stigma around mental health, advances in treatments). These factors can span across space and time to include geographical regions, time, historical events, and political ethos.

Current and emerging leaders in cultural psychiatry examine institutions and larger concepts, including community and population health, systems of care, and models of healthcare delivery. Cultural factors affect access to and quality of care in nearly every country, such that minority groups are subject to lower standards of care. By attending to these larger contextual factors, there is a call for focus on equity, appropriate service delivery models, and contribution to political justice [9]. Table 1.1 outlines key constructs related to cultural psychiatry. Additionally, scholars posit the importance of a historical and politically informed perspective to better

Table 1.1 Key constructs of cultural psychiatry

Cultural psychiatry constructs
Public and community systems of care
Cultural variability in expression and understanding of symptoms
Culturally competent care and adaptations to delivery of services
Mental health inequities
Globalization

inform global mental health as the world further shrinks and diversity in those that we care for becomes the norm [10, 11]. The importance of these issues cannot be overstated when evaluating how to best care for our patients. As mental health professionals, we are often relied on to know about behavioral health insurance coverage, available social supports in a community, how to best navigate a complicated behavioral health network, and patients' legal environment. Some may argue that these elements are not within a psychiatrist's scope. However, the reality is that our patient's clinical presentation and the best treatment modalities exist in the context of the larger cultural constructs that surround them. A patient in a primary care setting, for example, may present their psychiatric symptoms differently than in a psychiatric environment. An active duty military patient may understand their symptoms differently and mistrust civilian medical providers. Interaction with the legal system in context of asylum seeking process may change the ways in which a torture victim expresses their distress. Patients living in two different countries likely differ in the resources available for their care. As we intersect with colleagues, we also need to be mindful of how to best communicate and collaborate within their cultural norms. A psychiatrist's interactions with chaplains or patients with strong religious beliefs will likely vary significantly from how one would best provide care in a largely primary care delivery environment. By understanding the importance of different cultural constructs in which care is being delivered, we can best tailor the approach to benefit our patients.

Culture and Mental Health Conceptual Model

Culture affects the manifestation, development, and treatment response of mental health illness via multiple pathways. Generally, cultural factors are not considered "etiological agents of mental illness," or direct causes of psychiatric disorders, but instead pathogenic factors or etiopathogenic interactions which fit within our biopsychosocial framework [1]. It has been well documented that mental health inequities are present and influenced by a combination of systemic and structural systems, as well as exposure to adverse childhood experiences and environmental stressors. While the geopolitical and cultural context of where these stressors take place may affect the development of mental health symptoms, exposure to traumatic situations or chronic stress are universal triggers. Furthermore, culture affects more than just the prevalence of psychiatric illnesses. Stigmatization of mental health, or disapproval and discrimination toward the individual, greatly

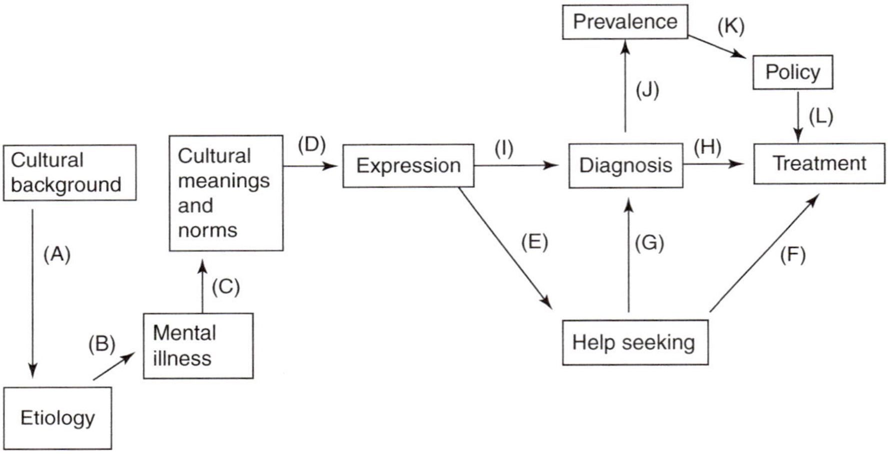

Fig. 1.2 Hwang and colleagues Cultural Influences on Mental Health (CIMH) model. (*Reproduced with permission from:* Hwang et al. [12])

affects the severity of illness and treatment outcomes. Identified supported means of healing can affect outcomes in both positive and negative ways. Given the broad, complex, and variable definitions of culture, few models have been posited to establish and understand the directionality and intersectionality between psychopathology and culture.

The Cultural Influences on Mental Health (CIMH) model provides a framework for how culture permeates and influences several core domains of the psychiatric illness process. Hwang and colleagues suggest several pathways relating how cultural background affects etiology of mental illness and how cultural meanings and norms influence expression of illness. They then relate symptom expression to both diagnosis and help-seeking behaviors, and how both issues, along with prevalence and policy, ultimately affect treatment outcomes [12]. The CIMH model is depicted in Fig. 1.2. The model considers the effects of generational traumas and acculturative stress (e.g., linguistic difficulties, pressures to assimilate, separation from family, experiences with discrimination) [12]. Conceptualization of the many complex ways that culture can impact mental health expression, identification, diagnosis, treatment, and outcomes is essential for the field of psychiatry.

Training and Education

Cultural competence is a journey, not a destination [13, 14]. No one can ever truly reach terminal "competence" in appreciating, integrating, and understanding cultural differences for all people and settings. Instead, as Cross and colleagues wrote, "becoming culturally competent is a developmental process for the individual and for the system. It is not something that happens because one reads a book, attends a workshop, or happens to be a member of a minority group. It is a process born of a commitment to provide quality services to all" [13]. Exposure to diverse groups including patients, colleagues, and faculty is essential to training and education. Additional strategies for increasing clinicians' cultural competence are presented throughout several chapters in the book, and key strategies and tools are outlined in Table 1.2.

Medical trainees and clinicians should also reflect on their own cultural identities, assumptions, and interactions with patients. They should evaluate weaknesses in their knowledge and willingness to collaborate with cultural brokers and people with lived experience to enhance clinical delivery and care. Additionally, "it is best to frame issues of cultural difference not simply in terms of the characteristics of patients or communities, but in terms of differences in the perspectives of patient and clinician in what is always, to some degree, an intercultural encounter" [4]. Every interaction with a patient is an interpersonal exchange and involves cultural

Table 1.2 Strategies and tools for trainees and clinicians to increase cultural-competence and humility

Strategies and tools	Definition
DSM-5 Cultural Formulation Interview (CFI)	Training and practice with the DSM-5 CFI [5] can be used to enhance clinical understanding and decision-making related to diagnosis and treatment. Sections include cultural definition of the problem; cultural perceptions of cause, context, and support; cultural factors affecting self-coping and past help seeking; and cultural factors affecting current help seeking
Cultural consultation/ brokers	Consult-liaison with cultural brokers or leaders/experts in their cultural group to improve patient-provider communication and understanding. The broker should be trusted in the cultural community and well versed with local knowledge, values, beliefs, and practices
Knowledge and education	Cultural competence training for healthcare providers is important to increase knowledge and sensitivity regarding systemic/structural issues, culture-specific considerations, and social determinants of health. It can also be used to teach skills, such as working with interpreters, cultivating cultural humility, and avoiding overgeneralizations
Self-reflection and awareness	Considering one's own personal identity, experience with people from diverse backgrounds, and knowledge of stereotypes/overgeneralizations. Clinicians can learn to slow down when assessing patients from different backgrounds and try to evaluate each person as an individual. This is an important topic to discuss in supervision
Implicit bias training	Taking implicit association tests, practicing self-awareness, and challenging internalized assumptions
Cultural adaptations to healthcare	Learning healthcare and psychosocial assessments and treatments tailored to specific cultural groups. For example, this may include adapting patient materials to reflect patients' culture, language, or literacy skills [15]
Exposure working with diverse patient populations	Medical education and training that offers rotations or tracks to underserved and diverse populations, such as uninsured, underinsured, migrants, rural populations, LGBTQIA+, physical disabilities, etc.
Diversity in cohort and leadership	Trainees benefit from working with colleagues, supervisors, and faculty from different cultural backgrounds and experiences
Trauma-informed care	Framework adopted at an organizational level to reflect an understanding of the widespread impact of trauma and actively seeking to prevent re-traumatization [16]. Strategies may include trauma screening, providing a safe space, and shared decision-making with patients [17]

contributions from different community groups and larger institutions. Recognizing the history and exercising cultural sensitivity is paramount to demonstrating cultural competence [18].

Lastly, equitable care relies heavily on clinicians' awareness of the limitations of psychiatric diagnosis, assessment, and treatment. There are many issues with validity of categorical psychiatric diagnoses and challenges in measurement and methodology, which may disproportionately disadvantage certain cultural groups. This may include overdiagnosing, underdiagnosing, or misdiagnosing. To improve diagnostic accuracy, Marsella and Kaplan recommend considering the following factors when choosing diagnostic screening instruments: (1) appropriate items and questions, including idioms of distress; (2) opportunities to index frequency, severity, and duration of symptoms since groups vary in their reporting within certain modes; (3) establishment of culturally relevant baselines in symptom parameters; (4) sensitivity to the mode and context of response (i.e., self-report, interview, translation issues); (5) awareness of normal behavior patterns; and (6) symptom scales should be normed and factor-analyzed for specific cultural groups [7]. Accurate screening, identification, and diagnosis are often the first step to providing equitable mental health care. Additionally, behavioral interventions are often studied in majority populations and may need to be tailored or individualized to be sensitive to the culture of an individual patient. Culturally informed adaptations to empirically supported treatments to modify language, metaphors, values, and context (while maintaining active components of interventions) have proven important to increase acceptability and efficacy of treatments [19, 20].

Survivors, Special Populations, and Systems and Settings

Throughout these chapters, authors aim to define the culture of their setting, patient population, and subspecialties within the field of psychiatry. Part I of this book covers the special population of survivors of trauma. The term *survivors* is used here rather than *victims*, denoting the cultural landscape (i.e., the term *survivors* or *victim-survivors* is often used in recovery settings, while the term *victim* is regularly used in the criminal justice system). In Chap. 2, Dr. Ojha details the experience of survivors of torture, particularly of asylees, and highlights the critical components of trauma-informed care. Next, in Chap. 3, authors Ortega, Gordon, Gordon-Achebe, and Robitz present on survivors of human trafficking, including the interconnection of structural and individual factors affecting the psychiatric illness process, such as socioeconomic status, family structure, race, gender, criminal justice, and experience of adverse childhood experiences. Finally in Chap. 4, Drs. Woodward and Nissan describe military culture, changes throughout service eras, and posttraumatic stress disorder in survivors of combat military trauma. Data on pharmacotherapy monotherapy and augmentation, as well as psychotherapy, are presented. By examining the experiences of a range of survivors of traumatic experiences, it is hoped that the reader can better understand the shared factors of etiology, trauma response, and evidence based practices, as well as the collective and unique cultural elements that comprise survivors of torture, human trafficking, and combat trauma.

The purpose of Part II of this volume is to examine special populations that often present with mental health challenges related to specific group factors or experiences. In order to optimally treat these populations, foundational knowledge and a conceptual framework for establishing assessment and treatment is required. Meyer, Mejia, and Gould present the latest research on patients with concurrent substance use and mental illness disorders. In Chap. 5, they discuss factors affecting treatment, including experienced, perceived, and internalized stigma, as well as criminalization of substances and challenges receiving appropriate treatments, such as medication-assisted therapies. In Chap. 6, Drs. Evangelatos, Valasquez, Le, Sosa, Thackaberry, and Hilty present essential components to consider when delivering telepsychiatry services to rural populations and strategies for enhancing tele modalities. Sweet and Paul discuss the role of religion and spirituality in diagnosis and treatment of patients, including positive and protective factors, in Chap. 7. They also share research on the changing role of religion in the USA and among psychiatrists. Lastly, Drs. Ng and Colimon present the historical and cultural constructs related to bicultural groups, specifically Mexicans and Americans. Research and models comparing and contrasting the two countries on religion, socioeconomic status, and the shared border regions are presented alongside a theoretical framework to understand and predict future development of biculturalism and bilingualism.

The final section of this volume, Part III, covers systems and settings that produce their own cultural environments. Patients that are treated within these larger institutions are often exposed to new cultural elements that intersect with their identities. Additionally, two of the chapters in this section discuss attempts at widespread organizational cultural change movements within healthcare systems, specifically the movement toward patient-centered care. In Chap. 9, Drs. Kumar and Candilis outline the unique challenges present while attempting to deliver optimal psychiatric care in correctional settings where the penal system's need for punishment and security must be balanced with the physician's oath to treat and rehabilitate. The authors also dissect the effects of structural racism and how to combat the continuous overrepresentation of people of color in these settings. In the case of Chap. 10, the cultural transformation of primary care is described as a shift from a traditional medical model to a collaborative care model. Drs. Pan, Lauhan, Maglione, and Hsu outline a psychiatrist's role in facilitating this model with primary care providers and how this model allows for increased shared decision-making with patients and better treatment outcomes. Lastly, in Chap. 11 Drs. Ghosn, Huege, and Sewell outline the unique cultural challenges present across the various residential care environments and the framework necessary when providing care to these older adults. They provide recommendations on how to best accommodate and integrate the patient's cultural identity within the parameters of long-term living facilities.

Clinical Case Vignettes

To help contextualize the dynamic nature that the broader culture plays in clinical practice, every chapter has one to two clinical case vignettes depicting critical aspects of a special setting, population, or experience. Across all cultures, storytelling and sharing narratives are a common and effective mode of communication. Sharing of clinical vignettes is common in scientific journals, national and international conferences, and used in training textbooks, classrooms, and exams. In addition to providing a glimpse into real-world application, personal cases are compelling and memorable. They are useful in demonstrating similarities and differences, as well as provoking critical examination and discussion across a range of issues. It is hoped that the clinical case vignette(s) and subsequent discussion in each chapter will serve as an effective tool in (1) identifying cultural context; (2) examining implications of culturally sensitive, or nonsensitive, assessment and treatment practices; and (3) creating a deeper appreciation for these special topics as they relate to patient outcomes and well-being.

From our clinical experience, a larger understanding of culture that is not limited to just the psychiatrist and the patient is required. By having a perspective of the whole person and the cultural constructs in which that patient presents in, we believe that richer and more comprehensive clinical care can be delivered. It is not simply a matter of correctly diagnosing and recommending a specific medication or type of therapy. By considering the full sum of the care delivery transaction within a cultural context, a clinician can provide a sustainable care plan that will last beyond the appointment. It allows us to be dynamic and adaptable in our clinical approach to all patients who seek help.

Conclusion and Future Directions

The clinical applications of cultural psychiatry are multifaceted. First and foremost, cultural competency and humility are fundamental in treating patients. Consideration of cultural factors should not be overly reductionistic but rather appreciated in its possible effect on a multitude of mental healthcare aspects, including idiosyncratic presentations, explanatory models of illness, and help-seeking behaviors. The historical emphasis on westernized cultures in clinical and research practices ought not to be forgotten. Secondly, appreciation for a broad view of culture beyond country of origin and race/ethnicity is recommended. Recognition that even within the field of psychiatry, there are cultural practices with traditions, orientations, and language. Interactions with mental health professionals are cultural exchanges and ultimately affect patient outcomes. Lastly, while psychiatric care is typically centered around the individual, patient's clinical presentation and the best treatment modalities are in context of the larger cultural construct that they find themselves in. Context within and between intersecting cultural groups matters. Shared experiences and generational factors may also be relevant. Systems that oppress marginalized groups and perpetuate mental illness should be identified. As globalization and institutions continue to shape the local, national, and worldwide landscape, contributions from community and population health, systems of care, and models of healthcare delivery will be critical in expanding the field of cultural psychiatry.

References

1. Alarcón RD. Cultural Psychiatry: A general perspective. In: Alarcón RD. (Ed.) Cultural Psychiatry. Basel: Karger; 2013:1–14. https://doi.org/10.1159/000348722.
2. Greene-Moton E, Minkler M. Cultural competence or cultural humility? Moving beyond the debate. Health promotion practice. 2020;21(1):142–5.
3. Shim RS. The evolution of cultural psychiatry. Psychiatr Ann. 2018;48(3):134–6.
4. Kirmayer LJ. Cultural variations in the clinical presentation of depression and anxiety: implications for diagnosis and treatment. Journal of clinical psychiatry. 2001;62:22–30.
5. American Psychiatric Association. Diagnostic and Statistical Manual of Mental Disorders. American Psychiatric Association; 2013. https://doi.org/10.1176/appi.books.9780890425596.
6. Kirmayer LJ, Ban L. Cultural psychiatry: research strategies and future directions. Cultural psychiatry. 2013;33:97–114.
7. Marsella AJ, Kaplan A. Cultural considerations for understanding, assessing, and treating depressive experience and disorder. Comparative treatments of depression. 2002:47–78.
8. Luhrmann TM. Of two minds: the growing disorder in American psychiatry. New York: Knopf; 2000.
9. Kirmayer LJ, Minas H. The future of cultural psychiatry: an international perspective. Can J Psychiatry. 2000;45(5):438–46.
10. Fassin D, Rechtman R. An anthropological hybrid: the pragmatic arrangement of universalism and culturalism in French mental health. Transcult Psychiatry. 2005;42(3):347–66.
11. Beneduce R. "Madness and despair are a force": global mental health, and how people and cultures challenge the hegemony of western psychiatry. Cult Med Psychiatry. 2019;43(4):710–23.
12. Hwang WC, Myers HF, Abe-Kim J, Ting JY. A conceptual paradigm for understanding culture's impact on mental health: the cultural influences on mental health (CIMH) model. Clin Psychol Rev. 2008;28(2):211–27.
13. Cross T, Bazron BJ, Dennis KW, Isaacs MR. Towards a culturally competent system of care. Vol. 1: Monograph on effective services for minority children who are severely emotionally disturbed. Washington: Georgetown University Child Development Center, CASSP Technical Assistance Center; 1989.
14. Sue DW, Bernier JB, Duran M, Feinberg L, Pedersen P, et al. Position paper: cross-cultural counseling competencies. Couns Psychol. 1982;10(2):45–52.
15. Pottie K, Hadi A, Chen J, Welch V, Hawthorne K. Realist review to understand the efficacy of culturally appropriate diabetes education programmes. Diabet Med. 2013;30(9):1017–25.
16. Substance Abuse and Mental Health Services Administration. SAMHSA's concept of trauma and guidance for a trauma-informed approach. HHS publication no. (SMA) 14-4884. 2014. https://store.samhsa.gov/system/files/sma14-4884.pdf.
17. Hostetter M, Klein S. Recognizing trauma as a means of engaging patients. Improving health care quality. The Commonwealth Fund. 2016 Jun 24. https://www.commonwealthfund.org/publications/2016/jun/focus-recognizing-trauma-means-engaging-patients.
18. Ahluwalia J, Baranowski T, Braithwaite R, Resnicow K. Cultural sensitivity in public health: defined and demystified. Ethn Dis. 1999;9(1):10–21.
19. Bernal G, Jiménez-Chafey MI, Domenech Rodríguez MM. Cultural adaptation of treatments: a resource for considering culture in evidence-based practice. Prof Psychol Res Pract. 2009;40(4):361.
20. Miranda J, Bernal G, Lau A, Kohn L, Hwang WC, LaFromboise T. State of the science on psychosocial interventions for ethnic minorities. Annu Rev Clin Psychol. 2005;1:113–42.

Part I

Survivors

Survivors of Torture

2

Priti Ojha

Vignette

Ms. A is a 34-year-old woman with no known psychiatric history who was tortured in Guatemala due to her family's indigenous roots. During her 12-month imprisonment, she was subjected to psychophysical torture. In addition to being placed in isolation, she was raped several times by multiple people and physically beaten, ultimately resulting in a need for medical intervention. During her hospitalization, Ms. A escaped her country of origin. After a long, lonely, distressing journey, she arrived in the USA where she applied for asylum. She was detained for six weeks and was released to the community with an ankle monitor. She was referred to a local community nonprofit organization that works with survivors of torture. With their assistance, Ms. A identified shelter and began to develop a sense of her new community. She was referred to an outpatient medical clinic for evaluation of chronic headaches and insomnia. The nonprofit organization also referred her to psychiatry.

P. Ojha (✉)
Department of Psychiatry, University of California San Diego, San Diego, CA, USA
e-mail: pojha@health.ucsd.edu

S. H. Koh et al. (eds.), *Diversity in Action*,
https://doi.org/10.1007/978-3-030-85401-0_2

Prior to her appointment with psychiatry, screening tools including the Hopkins Symptom Checklist and the Harvard Trauma Questionnaire were administered. A 90-min psychiatric intake was scheduled for Ms. A. A Spanish-speaking female interpreter was present and introduced to the patient prior to the appointment. During the appointment, the interpreter sat adjacent to the patient. Limitations of confidentiality were outlined early in the interview. In reviewing Ms. A's history, her life before her primary trauma was discussed; details related to her trauma history were explored only to the degree she felt comfortable. Her short-term and long-term goals were identified. A comprehensive review of symptoms including a detailed sleep history was taken.

Over the course of the first several appointments with the psychiatrist, various components of the patient's history were explored. The provider developed an understanding of how Ms. A's culture defined her sense of self and how her life was shattered by the traumas. As Ms. A became more comfortable with the psychiatrist, she endorsed additional symptoms that included irritability, nightmares, crying episodes, and dyspareunia. Ms. A described intrusive memories, negative cognitions, hypervigilance, and avoidance of public settings due to fears of deportation. She had significant pain associated with sexual activity; this led to anticipatory anxiety and resentment related to intimacy with her husband.

Ms. A was diagnosed with posttraumatic stress disorder (PTSD). She was started on sertraline 25 mg by mouth daily that, over time, was titrated to 100 mg to target mood symptoms associated with PTSD. She was also started on prazosin for management of nightmares. In addition to supportive psychotherapy during each psychiatric visit, she was referred for individual psychotherapy and engaged in 12 weekly sessions of trauma-focused psychotherapy. Eight months into psychiatric treatment, Ms. A's symptoms had fully resolved. Prazosin was slowly tapered and then discontinued. She transitioned to quarterly appointments and eventually gained employment and became pregnant. The frequency of her scheduled visits increased during the peripartum period as a preventative measure. She was continued on sertraline throughout her pregnancy. A letter in support of her asylum application was submitted to her attorney. Eighteen months after arriving in the USA, Ms. A's asylum petition was approved.

Introduction

Torture, derived from the Latin word *torquere*, "to twist," has been a means of corporal punishment and extraction of information as far back as Mesopotamia. The earliest documented description relates to an Egyptian pharaoh in 1300 BC who used torture to collect information regarding enemies during an invasion. Prisoners of war were held captive as slaves, deeming them "fit for torture." In ancient Greece and under Roman law, torture was permitted in slaves and foreigners and prohibited amongst the native free citizens [2]. Slaves were often tortured as a means to obtain incriminating evidence related to their owners. Around 200 AD, torture permissions extended to the lower class citizens as penalties [3].

In the last half-century, there have been multiple international treaties developed that prohibit torture; these include the Universal Declaration of Human Rights, the Geneva Convention, and the United Nations Convention against Torture and Other Cruel, Inhuman or Degrading Treatment or Punishment [1]. Despite recognition as a human rights violation, torture continues to be practiced today. According to Amnesty International, 141 countries reported cases of torture between 2009 and 2013 [4]. Worldwide, two-thirds of all refugees come from Syria, Afghanistan, South Sudan, Myanmar, and Somalia [5]. Human rights advocates argue that even countries who have signed the aforementioned treaties participate in torture, often amidst times of war. In recent years, concern has grown that what US government officials have described as "enhanced interrogation techniques" of prisoners in Guantanamo are in fact acts of torture. Prisoners have been victims to activities such as waterboarding, single cell operation, forcible cell extraction, and second-degree torture (a form of psychological torture in which family members are threatened).

Torture is typically utilized as a means of extracting enemy information during times of war. With the refugee population, torture can also be punishment for certain religious beliefs, political affiliations, and/or sexual orientation. Types of torture vary, and no list is truly comprehensive as methods of torture are invented regularly. Variations in types of torture are often region-specific. Psychological torture is nearly always present and varies in its form. Examples include observing a friend or family member being physically or sexually assaulted or sensory deprivation or overloading (e.g., music torture). The psychological impact this can have on individuals is profound. Many survivors recount that it is the psychological torture that has longer lasting consequences than the physical pain they endure. The fear of threats to loved ones or witnessing family members being tortured haunts some patients for a lifetime. Often, these concerns persist when refugees leave the country in which the torture was committed as they are separated from their contacts and struggle with the unknown state of their loved ones. Feelings of guilt and remorse, coupled with fear, contribute to the development of psychiatric illnesses including PTSD, depression, and anxiety. As court proceedings to obtain refugee/asylee status begin, the retelling of past painful experiences can lead to frequent triggers and experiences of reliving the trauma. The plight of torture survivors warrants identification and intervention by professionals providing their medical care. Effective care can only begin with awareness.

Definitions

The Torture Victims Relief Act of 1998 defines torture as [6]:

1. an act committed by a public official intended to inflict severe physical or mental pain or suffering (other than pain or suffering incidental to lawful sanctions) upon another person within his custody or physical control;
2. "severe mental pain or suffering" means the prolonged mental harm caused by or resulting from—
   (a) the intentional infliction or threatened infliction of severe physical pain or suffering;
   (b) the administration or application, or threatened administration or application, of mind-altering substances or other procedures calculated to disrupt profoundly the senses or the personality;
   (c) the threat of imminent death; or
   (d) the threat that another person will imminently be subjected to death, severe physical pain or suffering, or the administration or application of mind-altering substances or other procedures calculated to disrupt profoundly the senses or personality.

Refugees and *asylees* are unable or unwilling to reside in their country of nationality due to fear of persecution, war, or violence. Reasons for persecution include race, religion, nationality, and political opinion or social affiliation. Upon departure from their country of origin, refugees do not choose in which country they will reside. After leaving the country of nationality, they enter a neutral country until the United Nations High Commissioner for Refugees (UNHCR) recognizes them as refugees. Upon approval, refugees are flown to the host country, and resettlement is facilitated with subsidiary organizations in conjunction with the federal government. Resettlement agencies aid in the process, which can take up to 2 years.

Asylees are types of refugees. Unlike other refugees, *asylees* apply for humanitarian protection at the port of entry or within 1 year of arriving in the host country. The burden of proof of fear of persecution rests with the asylum seekers. They typically endure long, arduous journeys en route to the host country. Upon arrival and application for asylee status, claims are reviewed over a lengthy waiting period during which basic services are not permitted. Some applicants are deported immediately, while others may be detained for the duration of their legal proceedings. Applicants typically live under the threat of forced repatriation. Once asylee status is granted, applicants can become legal, permanent residents of the host country. Table 2.1 outlines the differences in application process for refugees and asylees.

Of the 22.5 million refugees worldwide, over a third identify as survivors of torture [7]. The majority of refugees come from Syria, Afghanistan, South Sudan,

Table 2.1 Application differences in the USA between refugees and asylees

	Refugee	Asylee
Location at time of application	Permission to enter the USA is granted while outside the country	Application for protection submitted upon arrival to the USA or point of entry
Agency responsible for reviewing application	United Nations High Commissioner for Refugees	Department of Homeland Security; United States Citizenship and Immigration Services
Application assistance	Application assistance with refugee resettlement agency	Burden of proof of persecution fear rests with applicant with limited assistance

Myanmar, and Somalia. For the last several years, the country hosting the most refugees has been Turkey. Since 1975, three million refugees have resettled in the USA. Of these, approximately 1.3 million are survivors of torture [5]. The number of applications which have been accepted in the USA has been decreasing, with the lowest in 2018 at 22,900. In FY 2017, asylum status was granted to 26,568 individuals in the USA, approximately 10% of those who applied [8]. Of these, 60% were approved by the Department of Homeland Security (affirmative asylum) and 40% by the Department of Justice (defensive asylum). Affirmative asylum applications are directly routed to USCIS. If that application is denied, an individual can apply for a defensive asylum application that goes through an immigration judge. The defensive process is much more laborious with a higher likelihood of rejection; 119,303 defensive applications were filed in 2017 of which 10,523 were granted (8%). There were 139,801 affirmative applications in 2017 of which 16,045 were granted (11%). Forty-five percent of those who were granted asylum came from China, El Salvador, or Guatemala. In recent years, the number of applications from people from the Northern Triangle (El Salvador, Guatemala, and Honduras) has steadily increased. The majority of these applicants are minors. The number and type of applicants granted asylum status is affected by political and other factors.

The journey of migration can be prolonged and demanding. Traditionally, a refugee's migration experience is divided into three categories: pre-migration, migration, and post-migration or resettlement. This collectively can be referred to as the "triple trauma paradigm" as each segment of this journey can harbor its own traumas [9]. The *pre-migration* period includes the primary trauma related to fear of persecution that motivates individuals to flee their native country. The *migration* period refers to the travel to the final host country. Often this may include passing through transit countries en route to the destination. This period can be met with uncertainty and unanticipated dangers with limited resources. The *post-migration* period reflects resettlement in a new country amassed with a new culture including social norms and practicalities of daily living. Initial relief of arriving to the host country can quickly be tempered by insecurity. Individuals may experience facets of racism and xenophobia as they transition to living in a new environment. Factors which impact this include prolonged detention periods, insecure immigration status with fear of expatriation, and limitations on work and education opportunities. Detention can be a particularly triggering time during which fear of authorities can compound environmental similarities to where people were tortured. Similarly when people are released from detention with ankle monitors, they may experience significant distress as there is a constant physical reminder on their bodies of the traumas they have endured. Additional resettlement stressors can include prolonged legal proceedings, limited knowledge of and poor access to services, and insecure unstable housing. Language and cultural barriers can be hard to overcome. Refugees also have varying levels of literacy, from being preliterate to possessing advanced educations. Many leave successful careers only to later face poverty and unemployment in the host country. These types of insecurities make individuals more vulnerable to forms of exploitation such as human trafficking for labor or sex.

When confronted with so many changes, an individual's sense of self may waiver and feelings of grief may surface. Individuals are often socially isolated during the resettlement period. For those that come from cultures that embrace multigenerational households, this solitude can be a harrowing experience. Patients are often separated from their families who may be scattered around the world. Other times, family members may still be in unsafe circumstances in the country of origin. In these scenarios, patients often express feelings of worry, in addition to guilt, for escaping their traumatic environments, while other family members may still be at risk.

Intersection with Healthcare

Physical symptoms tend to be what prompts torture survivors to seek care. Somatic complaints at presentation may include sleep impairment, headache, nausea, and chronic pain. Memory and concentration impairments also arise as a result of traumatic brain injuries. Physical injuries vary based on the type of torture endured, including blunt trauma with subsequent bruising and potential internal injuries, injuries from bodies being placed in stress positions during prolonged suspension and electrical and thermal injury [10]. Sexual trauma, including rape and genital mutilation, can lead to dyspareunia, urinary tract infections, menstrual irregularities, and infertility [11]. Certain physical injuries may not be visible as torturers often employ strategies to minimize evidence. For example, they may place a sheet on the victim's skin during a whipping.

There is also a correlation between physical and mental health illnesses. In an age- and sex-matched study of 1052 refugees in Nepal, those who were tortured (half of the study population) had higher rates of PTSD, depression, and anxiety [12]. These refugees also reported more respiratory and musculoskeletal symptoms. Back pain, disrupted sleep, decreased appetite and libido, and hearing and vision impairments were all reported more often by those who had been tortured [12]. Higher rates of medical conditions have been identified in survivors with comorbid PTSD with depression than with either mental illness alone [13]. Studies use various tools to screen and diagnose depression, anxiety, and PTSD; these include the Hopkins Symptoms Checklist, PTSD Checklist for Civilians, Harvard Trauma Questionnaire, Beck Depression and Anxiety Inventories, and DSM criteria assessed via clinical interview.

Several studies suggest increased rates of PTSD in survivors of torture, though actual prevalence is variable. Depression and anxiety are also common. Mental health diagnoses are likely underreported due to limited access to care and screening of torture survivors. Factors which may predict onset of mental illness include the type and severity of torture endured; post-migration stressors, especially unstable living environments; and length of time to accessing healthcare services. Population sizes in studies range from 30 survivors to over 1200 people; in these studies, rates of mental illness vary between different populations. For example, in one study of 91 Syrian Kurdish refugees, 38% screened positive for symptoms of PTSD [14]. In another study of 278 torture survivors from the Middle East who resettled in the USA, 56.9% screened positive for PTSD, 83.8% for depression, and 81.3% for anxiety. In a study of 131 torture survivors from Africa, 94.7% screened positive for depression and 57.3% for PTSD [15]. In a study of almost 80 survivors from various regions including the Middle East, South Asia, Central Africa, and Southeastern Europe, 78% screened positively for depression and anxiety, and 88% screened positively for PTSD [16]. In a study of 720 survivors in Nepal, under 10% screened positive for PTSD, 27.5% screened positive for depression, and nearly 23% screened positive for anxiety [17]. In one of the larger studies with over 1200 Syrian refugees who resettled in Sweden, 40% were diagnosed with depression, approximately 32% with anxiety, and almost 30% with PTSD [18].

Some studies have looked at mediators and moderators that may predict or protect from certain mental health outcomes. Many report a relationship between severity of torture endured and a diagnosis of PTSD. Those who were tortured for longer periods of time were more likely to be symptomatic. For many, the psychological trauma is more disturbing than the physical pain they weather. Additionally, the stress response can be mediated by a number of factors and demographic characteristics including preexisting mental and medical conditions and an individual's strengths and vulnerabilities, characterological qualities, and resiliency. Those with childhood trauma are more likely to have functional impairments [19]. In one study of survivors who settled in the USA, female sex and older age were predictive factors of later receiving PTSD and depression diagnoses. A similar finding was noted in the study of 720 survivors in Nepal and also found higher rates of anxiety in women and those of Islamic religion [7]. The gender difference with anxiety disorders is consistent with data from the general population [20].

As a form of interpersonal trauma, torture increases the risk of psychological stress. The severity of traumatic experiences coupled with the frequency of traumatic occurrences can reflect the likelihood of developing a mental health disorder. The migration journey and resettlement experiences can further compound psychiatric symptoms. As an example, survivors may fear re-experiencing symptoms while sharing their torture experience during the asylum application process that can include medical and psychological interviews. Sharing vivid memories of what they endured can exacerbate symptoms including nightmares, flashbacks, low mood, and episodes of panic. Once settled, symptoms of stress can also be triggered and further compounded by news, social media, current events, and the political climate as they are reminded of what they survived and from what their friends and family who are still in the country of origin may continue to suffer. In a study of 134 survivors, those who endured post-migration obstacles were more likely to meet criteria for multiple psychiatric illness than those who did not face as many migration complications [21]. Other studies have shown that torture survivors that experience financial and legal insecurities had higher rates of PTSD [22].

As a result of these known associations, one can observe social predictors of patient outcomes. For example, in a study of Iraqi asylum seekers in the Netherlands, patients who had a longer asylum period were more likely to develop a mental illness than those who recently arrived in the host country. PTSD rates were 10% higher in those whose asylum cases took longer than 2 years versus those who had arrived within the previous 6 months [23]. In another study, survivors who accessed clinical services after 1 year of arrival in the USA were more likely to be diagnosed with depression and PTSD compared to those that accessed services within the first year of resettlement [24]. Symptoms of depression and PTSD improved as immigration status was secured in a study of torture survivors who resettled in New York City [25]. All of these studies are correlational, and it is likely that psychiatric illness and assimilation challenges can affect one another bidirectionally. Experiencing symptoms of depression, anxiety, and PTSD likely further exacerbates assimilation difficulties. As such, it is imperative that social determinants of health and referrals to social and legal services are addressed by the treatment team.

Screening and Assessment

Estimates suggest up to 10% of immigrant patients in urban medical clinics in the USA are survivors of torture [26]. This likely underrepresents the number of patients who present to clinics in which providers are not asking about torture history. Feelings of guilt, shame, and mistrust may limit how much history a survivor of torture volunteers without being asked. Some patients expect medical providers to inquire about trauma, so it may not be disclosed without screening. Implementing screening tools can identify survivors and expedite their access to treatment and social services. One example of a screening tool is the Detection of Torture Survivor Survey (see Table 2.2) that is recommended to be conducted at a patient's second appointment once a doctor-patient relationship has already been established [27].

It may be that the patient's experience with torture is only one component of their trauma history, so it is important to inquire about a patient's life more holistically. A biopsychosocial formulation and treatment plan that encompasses a team-based approach with collaboration between the psychiatrist, therapist, and case manager is ideal. If the patient speaks a different language, all communication should be through a trained interpreter with as close to the patient's preferred dialect as possible. Consents and confidentiality should be highlighted throughout the treatment course and especially in the beginning, prior to establishing strong rapport.

Table 2.2 Detection of torture survivors survey (DOTSS) items from Eisenman (2007) [27]

Introduction: In this clinic we see many patients who have been forced to leave their countries because of violence or threats to the health and safety of patients and their families. I am going to ask you some questions about this:

1. In (your former country), did you ever have problems because of religion, political beliefs, culture, or any other reason?
2. Did you have any problems with persons working for the government, military, police, or any other group?
3. Were you ever a victim of violence in (your former country)?
4. Were you ever a victim of torture in (your former country)?

Adapted from Eisenman [27]

The assessment and subsequent treatment of psychiatric illness in survivors of torture should take a trauma-informed approach. In doing so, a provider recognizes the impact trauma may have on the individual and actively encourages recovery that limits re-traumatization. Paramount to trauma-informed treatment is trust building and psychoeducation. It may be difficult for patients to share details of their lives with anyone, especially someone they recently met. It takes time to develop a trusting doctor-patient relationship, and in the trauma-informed setting, providers should highlight collaboration and the patient's voice and choice, further fostering the patient's underlying resilience. For many torture survivors, engagement with medical care, especially mental health care, is novel. Open-ended questions are recommended, though some patients may need guidance of what to share if they have limited experience engaging in medical care. As an example, they may not correlate their chronic headaches or abdominal pain and disrupted sleep pattern to their emotional state.

Assessments should consider the cultural contributions of a patient's presentation, recognizing that patients may be reluctant to share details of their trauma history with providers. It can be prudent to research the political atmosphere and sociocultural norms of the patient's country of origin if it is known prior to the first appointment. Many torture survivors come from societies that discourage mental health services. As a result, there may be a component of stigma or limited knowledge about mental health that delays a patient's engagement in treatment. Feelings of guilt and shame may also impact a patient's reception to psychiatric diagnoses and care. Some may feel that they deserve to suffer. Reluctance may also be attributed to a fear of legal ramifications subsequent to disclosure so reviewing limits of confidentiality is especially important [28].

One resource that may assist a provider in gaining a better understanding of a patient's cultural background and impact that has on their engagement with mental health is the Cultural Formulation Interview in the Diagnostic and Statistical Manual of Mental Disorders (DSM-5) [29]. Through a series of questions, a provider can gain insight into a patient's perspective of the cultural meaning of their symptoms and treatment. Since cultural sensitivity can help inform subsequent treatment planning, using this evidence-based tool can help guide providers while developing the doctor-patient relationship.

Treatment

A patient-centered, strengths-based environment promotes empowerment and the development of a trusting relationship. This, of course, takes time as trust is often shattered when an individual is tortured. It is important for the provider to respect patients' boundaries in how much they share at initial visits. For those patients whose legal proceedings are underway, reviewing the affidavit prior to the intake can be particularly helpful to understand the patient's previous experiences.

When a patient screens positively for a history of torture, providers can share their familiarity and training in the topic to help normalize the patient's experiences. Connecting a patient's torture history to their physical and mental health can help bridge their history to their current presentation. Sometimes describing a cause-and-effect relationship can address some of the stigma issues that concern patients. If possible, refer the patient to appropriate local resources and services that have experience working with the tortured population. Some of these organizations provide more specialized treatment options including psychotherapy and medication management. If a patient reports psychiatric symptoms, treatment plans are typically multipronged with the core components being trauma-informed psychotherapy with concurrent pharmacologic intervention. It is imperative that patients actively participate in treatment planning and that psychoeducation is consistently reviewed. The teach back method is an effective way to ensure patients understand the treatment plan and reinforces an open line of communication.

Psychotherapy Treatments

Evidence-based psychotherapies for PTSD often include structured, time-limited sessions that involve components of exposure and/or changing patterns of cognitions, behaviors, and emotions that lead to difficulties in functioning related to the trauma. PTSD-specific psychotherapy should not occur if patients are currently unstable, suicidal, a danger to self or others, in need of urgent medical attention, or in an unsafe environment. Evidence-based modalities to treat PTSD include trauma-informed cognitive behavioral therapy including prolonged exposure and cognitive processing therapy. There is growing body of evidence that supports the utility of eye movement desensitization and reprocessing therapy and narrative exposures.

Through cognitive restructuring and *in vivo* or imaginal exposures, *cognitive behavioral therapy* (CBT) for PTSD evaluates negative appraisals related to the trauma. *Prolonged exposure*, which is rooted in the emotional processing theory, guides individuals through *in vivo* and imaginal exposures in an effort to recondition their fear response. *Cognitive processing therapy* (CPT) challenges distorted cognitions related to trauma and leads to altering beliefs to accommodate for more adaptive experiences [30]. In *narrative exposure therapy* (NET), patients develop a detailed chronological account of their life experiences while being grounded in the present time. *Eye movement desensitization and reprocessing* (EMDR) helps patients process trauma by focusing on saccadic eye movements while engaging in imaginal exposure to the trauma. Through this process, the traumatic experience is reformulated, making the memory less distressing. In the limited number of studies comparing these various modalities in refugee and asylum seeking populations, CBT, NET, and EMDR, when conducted in a culturally informed manner, have demonstrated to be efficacious [31, 32].

It is important to note that studies specifically researching trauma in the torture survivor are extremely limited and symptoms of comorbidities such as depression or anxiety may not be addressed by these specific psychotherapies. The National Institute for Clinical Excellence recommends that initial treatments should focus on acute symptomology and the development of adaptive coping skills prior to introducing trauma-informed therapies. Furthermore, awareness of ineffective or harmful treatments is important. For example, psychological debriefing immediately following a traumatic event has shown to be ineffective and may actually increase the likelihood of individuals developing PTSD symptoms [25].

Pharmacologic Treatments

Similar to psychotherapeutic interventions, psychotropic medications have not been extensively studied in the tortured population. Evidence from veteran and civilian trauma is applicable, though it is important to note that mental health cannot be treated in isolation of social, legal, medical, and spiritual needs of these patients. There is currently no evidence to support use of a pharmacological agent to prevent the development of PTSD. It is also necessary to screen for patients' use of traditional culturally appropriate remedies such as supplements or homeopathic therapies.

The Federal Drug Administration (FDA) has approved two selective serotonin reuptake inhibitors (SSRIs), paroxetine and sertraline, for the treatment of PTSD. Additionally, fluoxetine and venlafaxine, serotonin-norepinephrine reuptake inhibitors (SNRIs), have been shown to be effective options. In addition to treating the symptoms of PTSD, SSRIs and SNRIs can also treat mental health comorbidities and suicidal or aggressive behaviors [33]. While these medications are generally well-tolerated, considerations in medication selection should include potential drug-drug interactions (i.e., via CYP P450 2D6 inhibition), side effect profiles/tolerability, comorbidities such as chronic pain, and patient adherence. As an example, if a notable component of the patient's presenting problems include chronic pain, the SNRI duloxetine, which is FDA approved for the management of pain, may be a more appropriate choice than a SSRI. Since most survivors of torture are psychotropic medication naïve, the recommendation is to start at low doses and titrate to effectiveness.

A common symptom associated with torture is nightmares. Clinicians and researchers speculate autonomic nervous system hyperactivity leads to hyperarousal symptoms, agitation, and nightmares. The alpha-adrenergic antagonist prazosin has been shown to be effective for reducing nightmares [34]. Patients should be advised of its FDA off-label use and to monitor for dizziness/lightheadedness, to rise slowly, and to maintain adequate oral hydration. Providers should also monitor for orthostatic hypotension. Doses start at 1 mg at bedtime and should be titrated with provider check-ins to ensure tolerability. Patients typically report either the intensity or the frequency of the nightmares starts to improve as one gets closer to the optimal dosing. Anecdotally, some patients also report dreams become more vivid in nature prior to improvement. Ultimately the goal is for patients to sleep through the night uninterrupted. Daytime dosing, if tolerated, may be appropriate to target hypervigilance symptoms.

Benzodiazepines are the one class of medications thought to be contraindicated in the treatment of PTSD. Evidence shows that they are ineffective at treating PTSD symptomatology likely due to the differing pathophysiology of PTSD as compared to other anxiety disorders. Because benzodiazepines affect the brain globally, rather than specific structures, their effects can potentiate already hypoactive parts of the brain in the setting of PTSD. They can inhibit cognitive processing and induce emotional numbing that can interfere in the consolidation of memory that assists in the recovery from trauma. Some studies suggest benzodiazepine administration after a traumatic event can increase the likelihood of developing PTSD by promoting avoidance [35]. Discontinuation of this type of medication can lead to withdrawal symptoms that can mimic symptoms of PTSD such as insomnia and irritability [36]. Further, it may negatively impact psychotherapy outcomes by dulling the patient's emotional experiences during exposure exercises and increasing their avoidance of negative emotional states [37]. Figure 2.1 highlights recommended treatment approaches in survivors of torture with PTSD.

Treatment approaches typically target the most distressing symptoms first. For example, for someone with low mood and daily nightmares, focusing on the sleep disturbance can help provide relief as the patient becomes increasingly engaged in treatment. Limited adherence to medications is common in this patient population. It is important for patients to understand the anticipated treatment course including length of time it may take to see any response. For example, patients may self-discontinue an antidepressant after 2 weeks of seeing no benefit. Alternatively, patients may begin to feel better after 3 months on an antidepressant and think that they no

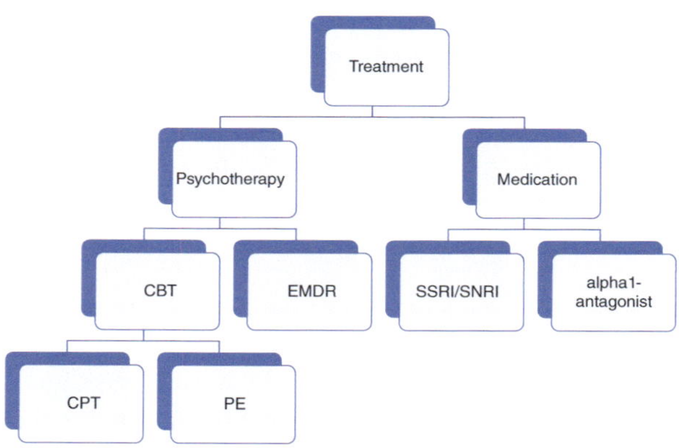

Fig. 2.1 Psychotherapy and medication treatments for PTSD. *CBT* cognitive behavioral therapy (trauma-informed), *CPT* cognitive processing therapy, *PE* prolonged exposure, *EMDR* eye movement desensitization and reprocessing, *SSRI* selective-serotonin reuptake inhibitor, *SNRI* selective-norepinephrine reuptake inhibitor

longer require medication. Frequent follow-up with discussions regarding medication administration are imperative to ensuring adequate adherence, as for many patients, medical literacy may be low. Also, while the psychological wounds are often most distressing, physical symptoms must not be overlooked in survivors of torture. If physical pain persists, it may interfere with resolution of psychological pain as they trigger one another and can exist in a cycle. Collaborating with primary care and referrals for acupuncture, massage, and physical therapy should be considered.

Social and Legal Services

Care coordination with social and legal services can greatly impact patients' progress. Many patients face financial uncertainty; support securing shelter and access to food, clothing, and hygiene products are necessary components in these patients' post-migration journeys. Patients also benefit from assistance to navigate the healthcare system and enroll in health insurance. Additionally, social services can coordinate transportation services so patients can attend their various appointments. They may offer assistance in enrolling patients in English classes, job training, and higher education, which can facilitate a rebuilding of one's sense of self in a new country. Since many torture survivors come from cultures that are based on interdependence, re-establishing a sense of community can be particularly constructive. Often social services introduce patients to fellow immigrants from their country of origin.

One of the primary stressors survivors of torture face are legal challenges. A lack of understanding of the US judicial system coupled with language barriers and financial pressure make it difficult for survivors to secure legal representation for their petition. Even if they are able to access legal services, it can be difficult to engage with them as recounting the details of their torture experiences can be triggering, and any underlying mental health issues such as depression, anxiety, or PTSD can further interfere with their ability to optimally utilize services. For those patients that do have attorneys, coordination between the legal and clinical teams can be instrumental to an asylee's application. In one study of 2400 asylum seekers, 37% were granted asylum without medical documentation. In contrast, of those who had medical documentation supporting their history and symptoms, 90% had their petition approved [38]. Clinically it is important to recognize the impact legal stress has on patients' mental health. It is often difficult for applicants to gather the evidence necessary for their asylum petitions, and the process of application can be quite lengthy. These components of the unknown can increase undue stress on patients and negatively impact the trajectory of their mental health.

Children and Adolescents

Whether a child has directly or indirectly been impacted by torture, the downstream effects can be substantial. Trauma can range from witnessing war zone areas to intergenerational trauma such as residing with parents who struggle in post-torture times. When treating parents, it is important to note how their wellbeing impacts their children. Youth who have been exposed to torture (directly or indirectly via parents' experiences) can develop PTSD and may present with sleep disturbances, poor concentration, irritability, and avoidant behaviors [39]. Children infrequently volunteer these symptoms, so it is important for caregivers to inquire. Given the limited set of coping skills one has at a young age, children may have more disruptive behavior that is characterized as acting out that can impact school performance. Additional signs can include, but are not limited to, crying episodes, sleep disturbances, developmental regressions (e.g., language and toileting skills), engaging in post-traumatic play, somatic complaints (e.g., headaches, stomachaches), irritability, separation anxiety, and poor school performance [40].

Direct traumas children often encounter are in the migration process, such as exposure to physical violence and shelter and food insecurity. The journey is often emotionally and physically draining. Parents' ability to tend to children's emotional needs during this time may be severely limited as priorities may shift to ensuring basic needs of food and shelter are safely acquired during the journey. In the post-migration period, children may struggle with assimilation. Having left behind friends and family, rebuilding a community is particularly important for children. Because they are more likely to quickly learn the host country's language, children also often serve as the family's interpreter for daily activities. While many will adapt without much difficulty those that show concerning signs (as described above) should be offered prompt intervention.

Pregnancy

For some survivors of torture, sexual activity can be a challenging experience. Dyspareunia is a common symptom that is seldom discussed but can have significant impact on a patient's mental health and relationships. For those with histories of sexual assault, obstetric/gynecologic exams can be particularly triggering. It is important to weigh risks versus benefits in the management of mental health issues when a patient becomes pregnant. In some cases, it may be detrimental to cease previously helpful medications during pregnancy. For example, antenatal in utero exposure to untreated depression is known to be associated with increased rates of prematurity and low birth weight and can have long-term negative outcomes including depression, anxiety, ADHD, and physical illnesses. Postpartum depression occurs more frequently in those who had prepartum depression that discontinued treatment during pregnancy [41]. Certainly each woman must be evaluated individually with a thorough discussion of potential consequences on fetal development so an informed decision can be made.

Conclusion

Well into the twenty-first century, torture continues to plague society. Survivors develop long-term physical and mental health sequelae. Utilization of evidence-based screening tools can help providers identify at risk patients. A resilience-based and strengths-focused approach to treatment that encompasses a multi-prolonged treatment approach – psychotherapy, pharmacotherapy, and social/legal services – can foster a survivor's recovery.

Summary of High-Yield Points

- As the number of survivors of torture who seek refugee and asylum status continues to grow worldwide, medical providers must recognize that they are at high risk for mental illness.
- Torture survivors can endure traumas throughout their migration experience: pre-migration, migration, and post-migration.
- Predictors of mental illness can include survivors' age, sex, type and severity of torture endured, post-migration obstacles, length of time to legal status resolution, and length of time to accessing healthcare.
- Providers can screen refugee patients for torture histories as many may not self-disclose if not prompted.
- While presenting symptoms are usually somatic in nature, PTSD, depression, and anxiety are common mental health disorders in survivors of torture.
- A trauma-informed approach should guide assessment and treatment that includes trauma-informed psychotherapies and psychotropic medications as well as coordination of care with social and legal services.

References

1. Innes B. The history of torture. Amber Books Ltd; 2012.
2. Peters E. Torture. University of Pennsylvania Press; 2018.
3. Ozkalipci O, Schlar C. The Istanbul protocol: international standards for the effective investigation and documentation of torture and ill treatment. The Lancet. 1999;354(9184):1117.
4. amnesty.org/en/what-we-do/torture/.
5. UNHCR Global Trends, Forced Displacement in 2018. https://www.unhcr.org/globaltrends2018/#:~:text=As%20in%202017%2C%20over%20two,South%20Sudan%2C%20Myanmar%20and%20Somalia.&text=Turkey%20continued%20to%20host%20the,the%20end%20of%20the%20year.
6. Section 2340(1) of title 18, United States Code.
7. Abu Suhaiban H, Grasser LR, Javanbakht A. Mental health of refugees and torture survivors: a critical review of prevalence, predictors, and integrated care. Int J Environ Res Public Health. 2019;16(13):2309.
8. Migrationpolicy.org.
9. Jackson JC, Haider M, Wilson Owens C, Ahrenholz N, Molnar A, Farmer B, Terasaki G. Healthcare recommendations for recently arrived refugees: observations from EthnoMed. Harv Public Health Rev. 2016;9:1–18. Available at http://harvardpublichealthreview.org/vol/special-commentary-2/. Verified 23 Dec 2018.
10. Pollanen MS. The pathology of torture. Forensic Sci Int. 2018;284:85–96.
11. Reisel D, Creighton SM. Long term health consequences of Female Genital Mutilation (FGM). Maturitas. 2015;80(1):48–51.
12. Shrestha NM, Sharma B, Van Ommeren M, Regmi S, Makaju R, Komproe I, Shrestha GB, de Jong JT. Impact of torture on refugees displaced within the developing world: symptomatology among Bhutanese refugees in Nepal. JAMA. 1998;280(5):443–8.

13. Berthold SM, Kong S, Mollica RF, Kuoch T, Scully M, Franke T. Comorbid mental and physical health and health access in Cambodian refugees in the US. J Community Health. 2014;39(6):1045–52.
14. Ibrahim H, Hassan CQ. Post-traumatic stress disorder symptoms resulting from torture and other traumatic events among Syrian Kurdish refugees in Kurdistan Region, Iraq. Front Psychol. 2017;8:241.
15. Leaman SC, Gee CB. Religious coping and risk factors for psychological distress among African torture survivors. Psychol Trauma Theory Res Pract Policy. 2012;4(5):457.
16. Schubert CC, Punamäki RL. Mental health among torture survivors: cultural background, refugee status and gender. Nord J Psychiatry. 2011;65(3):175–82.
17. Luitel NP, Jordans MJ, Sapkota RP, Tol WA, Kohrt BA, Thapa SB, Komproe IH, Sharma B. Conflict and mental health: a cross-sectional epidemiological study in Nepal. Soc Psychiatry Psychiatr Epidemiol. 2013;48(2):183–93.
18. Tinghög P, Malm A, Arwidson C, Sigvardsdotter E, Lundin A, Saboonchi F. Prevalence of mental ill health, traumas and postmigration stress among refugees from Syria resettled in Sweden after 2011: a population-based survey. BMJ Open. 2017;7(12):e018899.
19. La P. Healing the hurt. The Center for Victims of Torture; 2005.
20. McLean CP, Asnaani A, Litz BT, Hofmann SG. Gender differences in anxiety disorders: prevalence, course of illness, comorbidity and burden of illness. J Psychiatr Res. 2011;45(8):1027–35. https://doi.org/10.1016/j.jpsychires.2011.03.006.
21. Nickerson A, Schick M, Schnyder U, Bryant RA, Morina N. Comorbidity of posttraumatic stress disorder and depression in tortured, treatment-seeking refugees. J Trauma Stress. 2017;30(4):409–15.
22. Chu T, Keller AS, Rasmussen A. Effects of post-migration factors on PTSD outcomes among immigrant survivors of political violence. J Immigr Minor Health. 2013;15(5):890–7.
23. Laban CJ, Gernaat HB, Komproe IH, Schreuders BA, De Jong JT. Impact of a long asylum procedure on the prevalence of psychiatric disorders in Iraqi asylum seekers in The Netherlands. J Nerv Ment Dis. 2004;192(12):843–51.
24. Song SJ, Kaplan C, Tol WA, Subica A, de Jong J. Psychological distress in torture survivors: pre-and post-migration risk factors in a US sample. Soc Psychiatry Psychiatr Epidemiol. 2015;50(4):549–60.
25. Raghavan S, Rasmussen A, Rosenfeld B, Keller AS. Correlates of symptom reduction in treatment-seeking survivors of torture. Psychol Trauma Theory Res Pract Policy. 2013;5(4):377.
26. Eisenman DP, Keller AS, Kim G. Survivors of torture in a general medical setting: how often have patients been tortured, and how often is it missed? West J Med. 2000;172(5):301.
27. Eisenman D. Screening for mental health problems and history of torture. In: Immigrant medicine. Elsevier; 2007. p. 633–8.
28. Gorman W. Refugee survivors of torture: trauma and treatment. Prof Psychol Res Pract. 2001;32(5):443.
29. American Psychiatric Association. Diagnostic and statistical manual of mental disorders. 5th ed; 2013.
30. Watkins LE, Sprang KR, Rothbaum BO. Treating PTSD: a review of evidence-based psychotherapy interventions. Front Behav Neurosci. 2018;12:258.
31. Slobodin O, de Jong JT. Mental health interventions for traumatized asylum seekers and refugees: what do we know about their efficacy? Int J Soc Psychiatry. 2015;61(1):17–26.
32. Coetzee RH, Regel S. Eye movement desensitisation and reprocessing: an update. Adv Psychiatr Treat. 2005;11(5):347–54.
33. Alexander W. Pharmacotherapy for post-traumatic stress disorder in combat veterans: focus on antidepressants and atypical antipsychotic agents. Pharm Therap. 2012;37(1):32.
34. Boynton L, Bentley J, Strachan E, Barbato A, Raskind M. Preliminary findings concerning the use of prazosin for the treatment of posttraumatic nightmares in a refugee population. J Psychiatr Pract. 2009;15(6):454–9.

35. (a) Guina J, Rossetter SR, DeRhodes BJ, Nahhas RW, Welton RS. Benzodiazepines for PTSD: a systematic review and meta-analysis. J Psychiatr Pract. 2015;21(4):281–303; (b) notorture.org; (c) Forneris CA, Gartlehner G, Brownley KA, et al. Interventions to prevent post-traumatic stress disorder: a systematic review. Am J Prev Med. 2013;44(6):635–50.
36. Guina J, Rossetter SR, DeRhodes BJ, Nahhas RW, Welton RS. Benzodiazepines for PTSD. J Psychiatr Pract. 2015;21(4):281–303.
37. Cain CK, Maynard GD, Kehne JH. Targeting memory processes with drugs to prevent or cure PTSD. Expert Opin Investig Drugs. 2012;21(9):1323–50.
38. Miles SH, Garcia-Peltoniemi RE. Torture survivors: what to ask, how to document. J Fam Pract. 2012;61(4):E1–5.
39. Pynoos RS, Kinzie JD, Gordon M. Children, adolescents, and families exposed to torture and related trauma. In: The mental health consequences of torture. Boston: Springer; 2001. p. 211–25.
40. Smith HE, Keller AS, Lhewa DW. … Like a refugee camp on first avenue. New York: Bellevue/NYU Program for Survivors of Torture; 2007.
41. Pilowsky DJ, et al. Children of depressed mothers 1 year after the initiation of maternal treatment: findings from the STAR* D-Child Study. Am J Psychiatr. 2008;165(9):1136–47.

Survivors of Human Trafficking

3

Joanna Ortega, Mollie Gordon, Kimberly Gordon-Achebe, and Rachel Robitz

Introduction

Human trafficking is an egregious human rights violation and public health issue. Human trafficking is defined by the United Nation's Palermo Protocol (2000) as:

> the recruitment, transportation, transfer, harboring or receipt of persons, by means of the threat or use of force or other forms of coercion, of abduction, of fraud, of deception, of the abuse of power or of a position of vulnerability or of the giving or receiving of payments or benefits to achieve the consent of a person having control over another person, for the purpose of exploitation. Exploitation shall include, at a minimum, the exploitation of the prostitution of others or other forms of sexual exploitation, forced labor or services, slavery or practices similar to slavery, servitude or the removal of organs [93].

Human trafficking is composed of three elements: the *act* (what is done), the *means* (how it is done), and the *purpose* (why it is done). The act is either labor or commercial sex acts. The means is through force, fraud, or coercion. The purpose is for the benefit of the trafficker. Human trafficking is different than smuggling.

J. Ortega · R. Robitz (✉)
Department of Psychiatry and Behavioral Sciences, University of California Davis, Sacramento, CA, USA
e-mail: jcortega@ucdavis.edu; rarobitz@ucdavis.edu

M. Gordon
Menninger Department of Psychiatry and Behavioral Sciences, Baylor College of Medicine, Bellaire, TX, USA
e-mail: mrgordon@bcm.edu

K. Gordon-Achebe
Department of Psychiatry & Behavioral Sciences, Tulane University School of Medicine, New Orleans, LA, USA

University of Maryland, New Orleans, LA, USA
e-mail: kagordon@som.umaryland.edu

S. H. Koh et al. (eds.), *Diversity in Action*,
https://doi.org/10.1007/978-3-030-85401-0_3

Smuggling is the movement of people across borders. Humans who are smuggled may be trafficked, but not all smuggled persons are human trafficking victims. Smuggling is an illegal crime against a border, while trafficking is an illegal crime against a person. Smuggling may be voluntary, as individuals may pay their smuggler for an exchange of services. Human trafficking victims, by definition, are coerced or forced into their circumstances and economically exploited by another.

Because of its underground nature, it is difficult to collect data on human trafficking. Most information available is only on identified cases, so it is unclear if this data represents all or most trafficked people. Unlike drugs and weapons, humans can be trafficked, repeatedly, increasing the value of their commodity. Additionally, to be prosecuted, often victims must testify against their traffickers. Victims may be hesitant to testify against traffickers due to fear or trauma bonding that can occur with the trafficker.

Globally, there are an estimated 40 million people trapped in human trafficking and forced marriages. It is estimated that one in four victims of human trafficking are children, or about ten million children across the world [45]. In the USA, human trafficking has been reported in all 50 states [54]. In 2015, US attorneys prosecuted 1049 suspects for human trafficking offenses [11]. Trafficking can occur across race/ethnicities; however, African-Americans are disproportionately affected with 40% of identified trafficking cases from 2008 to 2010 being African-Americans [10]. In the USA over 25 different types of labor and sex trafficking have been described, including but not limited to workers in domestic, food service, traveling sales, agriculture, and massage settings [70].

The Victims of Trafficking and Violence Protection Act of 2000 [94] (TVPA) is a US federal statute passed into law in 2000 and signed by President Bill Clinton. It has the ability to authorize protections for undocumented immigrants and US citizens who are victims of severe forms of all types of trafficking. In 2000, the Palermo Protocols were adopted by the United Nations (UN) to supplement the Convention against Transnational Organized Crime. These protocols include (1) the Protocol to Prevent, Suppress and Punish Trafficking in Persons, especially Women and Children; (2) the Protocol against the Smuggling of Migrants by Land, Sea and Air; and (3) the Protocol against the Illicit Manufacturing and Trafficking in Firearms, their Parts and Components and Ammunition [93].

Around this same time, in order to further protect trafficked children, individual states began adopting safe harbor laws. New York was the first state to adopt a safe harbor law, which went into effect in 2010. As of 2015, 34 states had passed safe harbor laws. Safe harbor laws are designed to protect minors who have been exploited for labor services or commercial sex. Children being trafficked are often forced or coerced into engaging in illegal activities such as prostitution or selling drugs, and many are prosecuted as criminals as a result. Arrest and prosecution can cause additional trauma and distrust in law enforcement that may prevent children from seeking assistance [68]. The aim of safe harbor laws is to ensure that instead of being arrested and punished, exploited children are treated as victims and provided with needed services. Although state laws vary substantially, in general, safe harbor laws have two main components: provision of services and legal protection.

The legal protection component provides trafficked children with immunity for certain types of offenses or establishes diversion programs for the dismissal of certain charges under the condition that children participate in designated programs or services [68]; however, these systems may not mitigate recidivism and trauma as they were designed. The services component makes specialized services such as medical, psychological, housing, education assistance, job training, and legal services available for children who have been trafficked [68].

Healthcare professionals feel undertrained to recognize, evaluate, and manage patients who are trafficked [81]. The lack of confidence in responding appropriately to trafficked people includes how to ask about experiences of trafficking and how to make referrals [27]. However, even minimal training can increase the awareness and lead to improved treatment outcomes. Patients who are trafficked come to the attention of medical professionals in one of three ways: (1) the patient discloses their experience of exploitation either spontaneously or with proper screening by the provider, (2) the patient presents with signs or symptoms of abuse or exploitation that leads the professional to suspect trafficking, and (3) the healthcare worker is informed by another professional such as law enforcement, immigration, social services, voluntary sector, or consultation by other health professionals [101].

Cultural Considerations of Human Trafficking

The experience of a trafficked individual sits at the nexus of multiple structural factors, all of which contribute not only to an individual's risk of being trafficked but also to the ability of that individual to leave trafficking, and the way in which they recover from the various physical and psychological sequelae of trafficking [47]. In order to have some understanding of how trafficked individuals experience their exploitation, one must understand the structural and cultural frame that trafficking occurs within. Health professionals who embrace an intersectionality lens commit to understanding the systems, structures, policies, and practices that put individuals based on their intersecting identities, at increased risk for discrimination, prejudices, and oppression [23].

These factors will impact the way that a trafficked patient presents clinically and will also affect how we manage their psychiatric needs. Figure 3.1 depicts several structural factors that intersect to affect human trafficking survivors in the USA: the criminal justice system, socioeconomic status, family structure, race, gender, and experience of adverse childhood experiences.

Criminal Justice System

A Criminal Justice Approach to Trafficking

Anti-trafficking legislation in the USA is rooted in anti-prostitution laws and the historical debate around these laws. The historical debate around prostitution can be understood by looking at two main conflicting viewpoints on how to address

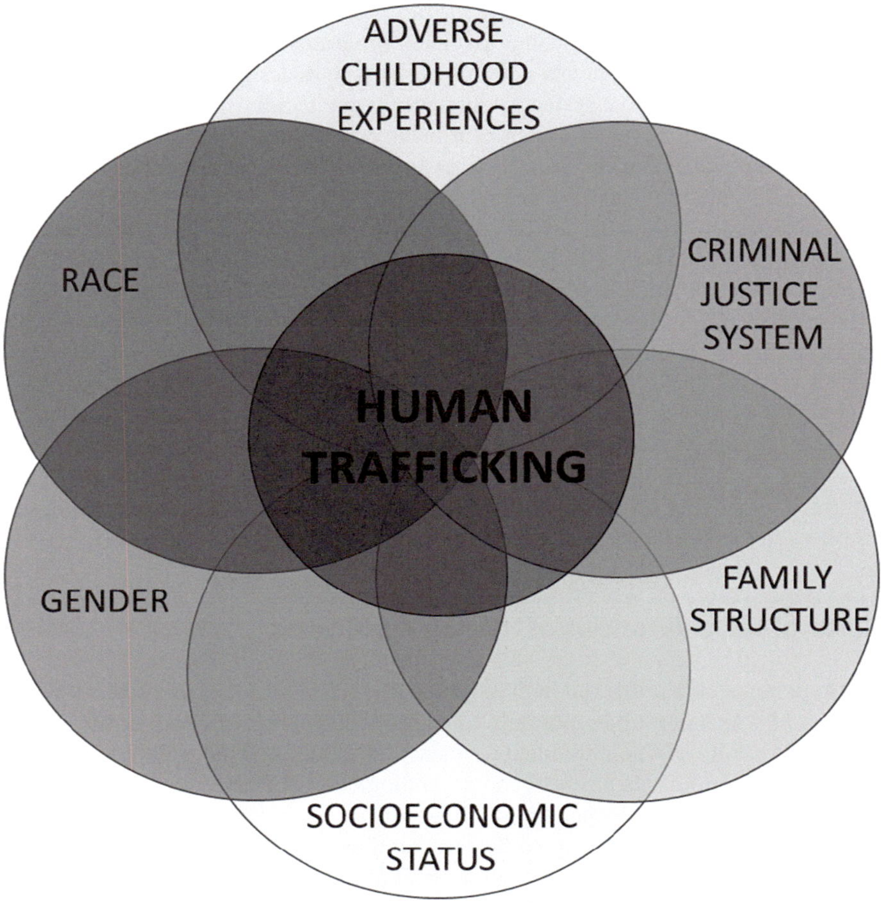

Fig. 3.1 Structural view of human trafficking

prostitution. The first position posits prostitution as a form of violence against women that is degrading, exploitative, and should be abolished. This point of view supports criminal law as a powerful method of combating prostitution [19]. Some refer to this stance as the "oppression paradigm" [98]. In contrast, the opposing position asserts that not all prostitution is exploitative, and some women voluntarily engage in prostitution. Some refer to this as the "empowerment paradigm" [98]. This stance rejects the criminalization of prostitution [19]. While there are many additional perspectives around prostitution that may not be classified within these two categories, these viewpoints serve the purpose of understanding the broader debate.

The oppression paradigm was, and in many ways continues to be, the driving force behind anti-trafficking legislation. Global anti-trafficking laws and policies have since been largely driven by anti-prostitution viewpoints that favor an aggressive criminal justice approach [19] and focus on the victimization of those in commercial sex while ignoring the root causes of the issue [98]. A criminal justice approach is one that is prosecution-oriented and focuses on cultivating victims as witnesses in order to prosecute and convict more traffickers [59]. This approach contrasts with a public health mission, which focuses on preventing the downstream health impacts of trafficking by addressing the needs of people who have been trafficked, empowering and supporting them, and acknowledging the impact of trafficking on individuals, families, and communities [15].

Although the approach to addressing trafficking in the USA today is rooted in a criminal justice framework, collaboration between the criminal justice system and nongovernmental organizations providing services to people who have been trafficked is increasing. Today, people who are identified as being trafficked or at risk for trafficking may receive a combination of services through both the criminal justice system and social services to address ongoing needs and provide support [59]. Efforts are needed to further a more comprehensive public health approach to human trafficking that focuses on the needs of trafficked people and how to best address these needs [15]. Services can include medical, psychological, housing, education, job training, and legal services among others.

Community and Police Relations

Traffickers rely on a trafficking survivor's fear of law enforcement to keep them hidden. Distrust of law enforcement officials deters trafficking survivors from reporting abuse and collaborating with legal efforts to prosecute traffickers [18, 20]. Furthermore, a trafficked individual may have been forced to commit a crime in the context of their exploitation [69]. In historically marginalized communities, this mistrust may be greater due to a history of mistreatment and poor relationships between law enforcement and BIPOC (black, indigenous, and people of color). This is particularly important as trafficking victims in the USA are disproportionately African-American and Latinx [10].

BIPOC are more likely to be stopped, arrested, and convicted of crimes. When convicted, they face harsher sentences [29]. The "War on Drugs" led to an increase in drug-related arrests [76], and these arrests disproportionately affected BIPOC. Black/African-American people make up 13% of the US population [95] but account for 27% of arrests for drug violations [32] and 38% of people incarcerated in prison for drug law violations [91]. Hispanic/Latinx people make up 18% of the population but account for 20% of arrests for drug abuse violations [32] and 37% of people incarcerated in prison for drug law violations [91].

Although drug-related arrests are higher among BIPOC, the Substance Abuse and Mental Health Services Administration (SAMHSA) reports similar proportions of illicit drug use among Blacks/African-Americans and Whites and slightly lower rates of illicit drug use among Hispanic/Latinxs compared to Whites [89]. Sentencing for drug-related offenses has disproportionately focused on drugs that are prevalent in Black and Latinx communities. For example, before the Fair Sentencing Act passed in 2010, there was a 100 to 1 disparity in sentencing between crack and powder cocaine, which have similar effects and addiction potential. Crack cocaine is more prevalent in Black and Latinx communities, and powder cocaine is more prevalent in White communities. This disproportionate sentencing led to greater numbers of Black people being incarcerated for drug offenses compared to Whites [2].

Young Black and Latino men also experience "aggressive policing," in which they are disproportionately stopped, searched, and detained based on suspicious behavior only later to be reported as innocent by police in eight out of ten cases [30]. Young Black and Latino males make up 5% of New York City's population yet accounted for 38% of reported stops between 2014 and 2017. Black and Latinx individuals were more likely to be frisked than White individuals, and among those who were frisked, they were less likely to be carrying a weapon [30]. Furthermore, Black, Native or Indigenous People, and Latinx individuals are disproportionately affected by police brutality. In 2017, Black people made up 25% of those killed by the police despite being only 13% of the population, and they were three times more likely to be killed by police than White people [13, 55]. The long history of structural racism and community and police interactions may also make BIPOC more reluctant to seek out legal support when they need it.

Immigration Policy

The immigrant population in the USA also faces unique challenges that increase their vulnerability to trafficking. Many immigrants and asylum seekers come to the USA fleeing violence or instability. Seeking a better life for their families, they often take jobs in some of the least desirable occupations. Current immigration and labor laws do not recognize the benefits that immigrant laborers bring to the USA and do not provide adequate protection to these individuals, leaving them vulnerable to exploitation [35]. Immigrant workers may fear the police and fear being deported, and those being trafficked for labor may be reluctant to provide information about their traffickers out of fear of punishment [64]. All of these factors can lead to increased exploitation of immigrant workers and underreporting of labor trafficking, leaving immigrant workers trapped and powerless in their situations.

Race

There are several aspects related to race that may increase vulnerability to sex and labor trafficking. Specifically, hypersexualized racial stereotypes, stereotypes of criminality, dehumanization, perception of less innocence, internalized racist beliefs, and limited resources and access to services all play a role in increased labor and sex trafficking in minoritized communities in the USA [37, 40].

Racial Stereotypes

Racial stereotyping and dehumanizing BIPOC have contributed to their sexual exploitation and trafficking in the USA. Many BIPOC have historically been stereotyped as hypersexual, impure, driven by sexual pleasure, and lacking autonomy [5, 62, 66, 67]. Racial stereotypes dehumanize and devalue BIPOC, contributing to the acceptability of their exploitation and increasing their vulnerability to human trafficking [9].

The stereotype of the Black woman as the "Jezebel," described as "seductive, alluring, worldly, beguiling, tempting, lewd, and innately promiscuous" [67] was first used during slavery to justify White men's unchecked, unpunished sexual abuse of Black women. After slavery, Jim Crow laws, and later the Mann Act, continued to enforce these negative stereotypes about Black women's sexuality in order to rationalize their continued rape and exploitation. This stereotype also shaped a culture in the USA that condoned and promoted the sexual exploitation of Black women [12].

In addition to using racial stereotypes to justify sexual exploitations of Black women, White settlers used stereotypes of Native American women's impurity to justify sexual assault, sexual mutilation, and prostitution [66]. The selling of Native American women began in the colonial era, and their exploitation continues today. Native American women experience alarmingly high rates of sexual and physical violence. In fact, 84% have experienced some type of violence in their lifetime, and 56% have experienced sexual violence [80]. There are notable gaps in data and research on trafficking of American Indian and Alaskan Native women [96]. In addition to stereotypes about their sexuality, their vulnerability to trafficking is reinforced by their "versatility," which allows traffickers and pimps to market Native American women as other races such as Mexican, Hawaiian, Asian, and others, to fit the desires of many different buyers [49].

Asian and Latina women also have been subject to being overly sexualized and objectified in US history. As a result of historical immigration laws that discriminated on the basis of race and gender, early Asian immigrants were primarily men. The few early Asian immigrant women in the USA were seen as sexual servants or extensions of their male counterparts with little autonomy [62]. The obedient, delicate "China Doll" and the aggressive yet sensual "Dragon Lady" are examples of American media stereotypes that dehumanize East Asian women and justify their dominance [51]. Latinas have a sexualized stereotype, the "hot Latina," defined as "exotic, sexual, and available, and as more in touch with their bodies and motivated by physical and sexual pleasure than white women" [5]. The stereotype of the "hot Latina" encourages the excessive use of makeup, perfume, clothing, and other associations affiliated with hypersexuality [5]. As a result of this stereotype, Latina women are more vulnerable to sexual harassment in the workplace [52] and may also be more vulnerable to trafficking.

Media

The media often misrepresents BIPOC as having qualities that are inferior to those of White people. News and media outlets often inaccurately and disproportionately portray Black families as socially unstable, living in poverty, and associated with criminality [26]. People who experience any type of racism are at risk for internalizing negative stereotypes about themselves, which can lead to shame and self-blaming behaviors. This type of internalized racism can lower BIPOC's feelings of self-worth and create a drive for external acceptance, making them more vulnerable to people who seek to exploit them [42].

Mental Health

Racism may also increase susceptibility to trafficking through its impact on mental health. Research shows that experiencing racial prejudice can cause feelings of emotional distress, and racism is associated with poorer mental health outcomes, including depression, anxiety, and posttraumatic stress [65]. These mental health impacts may be similar and intensify those experienced as a result of childhood trauma or maltreatment, which has been identified as a risk factor for childhood sexual exploitation [60].

The often tenuous migrant status of many people experiencing labor trafficking is associated with feelings of physical and cultural isolation, housing instability, inability to communicate in the dominant language, and a lack of familiarity with systems and institutions in the country where they are being trafficked. All of these factors can increase an individual's vulnerability and susceptibility to being trafficked for labor [24].

Access to Services and Legal Outcomes

Racial bias also affects the ability of people who have been trafficked to access supportive services. Identifying people who are being trafficked is the first step in providing these individuals with the supportive services they need. Many people who are trafficked go unidentified. Historically, the issue of trafficking has disproportionately focused on the White female experience [12]. When trafficking is viewed as an issue of White women, the experiences of BIPOC, LGBTQ populations, and trafficked men go overlooked, and fewer people in these groups are eligible for and receive needed services. Even when BIPOC are identified as having been trafficked, they may be poorly served or even harmed by the healthcare and legal system [77]. Decisions of judges and jurors are influenced by their own implicit and explicit biases, which have been shaped by a society that disproportionately associates BIPOC with criminality [77].

When BIPOC are identified as being trafficked and are connected to services, they may continue to confront bias that affects the quality of services they receive. In general, BIPOC receive lower-quality healthcare and are more likely to be diagnosed with severe mental health disorders [9, 58]. Unconscious racism and a lack of cultural awareness among service providers can lead to discrimination, the provision of lower-quality services, and early termination of services for BIPOC [9, 42].

People experiencing labor trafficking may also have limited access to supportive services due to limited knowledge and training among service providers about the issue of labor trafficking [1]. Most of the information designed for social workers who work with trafficked people is biased toward sex trafficking and neglects a discussion of labor trafficking or other forms of exploitation [1].

Adverse Childhood Experiences (ACEs)

Experiencing adverse events during childhood has been linked to an increased vulnerability to trafficking. Researchers at the Center for Disease Control and

Prevention (CDC) and Kaiser Permanente first used the adverse childhood experience (ACE) questionnaire in the early 1990s to study the effects of adverse childhood events on health risk behaviors, disability, disease, and premature mortality [33]. The ACE questionnaire has since been used by numerous researchers to investigate the relationship between ACEs and other health, behavioral, and social outcomes. The questionnaire consists of ten questions that address childhood trauma in the following categories: physical abuse, emotional abuse, sexual abuse, physical neglect, emotional neglect, household mental illness, household substance abuse, household domestic violence, incarcerated household member, and parental separation or divorce.

Several research studies have found associations between exposure to ACEs and sex trafficking in children and adolescents. In a study investigating the prevalence of ACEs among youth arrested for trading sex vs various other crimes, Naramore and colleagues found that sex-trafficked youth were more likely (81%) than non-sex-trafficked youth (50%) to have a high-risk ACE score (i.e., four or more ACEs) [60]. Specifically, sex-trafficked youth experienced high levels of parental separation or divorce (92%), household violence (90%), and household member incarceration (84%) [60]. They were also significantly more likely to have experienced physical neglect, sexual abuse, and parental separation or divorce in childhood [60, 75]. Childhood emotional abuse may reduce self-confidence and ability to manage emotions and lead to the use of survival strategies such as trading sex for necessities [88]. Emotional abuse during childhood is associated with a younger age of entry into commercial sexual exploitation [79].

Although less well-studied, histories of trauma and violence are also seen among people who experience labor trafficking. In a qualitative study exploring the characteristics and behaviors associated with labor trafficking, interviewees noted that many members of the migrant population experience domestic violence, child abuse, or past exploitation, and these experiences increase their vulnerability to further exploitation [24].

Family Structure

In addition to adverse childhood experiences, other family dynamics affect an individual's likelihood of being trafficked. Children who are involved in the foster care system, elope from home, or become homeless are more vulnerable to being trafficked [16]. Both running away from home and homelessness are associated with an increased risk of commercial sexual exploitation [22, 31]. Furthermore, youth who experience an unstable home environment may be less likely to have an adult in their life to provide guidance, protection, and support. In a study that explored the differences between youth experiencing homelessness who had been trafficked and youth experiencing homelessness who had not, the presence of one supportive adult was protective against being trafficked [16].

It is not uncommon for children and youth to be trafficked by members of their own family. In a survey that asked professionals working with sex-trafficked minors about the relationship of the person being trafficked to their trafficker, family member trafficking varied from 50% to 82% depending on the community setting [21]. Other studies have reported slightly lower estimates of family member trafficking; however, it is clear that family members play an important role in the trafficking of young people [7]. Research suggests that in over 60% of cases of familial trafficking, the trafficker is the mother [87]. In cases of familial trafficking, physical threats from caregivers, emotional threats of abandonment, intimidation, and parental authority are some of the tactics used to recruit and maintain youth in prostitution [87].

Youth who grow up in a household in which prostitution is the family business learn from a young age about the sense of control, power, and monetary benefits derived from work in prostitution or pimping. While not all pimps can be classified as traffickers, in a study exploring the experiences of ex-pimps, over half of which reported selling sex before pimping, many of the ex-pimps came from homes in which prostitution was the family business [73]. Some described how learning about the monetary benefits of the sex trade in their homes influenced their decision to participate. Others explained that their decision to enter the sex trade was driven by a desire to regain a sense of power and control in their environment [73].

Socioeconomic Factors

Individuals living in socioeconomically disadvantaged neighborhoods are more likely to experience adverse childhood events [84], have higher rates of posttraumatic stress disorder (PTSD) [36, 41], and have unstable housing [24], which all increase vulnerability to labor and sex trafficking [60]. Individuals experiencing poverty may be more likely to use survival strategies such as trading sex for necessities, which can put them at risk for future exploitation.

Wealth contributes to an individual's well-being and is protective against trafficking. Wealthier families have better healthcare and education, live in safer neighborhoods, secure higher-quality child care and supervision, have a greater financial ability to deal with emergency situations, and can afford higher-quality legal representation [39]. Wealth has historically been linked to race. The racial wealth gap has been widening since the Great Recession of 2008 and continues to grow. In 2013, the median wealth of White households was 13 times that of Black households and 10 times that of Hispanic households [48]. Some people have tried to explain the racial wealth gap by arguing that Black people are less frugal or are worse at managing their assets than White people; however, it has been shown that Black people actually have slightly higher savings rates than White people when accounting for household income and asset appreciation rates are similar among racial groups [39]. The historical, social, political, cultural, and economic factors that play into the racial wealth gap are complex. However, it is important to note the role that discriminatory credit practices have played in fueling this gap. For example, a 2009 report on race and mortgage lending in Twin Cities, Minnesota, found that Black residents earning over $150,000 were twice as likely to be denied a home loan in comparison to Whites earning below $40,000, and Black residents who were able to get loans were more than three times as likely to have a higher interest, subprime loan [44].

BIPOC face many disadvantages that lead them to experience higher rates of poverty, higher rates of adverse childhood events, lower rates of educational attainment, lower rates of employment, and worse access to healthcare in comparison to White people. These factors, along with other aspects of marginalization, structural racism, and bias, all increase BIPOC's vulnerability to human trafficking.

Gender

In the USA, trafficking has primarily been viewed as an issue affecting heterosexual cisgender women. As a result, the experiences of trafficked people of other gender identities and sexual orientations have been greatly overlooked. Although the exact percentage of men being trafficked in the USA is unknown, men and boys account for 29% of people being trafficked globally [45], and men have been shown to make up a large portion of labor trafficking [64]. Research exploring the sexual exploitation of youth indicates that gender is not associated with a trafficking experience [16].

Research on trafficking of men and boys is limited, although men and boys appear to share many of the same risk factors for trafficking as women and girls such as experiencing adverse childhood events, being kicked out of the house, and being homeless. However, as a result of male stereotypes, men and boys may be less likely to be identified as people being trafficked or to seek out help. LGBTQ trafficking is similarly overlooked and underreported [56]. A study on runaway/homeless youth found that youth involved in prostitution were more than five times as likely to report homosexual or bisexual identities compared to youth experiencing homelessness not involved in prostitution [100].

LGBTQ youth may face rejection from families who are unaccepting of their sexual orientation, and as a result, LGBTQ youth may run away and become homeless [99]. LGBTQ individuals make up about 7% of the general population, yet almost 40% of youth experiencing homelessness identify as LGBTQ [71]. Once homeless, LGBTQ youth are at a higher risk for mental health problems and victimization [61]. Homelessness puts all youth at risk for sexual exploitation, but LGBTQ youth report higher rates of sexual victimization. Close to 60% of LGBTQ youth experiencing homelessness report being sexually victimized compared to 33% of heterosexual youth experiencing homelessness, and LGBTQ youth experiencing homelessness are over seven times more likely to experience acts of sexual violence compared to heterosexual youth experiencing homelessness [61]. As a result of familial rejection and homelessness, LGBTQ youth may also be less likely to have a supportive adult, which has been identified as protective against trafficking [16].

LGBTQ people are more likely to experience mental health conditions and substance abuse compared to heterosexual individuals [57], which may further increase their risk for trafficking. Due to inadequate training of healthcare providers on the experiences and needs of the LGBTQ population, LGBTQ youth may have unmet medical, psychiatric, and psychological needs that also put them at risk for being trafficked [99].

There has been little research on the role of gender in trafficking. Overall, women may have increased vulnerability to trafficking and exploitation because they are more susceptible to oppression, subscribe to gender roles and social norms from their home country that differ from those in the USA, and may be considered subordinate as the result of a patriarchal culture [24]. Nevertheless, men make up a large proportion of people being trafficked for labor [64], and youth, regardless of gender, are often targeted for trafficking [16].

Vignette

Kerry, a 15-year-old African-American girl with a history of complex posttraumatic stress disorder and bipolar disorder was court-ordered for placement in a residential treatment center (RTC). She experienced a number of ACEs from a young age including physical abuse, verbal abuse, sexual abuse, emotional neglect, household mental illness, household substance abuse, household domestic violence, and parental separation. Upon admission, she was noted to have symptoms of non-suicidal self-injurious behaviors (SIB), physical and verbal aggression, and severe mood lability that made it unsafe for her to remain in the community. She presented with various high-risk behaviors including risky sexual behavior, falsifying/exaggerating information, and elopement that limited her response to community-based outpatient psychiatric care. Her caregivers were particularly concerned because they recently learned that she had been in contact with older men via social media.

Prior to Kerry's RTC admission, she had been living in a group home. She had previously been in her grandmother's custody but was placed in the group home due to behavioral difficulties. After a few days in the group home, she ran away and went missing for 12 days. Records indicated that a police officer found her at a motel meeting an older man for sex. She was residing with a couple in their early 20s who were allowing her to stay with them in exchange for money obtained through selling sex. She was admitted to a psychiatric hospital due to danger to self and was discharged with a treatment plan including lamotrigine and risperidone. Shortly after her discharge, she was readmitted to the psychiatric hospital after sharing her thoughts of suicide to group home staff. Following this second admission, the judge determined that she would benefit from placement at a RTC.

Kerry had a difficult time adjusting to the RTC and continued to engage in impulsive and dangerous behaviors. She had poor boundaries, was highly impulsive, and demonstrated a lack of insight and poor judgment. Additionally, she often engaged in attention-seeking behaviors, split staff and peers, and instigated fights amongst peers. Staff provided close supervision with regards to her phone, Internet, and social media use. She struggled to accept responsibility for her actions. On admission to the RTC, Kerry denied suicidal ideations, homicidal ideations, auditory hallucinations, or visual hallucinations. She denied any mood symptoms except for sadness related to her grandmother's depression.

Past Psychiatric Hx

Kerry has a history of four psychiatric hospitalizations, typically in the context of suicidal ideation and behavior. She has a history of two suicide attempts. At 11 years old, she attempted suicide by cutting her wrists. She more recently had an attempt at 14 years of age by overdosing on acetaminophen. She has been in and out of outpatient care and has never seen the same provider for more than 6 months. She has a history of admission to a group home for psychiatric and behavioral difficulties. Past diagnoses include oppositional defiant disorder, posttraumatic stress disorder, bipolar disorder, major depression, conduct disorder, and attention-deficit/hyperactivity disorder. She has been trialed on methylphenidate, clonidine, sertraline, fluoxetine, aripiprazole, risperidone, lamotrigine, carbamazepine, atomoxetine, guanfacine, and valproic acid. She never stayed on a medication for longer than 2 months, and she did not have a significant response to any of them.

Social History

The patient has lived with her grandparents since birth. On two separate occasions, she briefly lived with her biological mother. During both stays with her biological mother, the patient and her grandparents reported that she witnessed domestic violence and experienced physical abuse, emotional abuse, and neglect.

Educational History

The patient has been repeatedly suspended and expelled from three different schools. When she was 8 years old, the police were called to her school because she hit another student and was throwing objects at her teacher. She had an individualized education plan for grades 5–7 due to behavioral problems. She was last consistently enrolled in school in the seventh grade.

Family History

Both of her parents had substance use disorders. Her mother has a history of posttraumatic stress disorder. Her grandmother has depression. Her father had a significant cognitive impairment and resides in a rehabilitation facility for long-term care of individuals who cannot care for themselves.

Developmental History

Kerry was born full term to her 18-year-old biological mother and 21-year-old father. There were no complications with the pregnancy, and she reached all developmental milestones on time.

Substance Use History

The patient denied drug and alcohol use.

Past Medical History
History of hypokalemia requiring potassium supplementation, acne, and eczema.

Strengths
Kerry enjoys fashion, poetry, song writing, and discussing her feelings with adults whom she can trust and has a great deal of love and respect for her grandparents.

Psychiatric Assessment and Treatment of Human Trafficking Survivors

Assessment

In Kerry's situation, she was brought to the healthcare community due to her involvement with law enforcement. Identifying trafficked patients can be difficult. While there are no validated screening tools for human trafficking in psychiatric patients [6], screening tools have been developed in other patient populations including pediatric emergency rooms [38] and homeless youth shelters [17]. There are also nonspecific screening tools created for use by law enforcement, healthcare, and shelter workers [97]. Because these tools have not been validated in psychiatric patients, their utility is unclear. Moreover, because of lessons learned in the intimate partner violence literature, there is a shift away from using checkbox-based identification tools and moving more toward an approach of universal education [46]. This allows patients to discuss their experiences of violence in the way that they are most comfortable. It also shifts the conversation from one in which the goal is identification to one in which the goal is to meet the needs of the patient. One tool that helps providers do this is the PEARR (provide privacy, educate, ask, respect, and respond) tool [25].

It is also important that there is an identified protocol for managing clinical and safety needs if a patient is identified as being trafficked. Protocols should address how staff will be educated about trafficking, how patients will be screened, and what to do if a patient is identified as being trafficked. Protocols should address referrals to appropriate services, confidentiality, and mandatory reporting [3]. Involving law enforcement can be a complicated decision. Providers should be aware of their state's mandated reporting laws, and patients should be notified of limits to confidentiality. It is important to note that when there is no mandated reporting obligation, the decision to involve law enforcement should be a shared decision between patient and provider.

When managing the care of trafficked patients, providers should be cognizant that patients who are trafficked have a series of well-described psychiatric and medical sequelae [63]. Roughly 67% of trafficking victims report being seen by a medical provider at least once during trafficking [14]. Patients who are trafficked often suffer from neurological (e.g., cognitive, memory, headaches, dizziness), infectious (e.g., STI/HIV), cardiopulmonary, obstetric (e.g., foreign objects, pregnancy, pregnancy termination, abnormal pap smears, dysplasia requiring surgical excision), dermatological (e.g., burns, skin infections), and musculoskeletal (e.g., falls, back pain, traumatic injuries) disorders [28]. These presenting conditions may be driven by lack of access to care, neglect, crowding, exposure to infections during the trafficking process, forced drug or alcohol use, accidental injuries from unsafe working environments, or direct physical abuse. Patients often present to emergency rooms, obstetricians, and mental health providers for a combination of the above needs.

Trafficked patients suffer from a high prevalence of psychiatric sequelae including posttraumatic stress disorder, depression, self-harming behaviors, and suicidality [8, 63]. Longer periods of trafficking and more severe forms of violence toward the patient may increase the healthcare need. For example, victims who have been exploited for longer than 6 months report higher levels of depression and anxiety than those who were trafficked less than 3 months [63]. Psychological distress including shame, stigma, disrupted social identity, entrapment, religious discrimination, and cultural isolation exacerbates comorbid psychiatric and medical conditions [4]. Social stressors, such as waiting for documentation, further affect mental health. Longer duration of asylum procedures is also a risk factor for worsened psychiatric sequelae [53].

Treatment Recommendations

There are no identified treatment modalities specific to survivors of human trafficking, but a review of literature suggests that using cognitive modalities (e.g., cognitive processing therapy) to address symptoms is ideal [82]. Recommended treatment approaches include cultural responsiveness and trauma-informed care. Also, it is important that providers are aware of their potential implicit bias and how it may impact the care that they provide. Lastly, systems caring for trafficked persons must be aware of structural and cultural factors that can be adjusted to improve care.

Trauma-Informed Care

Addressing trauma is an important component of effective behavioral health services. Trauma-informed care is based on an understanding of the signs and symptoms of trauma, its pervasiveness, and its harmful impact. It also involves understanding the potential for re-traumatization and the potential for recovery [83]. There are six key principles to a trauma-informed approach: (1) safety, both staff members and the people they serve feel physically and psychologically safe; (2) trustworthiness and transparency, organizations operate with transparency and maintain trust with their clients and staff; (3) peer support, support from peers who have lived experiences of trauma; (4) collaboration and mutuality, addressing power differences between staff and clients and among staff members; (5) empowerment, voice, and choice, recognizing individuals' strengths and experiences and building upon them; (6) cultural, historical, and gender issues, moving past racial, cultural stereotypes, and biases, offering gender-responsive services, supporting healing through cultural connections, recognizing and addressing historical trauma and historical narratives, and responding to the racial, ethnic, and cultural needs of individuals [37, 83]. Qualitative studies indicate that these principals are important for working with individuals who have been sex trafficked. Useful key components of trauma-informed care identified by sex-trafficked youth include being nonjudgmental and allowing youth to share in their own time [78]. In Kerry's case, a nonjudgmental approach that allows Kerry to open up in her own time is critical.

Culturally Responsive Care

Understanding the cultural and structural factors that have positioned a youth to be trafficked may help providers have a more complete and trauma-informed understanding of why youth are trafficked. Clinicians who work with trafficked individuals should work to have a nonjudgmental stance. Cultural responsiveness refers to healthcare services that are respectful of, and relevant to, the health beliefs, health practices, culture, and linguistic needs of diverse consumer/patient populations and communities.

Moreover, cultural humility and responsiveness give us a frame for working with all populations. This frame involves taking an attitude of lifelong learning that includes frequent self-reflection, evaluation, and critique. Cultural humility also includes building mutually beneficial partnerships with communities and addressing the power imbalances between clinician and client [92].

Addressing Clinician Bias

Individuals from BIPOC groups are at a disproportionally increased risk of sex trafficking, and those who are trafficked may be treated differently once they have been identified resulting in further health disparities. These differences in treatment of BIPOC people impacted by sex trafficking and commercial sexual exploitation in the USA are due in part to historical and contemporary traumas of racism and racialized practices, policies, and ideologies. Treatment settings are often ill-equipped to manage diverse patient populations, particularly patients whose values and culture deviate from dominant cultural groups. Barriers to providing culturally responsive care include clinician's lack of awareness of the cultural and structural factors impacting patients and implicit and explicit biases. These biases may result in excessive use of involuntary commitment, biases in level of care, and excessive use of restraints in treatment settings [40, 86].

The ideal clinical encounter is one in which both the provider and the patient are keenly aware of the impact of racism and bias on mental health, and they are both able to freely discuss the experience and consequences of racism [90]. Oftentimes, clinicians are unaware of their own biases. Clinicians working with sex-trafficked individuals should commit to ongoing work to recognize and address their own implicit biases. Clinicians may consider starting by taking implicit association tests; tests validated to demonstrate where clinicians may have implicit biases [40, 50]. While more research must be done, some practices at reducing bias show some early promise. These strategies include exposing oneself to counter-stereotypical exemplars and ways to identify with the out-group [34]. As clinicians become more aware of their own biases, they will become better equipped to work with a diverse population.

Due to biases toward individuals who are sex-trafficked as well as against individuals from BIPOC groups, patients might be viewed by providers as "bad people" who have chosen to engage in "deviant" behavior. These attitudes can lead individuals to feel judged. Both sex-trafficked women and youth have expressed concerns about feeling judged by health providers [43, 74, 78]. In Kerry's case, clinicians should take the aforementioned considerations into account. Prior to beginning their clinical encounter with her, they may consider their own implicit biases about young African-American women and youth in the sex trade and how these biases may impact Kerry's care.

Systemic Changes

Apart from individual clinician interventions, there are systematic changes that can occur in order to improve the cultural responsiveness of care for sex-trafficked individuals from BIPOC groups. It is important to recognize that while clinicians may view the therapeutic space as "safe," the client may perceive that same space as "threatening." In most treatment settings, imbalanced emphasis on "protection" of victims of trafficking results in involuntary, locked, and judiciary involvement that further interferes with efforts to "prepare" survivors by incorporating community, family, mentorship, and culturally responsive programs. The foundations of the current anti-trafficking movement in a criminal justice response have resulted in what Musto classified as "carceral protectionism" [59]. At times trafficked people are treated as "victim-offenders," instead of victims. This approach can mimic the pattern of control that occurred between a trafficked person and their trafficker.

For example, victims of trafficking sometimes stay in shelters, but the shelters are locked down and have policies that resemble imprisonment. The blurring of rehabilitative and coercive approaches to domestic sex trafficking represents an extension of punitive tactics. This speaks to the tangible effects of an anti-trafficking ideology that has placed more emphasis on "saving victims" than on addressing the complex and systemic inequalities that create them. In the USA, such complexities and inequities are varied including factors previously discussed such as the criminal justice system, socioeconomic status, family structure, race, gender, and experience of adverse childhood experiences. Many of these are impacted by the persistent pipeline of resources from the welfare state into an expansive carceral state. Systems looking to create programs to care for trafficked individuals may consider embarking on a Racial Equity Impact Assessment (REIA). Race Forward: The Center for Racial Justice Innovation has created a toolkit to assist organizations in undergoing a REIA. An REIA systematically evaluates how a proposed program may impact racial and ethnic groups [72]. Beyond creating clinical spaces that are culturally responsive, there has been a recent call to engage mental health clinicians in changing social norms and improving public policies [85]. This work is necessary to improve the mental health of trafficked individuals, including those differentially affected by minoritized status or statuses.

The mental health system may consider whether less restrictive and culturally responsive community-based services are available for young people like Kerry. For example, a race-concordant outpatient provider delivering intensive case management services, peer mentorship services, and peer support groups focusing on distress tolerance, symptom self-management, racial injury, healthy relationships, education, and job skills may have been beneficial.

Conclusion

Human trafficking is a complex subject that is impacted by a variety of cultural and structural factors. Clinicians who are aware of these complexities can greatly improve the care of sex and labor trafficked patients, particularly those of BIPOC groups. Clinicians should provide care grounded in culturally responsive and trauma-informed approaches. Steps to providing this care include committing to a lifelong process of recognizing and minimizing one's own implicit and explicit biases, reducing the power imbalances in the therapeutic encounter, talking openly with patients about race and experiences of racism, working to eliminate structural racism embedded in existing mental health services, and working upstream to reduce risk factors that put people at risk of trafficking [92].

Summary of High-Yield Points

- Human trafficking is a serious human rights violation and public health issue. It is defined as the use of force, fraud, or coercion for the purpose of sexual exploitation or forced labor. Trafficking occurs across all races/ethnicities; however, African-Americans are disproportionately affected, making up nearly 40% of trafficking cases [10].
- In order to fully understand how trafficked individuals experience their exploitation, one must understand the structural and cultural frame that trafficking occurs within. The experience of a trafficked individual sits at the nexus of multiple structural factors including socioeconomic status, family structure, race, gender, the criminal justice system, and experience of adverse childhood experiences. These factors contribute to an individual's risk of trafficking, their ability to leave trafficking, and their recovery from the various physical and psychological sequelae of trafficking.
- People who are trafficked have a series of well-described psychiatric and medical sequelae. Roughly two-thirds of trafficking victims report being seen by a medical provider at least once during trafficking [14]. Healthcare professionals have a unique opportunity to provide services to people being trafficked, yet many feel undertrained to recognize, evaluate, and manage patients who are trafficked.
- In order to appropriately treat individuals experiencing trafficking, clinicians must identify and address their own biases, understand the cultural and structural factors impacting patients, and practice cultural humility as well as trauma-informed care.
- Systemic changes must also occur to improve the cultural responsiveness of care for individuals experiencing trafficking. Work must be done to eliminate structural racism embedded in existing mental health services and to reduce the upstream factors that put people at risk of trafficking.

References

1. Alvarez MB, Alessi EJ. Human trafficking is more than sex trafficking and prostitution: implications for social work. Affilia. 2012;27(2):142–52.
2. American Civil Liberties Union (ACLU). Racial disparities in sentencing, report to Inter-American Commission on Human Rights. 2014. Available via https://www.aclu.org/sites/default/files/assets/141027_iachr_racial_disparities_aclu_submission_0.pdf. Accessed 27 Dec 2019.
3. Baldwin SB, Barrows J, Stoklosa H. Protocol toolkit for developing a response to victims of human trafficking in health care settings. USA: Heal Trafficking and Hope for Justice; 2017.
4. Beck DC, Choi KR, Munro-Kramer ML, Lori JR. Human trafficking in Ethiopia: a scoping review to identify gaps in service delivery, research, and policy. Trauma Violence Abuse. 2017;18(5):532–43.
5. Beltran M. The Hollywood Latina body as site of social struggle: media constructions of stardom and Jennifer Lopez's "Cross-over Butt.". Quart Rev Film Video. 2002;19(1):71–86.
6. Bespalova N, Morgan J, Coverdale J. A pathway to freedom: an evaluation of screening tools for the identification of trafficking victims. Acad Psychiatry. 2016;40(1):124–8.
7. Bigelsen J, Vuotto S. Homelessness, survival sex and human trafficking: as experienced by the youth of Covenant House New York. Covenant House New York. 2013. Available via https://humantraffickinghotline.org/sites/default/files/Homelessness%2C%20Survival%20Sex%2C%20and%20Human%20Trafficking%20-%20Covenant%20House%20NY.pdf. Accessed 27 Dec 2019.
8. Borschmann R, Oram S, Kinner SA, Dutta R, Zimmerman C, Howard LM. Self-harm among adult victims of human trafficking who accessed secondary mental health services in England. Psychiatr Serv. 2017;68(2):207–10.
9. Bryant-Davis T, Tummala-Narra P. Cultural oppression and human trafficking: exploring the role of racism and ethnic bias. Women Ther. 2017;40(1–2):152–69.
10. Bureau of Justice (BOJ). Most suspected incidents of human trafficking involved allegations of prostitution of an adult or child. 2011. Available via https://www.bjs.gov/content/pub/press/cshti0810pr.cfm. Accessed 18 Feb 2020.
11. Bureau of Justice Statistics. Federal human trafficking prosecutions increased more than 40% from 2011 to 2015. 2018. Available via https://www.bjs.gov/content/pub/pdf/fphtc15pr.pdf. Accessed 15 Mar 2020.
12. Butler C. The racial roots of human trafficking. UCLA Law Rev. 2015;62:1464.
13. Center on Juvenile and Criminal Justice (CJCJ). Who are police killing. 2014. Available via http://www.cjcj.org/news/8113. Accessed 18 Feb 2020.
14. Chisolm-Straker M, Baldwin S, Gaïgbé-Togbé B, Ndukwe N, Johnson PN, Richardson LD. Health care and human trafficking: we are seeing the unseen. J Health Care Poor Underserved. 2016;27(3):1220–33.
15. Chisolm-Straker M, Stoklosa H, editors. Human trafficking is a public health issue: a paradigm expansion in the United States. Cham: Springer; 2017.
16. Chisolm-Straker M, Sze J, Einbond J, et al. A supportive adult may be the difference in homeless youth not being trafficked. Child Youth Serv Rev. 2018;91:115–20.
17. Chisolm-Straker M, Sze J, Einbond J, White J, Stoklosa H. Screening for human trafficking among homeless young adults. Child Youth Serv Rev. 2019;98:72–9.
18. Chuang J. The United States as global sheriff: using unilateral sanctions to combat human trafficking. Mich J Int Law. 2005;27:437.
19. Chuang JA. Rescuing trafficking from ideological capture: prostitution reform and anti-trafficking law and policy. Univ Pa Law Rev. 2009;158(6):1655–728.
20. Clawson HJ, Dutch N. Identifying victims of human trafficking: inherent challenges and promising strategies from the field. Washington, DC: US Department of Health and Human Services (HHS); 2008.

21. Cole J, Sprang G. Sex trafficking of minors in metropolitan, micropolitan, and rural communities. Child Abuse Negl. 2015;40:113–23.
22. Cole J, Sprang G, Lee R, et al. The trauma of commercial sexual exploitation of youth: a comparison of CSE victims to sexual abuse victims in a clinical sample. J Interpers Violence. 2016;31(1):122–46.
23. Crenshaw K. Mapping the margins: intersectionality, identity politics, and violence against women of color. Stanford Law Rev. 1993;43(6):1241–99.
24. Deckert JC, Warren S, Britton H. Midwestern service provider narratives of migrant experiences: legibility, vulnerability, and exploitation in human trafficking. Adv Soc Work. 2018;18(3):887–910.
25. Dignity Health. PEARR tool: trauma-informed approach to victim assistance in health care settings. 2018. Available via https://www.dignityhealth.org/-/media/Documents/PEARRToolm7.ashx?
26. Dixon TL. A dangerous distortion of our families: representations of families, by race, in news and opinion media. Color of Change and Family Story research report. December 2017. Available via https://colorofchange.org/dangerousdistortion. Accessed 27 Dec 2019.
27. Domoney J, Howard LM, Abas M, Broadbent M, Oram S. Mental health service responses to human trafficking: a qualitative study of professionals' experiences of providing care. BMC Psychiatry. 2015;15(1):289.
28. Dovydaitis T. Human trafficking: the role of the health care provider. J Midwifery Womens Health. 2010;55(5):462–7.
29. Drug Policy Alliance. The drug war, mass incarceration, and race. 2018. Available via http://www.drugpolicy.org/sites/default/files/drug-war-mass-incarceration-and-race_01_18_0.pdf. Accessed 27 Dec 2019.
30. Dunn C, Shames M. Stop-and-frisk in the De Blasio era. New York Civil Liberties Union (NYCLU). 2019. Available via https://www.nyclu.org/sites/default/files/field_documents/20190314_nyclu_stopfrisk_singles.pdf. Accessed 27 Dec 2019.
31. Estes RJ, Weiner NA. The commercial sexual exploitation of children in the US, Canada and Mexico. Philadelphia: University of Pennsylvania, School of Social Work, Center for the Study of Youth Policy; 2001.
32. Federal Bureau of Investigations (FBI). 2017 crime in the United States. Table 43A, Arrests by race and ethnicity, 2017. 2017. Available via https://ucr.fbi.gov/crime-in-the-u.s/2017/crime-in-the-u.s.-2017/tables/table-43. Accessed 27 Dec 2019.
33. Felitti VJ, Anda RF, Nordenberg D, et al. Relationship of childhood abuse and household dysfunction to many of the leading causes of death in adults: the Adverse Childhood Experiences (ACE) study. Am J Prev Med. 2019;56(6):774–86.
34. FitzGerald C, Martin A, Berner D, et al. Interventions designed to reduce implicit prejudices and implicit stereotypes in real world contexts: a systematic review. BMC Psychol. 2019;7(1):29. https://doi.org/10.1186/s40359-019-0299-7.
35. Freedom Network USA. Human trafficking and immigrant rights. 2015. Available via https://freedomnetworkusa.org/app/uploads/2018/07/HT-and-Immigrant-Rights.pdf. Accessed 27 Dec 2019.
36. Gapen MD, Cross K, Ortigo A, et al. Perceived neighborhood disorder, community cohesion, and PTSD symptoms among low-income African Americans in an urban health setting. Am J Orthopsychiat. 2011;81(1):31–7.
37. Gordon-Achebe K, Hairston DR, Miller S, Legha R, Starks S. Origins of racism in American medicine and psychiatry. In: Medlock M, Shtasel D, Trinh NH, Williams D, editors. Racism and psychiatry. Current clinical psychiatry. Cham: Humana Press; 2019. https://doi.org/10.1007/978-3-319-90197-8_1.
38. Greenbaum VJ, Dodd M, McCracken C. A short screening tool to identify victims of child sex trafficking in the health care setting. Pediatr Emerg Care. 2018;34(1):33–7.
39. Hamilton D, Darity W Jr. Race, wealth, and intergenerational poverty: there will never be a post-racial America if the wealth gap persists. Am Prospect. 2009;20(7):A10–2.

40. Hairston DR, Gibbs TA, Wong SS, Jordan A. Clinician bias in diagnosis and treatment. In: Medlock M, Shtasel D, Trinh NH, Williams D, editors. Racism and psychiatry. Current clinical psychiatry. Cham: Humana Press; 2019. https://doi.org/10.1007/978-3-319-90197-8_7.
41. Hong S, Burnett-Zeigler I. The frequency of PTSD and subthreshold PTSD among African-American women with depressive symptoms in a disadvantaged urban neighborhood: pilot study. J Racial Ethn Health Disparities. 2016;4(6):1069–73.
42. Hurst TE. Internalized racism and commercial sexual exploitation of children (CSEC). Race Gender Class. 2015;22(1–2):90–101.
43. Ijadi-Maghsoodi R, Bath E, Cook M, et al. Commercially sexually exploited youths' health care experiences, barriers, and recommendations: a qualitative analysis. Child Abuse Negl. 2018;76:334–41.
44. Institute on Metropolitan Opportunity. Communities in crisis: race and mortgage lending in the twin cities. University of Minnesota Law School. 2009. Available via https://scholarship.law.umn.edu/cgi/viewcontent.cgi?article=1093&context=imo_studies. Accessed 27 Dec 2019.
45. International Labour Organization (ILO). Global estimates of modern slavery: forced labour and forced marriage. Geneva: International Labour Office (ILO); 2017.
46. James L, Miller E. Beyond screening: a patient centered approach to intimate partner violence. Futures Without Violence. 2016. Available via https://www.futureswithoutviolence.org/beyond-screening-a-patient-centered-approach-to-domestic-violence/. Accessed 15 Sept 2020.
47. Kerr P. Treating trauma in the context of human trafficking: intersections of psychological, social and cultural factors. In: Ghafoori C, Smith, editors. International perspectives on traumatic stress: theory, access, and mental health services. Nova Science Publishers; 2016.
48. Kochhar R, Fry R. Wealth inequality has widened along racial, ethnic lines since end of great recession. Pew Res Cent. 2014;12(104):121–45.
49. Krol D. Identifying, tracking and preventing human trafficking in Indian country. Navajo-Hopi Observer. 2019. Available via https://www.nhonews.com/news/2019/mar/19/identifying-tracking-and-preventing-human-traffick/. Accessed 27 Dec 2019.
50. Lane KA, Banaji MR, Nosek BA, et al. Understanding and using the implicit association test: IV. In: Implicit measures of attitudes. The Guilford Press; 2007. p. 59–102.
51. Lee J. East Asian "China Doll" or "Dragon Lady"? Bridges Undergrad J Contemp Connect. 2018;3(1)
52. Lopez JP. Speaking with them or speaking for them: a conversation about the effect of stereotypes in the Latina/Hispanic women's experiences in the United States. New Horiz Adult Educ Human Resour Dev. 2013;25(2):99–106.
53. Lurie I. Psychiatric care in restricted conditions for work migrants, refugees and asylum seekers: experience of the open clinic for work migrants and refugees, Israel. Isr J Psychiatr Relat Sci. 2009;46(3):172–81.
54. Macias-Konstantopoulos W, et al. Human trafficking: the role of medicine in interrupting the cycle of abuse and violence. Ann Intern Med. 2016;165(8):582–58.
55. Mapping Police Violence. 2019. Available via http://mappingpoliceviolence.org. Accessed 27 Dec 2019.
56. Martinez O, Kelle G. Sex trafficking of LGBT individuals: a call for service provision, research, and action. Int Law News. 2013;42(4)
57. Medley G, Lipari RN, Bose J, et al. Sexual orientation and estimates of adult substance use and mental health: results from the 2015 National Survey on Drug Use and Health. NSDUH data review. 2016. Available via https://www.samhsa.gov/data/sites/default/files/NSDUH-SexualOrientation-2015/NSDUH-SexualOrientation-2015/NSDUH-SexualOrientation-2015.htm. Accessed 27 Dec 2019.
58. Metzl J. The protest psychosis: how schizophrenia became a Black disease. Boston: Beacon Press; 2009.

59. Musto J. Control and protect: collaboration, carceral protection, and domestic sex trafficking in the United States. Oakland: University of California Press; 2016.
60. Naramore R, Bright MA, Epps N, et al. Youth arrested for trading sex have the highest rates of childhood adversity: a statewide study of juvenile offenders. Sex Abus. 2017;29(4):396–410.
61. National Coalition for the Homeless. LGBT homelessness. 2017. Available via https://nationalhomeless.org/wp-content/uploads/2017/06/LGBTQ-Homelessness.pdf. Accessed 27 Dec 2019.
62. Okihiro GY. Margins and mainstreams: Asians in American history and culture. Seattle: University of Washington Press; 2014.
63. Oram S, Stöckl H, Busza J, Howard LM, Zimmerman C. Prevalence and risk of violence and the physical, mental, and sexual health problems associated with human trafficking: systematic review. PLoS Med. 2012;9(5):e1001224.
64. Owens C, Dank M, Breaux J, et al. Understanding the organization, operation, and victimization process of labor trafficking in the United States. Washington, DC: Urban Institute; 2014.
65. Paradies Y, Ben J, Denson N, et al. Racism as a determinant of health: a systematic review and meta-analysis. PLoS One. 2015;10(9):e0138511.
66. Pierce A, Koepplinger S. New language, old problem: sex trafficking of American Indian women and children. VAWnet, a project of the National Resource Center on Domestic Violence. 2011. Available via https://vawnet.org/material/new-language-old-problem-sex-trafficking-american-indian-women-and-children. Accessed 27 Dec 2019.
67. Pilgrim D. The Jezebel stereotype. 2002. Available via https://www.ferris.edu/jimcrow/Jezebel/. Accessed 27 Dec 2019.
68. Polaris. Human trafficking issue brief: safe harbor. 2015. Available via https://polarisproject.org/sites/default/files/2015%20Safe%20Harbor%20Issue%20Brief.pdf. Accessed 27 Dec 2019.
69. Polaris. Bill to clear human trafficking survivor criminal records introduced. 2016. Available via https://polarisproject.org/news/press-releases/bill-clear-human-trafficking-survivor-criminal-records-introduced. Accessed 27 Dec 2019.
70. Polaris. The typology of modern slavery: defining sex and labor trafficking in the United States. 2017. Available via https://polarisproject.org/the-typology-of-modern-slavery/. Accessed 15 Mar 2020.
71. Polaris. Sex trafficking and LGBTQ youth. 2019. Available via https://polarisproject.org/sites/default/files/LGBTQ-Sex-Trafficking.pdf. Accessed 27 Dec 2019.
72. Race Forward: The Center for Racial Justice Innovation. Racial equity impact assessment. 2009. Available via https://www.raceforward.org/sites/default/files/RacialJusticeImpactAssessment_v5.pdf. Accessed 27 Dec 2019.
73. Raphael J, Myers-Powell B. From victims to victimizers: interviews with 25 ex-pimps in Chicago. Chicago: Schiller DuCanto & Fleck Family Law Center of DePaul University College of Law; 2010.
74. Ravi A, Pfeiffer MR, Rosner Z, et al. Trafficking and trauma: insight and advice for the healthcare system from sex-trafficked women incarcerated on Rikers Island. Med Care. 2017;55(12):017–1022.
75. Reid JA. Risk and resiliency factors influencing onset and adolescence-limited commercial sexual exploitation of disadvantaged girls. Crim Behav Ment Health. 2014;24(5):332–44.
76. Reuter P. Why has US drug policy changed so little over 30 years? Crime Justice. 2013;42(1):75–140.
77. Richardson L. Systemic triage: implicit racial bias in the criminal courtroom. Yale Law J. 2017;126(3):862–93.
78. Robitz R, Ulloa EC, Salazar M, Ulibarri MD. Mental health service needs of commercially sexually exploited youth: voices of survivors and stakeholders. Violence Vict. 2020;35(3):354–62.
79. Roe-Sepowitz DE. Juvenile entry into prostitution: the role of emotional abuse. Violence Against Women. 2012;18(5):562–79.

80. Rosay AB. Violence against American Indian and Alaska Native women and men: 2010 findings from the National intimate partner and sexual violence survey. National Institute of Justice. 2016. Available via https://www.ncjrs.gov/pdffiles1/nij/249736.pdf. Accessed 27 Dec 2019.
81. Ross C, Dimitrova S, Howard LM, Dewey M, Zimmerman C, Oram S. Human trafficking and health: a cross-sectional survey of NHS professionals' contact with victims of human trafficking. BMJ Open. 2015;5(8):e008682.
82. Salami T, Gordon M, Coverdale J, Nguyen PT. What therapies are favored in the treatment of the psychological sequelae of trauma in human trafficking victims? J Psychiatr Pract. 2018;24(2):87–96.
83. Substance Abuse and Mental Health Services Administration (SAMHSA). SAMHSA's concept of trauma and guidance for a trauma-informed approach. 2014. Available via https://ncsacw.samhsa.gov/userfiles/files/SAMHSA_Trauma.pdf.
84. Schilling EA, Aseltine RH, Gore S. Adverse childhood experiences and mental health in young adults: a longitudinal survey. BMC Public Health. 2007;7(1):30.
85. Shim RS, Compton MT. Addressing the social determinants of mental health: if not now, when? If not us, who? Psychiatr Serv. 2018;69(8):844–6.
86. Spector R. Is there racial bias in clinicians' perceptions of the dangerousness of psychiatric patients? A review of the literature. J Ment Health. 2001;10(1):5–15. https://doi.org/10.1080/09638230020023570.
87. Sprang G, Cole J. Familial sex trafficking of minors: trafficking conditions, clinical presentation, and system involvement. J Fam Violence. 2018;33(3):185–95.
88. Stoltz JAM, Shannon K, Kerr T, et al. Associations between childhood maltreatment and sex work in a cohort of drug-using youth. Soc Sci Med. 2007;65(6):1214–21.
89. Substance Abuse and Mental Health Services Administration (SAMHSA) 2017 National Survey on Drug Use and Health: Detailed Tables. Table 1.30B Illicit drug use in past year among persons aged 12 or older, by Age Group and Demographic Characteristics: Percentages, 2016 and 2017. Available via https://www.samhsa.gov/data/sites/default/files/cbhsq-reports/NSDUHDetailedTabs2017/NSDUHDetailedTabs2017.pdf. Accessed 27 Dec 2019.
90. Sue DW, Sue D, Neville HA, Smith L. Counseling the culturally diverse: theory and practice. Wiley; 2019.
91. Taxy S, Samuels J, Adams W. Drug offenders in federal prison: estimates of characteristics based on linked data. Washington, DC: US Department of Justice, Office of Justice Programs, Bureau of Justice Statistics; 2015.
92. Tervalon M, Murray-Garcia J. Cultural humility versus cultural competence: a critical distinction in defining physician training outcomes in multicultural education. J Health Care Poor Underserved. 1998;9(2):117–25.
93. United Nations Office on Drugs and Crime (UNODC). Protocol to prevent, suppress and punish trafficking in persons, especially women and children, supplementing the United Nations convention against transnational organized crime. United Nations Office on Drugs and Crime. Vienna: United Nations Convention against Transnational Organized Crime and the Protocols Thereto; 2000.
94. United States. Victims of Trafficking and Violence Protection Act of 2000 (TVPA). US Government Printing Office; 2000.
95. U.S. Census Bureau. Quick facts. 2018. https://www.census.gov/quickfacts/fact/table/US/PST045218. Accessed 27 Dec 2019.
96. U.S. Department of Justice. Human trafficking (including sex trafficking) of American Indians and Alaska natives. 2017. Available via https://www.justice.gov/ovw/page/file/998081/download.
97. Vera Institute of Justice. Screening for human trafficking: guidelines for administering the Trafficking Victim Identification Tool (TVIT). 2014. Available via https://www.vera.org/downloads/publications/human-trafficking-identification-tool-and-user-guidelines.pdf.
98. Weitzer R. Sex trafficking and the sex industry: the need for evidence-based theory and legislation. J Crim Law Criminol. 2011;101:1337.

99. Xian K, Chock S, Dwiggins D. LGBTQ youth and vulnerability to sex trafficking. In: Chisolm-Straker M, Stoklosa H, editors. Human trafficking is a public health issue. Cham: Springer; 2017. p. 141–52.
100. Yates GL, MacKenzie RG, Pennbridge J, et al. A risk profile comparison of homeless youth involved in prostitution and homeless youth not involved. J Adolesc Health. 1991;12(7):545–8.
101. Cary M, Oram S, Howard LM et al. (2016) Human trafficking and severe mental illness: an economic analysis of survivors' use of psychiatric services. BMC Health Services Research 16(1):1–8.

Survivors of Combat Trauma

4

Savannah L. Woodward and David Nissan

When I'm asleep, dreaming and lulled warm,
They come, the homeless ones, the noiseless dead.
While the dim charging breakers of the storm
Bellow and drone and rumble overhead,
Out of the gloom they gather about my bed.
They whisper to my heart; their thoughts are mine.
"Why are you here with all your watches ended?
From Ypres to Frise we sought you in the Line."
In bitter safety I awake, unfriended;
And while the dawn begins with slashing rain
I think of the Battalion in the mud.
"When are you going out to them again?
Are they not still your brothers through our blood?"
Siegfried Sassoon, 1918

Introduction

It has long been recognized that one's cultural background contributes dramatically to the way that an individual interacts with the world around them and the way the world interacts with them in return. This is certainly true in medicine and particularly so in psychiatry where one's perception and background have a significant impact on diagnosis, conceptualization, treatment, and clinical outcomes. One distinct culture that is often under-recognized is that of military service members. In many societies, at least at the time of this writing, military service and direct

S. L. Woodward · D. Nissan (✉)
Department of Psychiatry, Naval Medical Center San Diego, San Diego, CA, USA
e-mail: david.a.nissan.mil@mail.mil

S. H. Koh et al. (eds.), *Diversity in Action*,
https://doi.org/10.1007/978-3-030-85401-0_4

exposure to combat have become increasingly infrequent, and only a small minority of citizens experiences the brutal reality of war firsthand. Most ancient civilizations had rituals to acknowledge the metamorphosis that occurs with or in preparation for combat. In Maori culture, the Haka, known as a war cry, is performed prior to war. In Jewish culture, laws mandated that those who killed or touched anyone who had killed must remain outside of the camp for 7 days [1]. Many early societies revered survivors of combat, extolling them as the "normals" who possessed a special knowledge unknown to those spared that exposure [2]. As time and technology have progressed, less and less of the population has been directly exposed to traditional combat.

Currently, only about 10% of the adult population in the United States has served in the military, and 80% of new military recruits have at least one family member who previously served [3]. The term "warrior caste" has been used to describe this hereditary phenomenon and to illustrate the smallness of the population with a military history [3]. As combat exposure becomes a rare experience, the divide between those who experienced war and those who have not grows more profound. Clinicians working with this population must recognize this chasm and make an effort to understand the nature of this barrier, within and out of military culture, in order to provide combat veterans with meaningful psychological support and treatment.

When assessing for any mental illness in a culturally informed way, it is important to consider three specific aspects (though it should be noted that not all three of these may be applicable to every culture) [4]:

1. Cultural-specific syndromes, clusters of symptoms (psychiatric and otherwise) common to members with the shared experience
2. Idioms of distress, or how members communicate, or may fail to communicate, his or her emotional suffering
3. Cultural explanations of perceived causes

With these factors in mind, the provider can then create a cultural formulation (see the "Cultural Formulation Interview" in the *Diagnostic and Statistical Manual of Mental Disorders, Fifth Edition*, DSM-5) [5] as a means of conceptualizing the patient and their presentation. This should incorporate the cultural identity of the individual, their cultural conceptualization of distress, psychosocial stressors and cultural features of vulnerability and distress, cultural features of the relationship between the individual and the clinician, and an overall cultural assessment for diagnosis and treatment.

This chapter aims to explore the specific cultural challenges that come with treating survivors of combat trauma. Key cultural characteristics of the military are discussed including stoicism, team orientation, stigma related to seeking mental health care, and an ingrained belief in an external locus of control, among others, and how they relate to the treatment of combat trauma in both active duty service members and veterans. Through a review of relevant background information and a case vignette, unique challenges and specific recommendations for providers working with this patient population are presented.

Background

Military Structure and Organization

To understand military culture, it is helpful to first understand military structure. The US military is divided into both active and reserve components. Said reserve component is comprised of the National Guard and the Reserves (each branch of the military has its own reserve service). The active component, on the other hand, is comprised of the five branches of the military: the US Navy, Marine Corps, Air Force, Army, and Coast Guard. Members of the active component are full-time military personnel who can be deployed (i.e., moved into position for military action) at any time, whereas members of the reserve component are not full-time employees and are typically only called into active duty during times of war or national emergency. During Operation Iraqi Freedom/Operation Enduring Freedom (OIF/OEF), reserves from all branches were heavily utilized, so it is important to not make assumptions about deployments based on reserve or active status.

All military members are either enlisted or hold officer rank in their respective branch. Enlisted personnel begin their service by going to a branch specific basic training (boot camp), between 7 and 12 weeks in duration. In basic training they are prepared for the military – physically, mentally, and emotionally – and they also learn about the culture and traditions of their respective service. Following basic training, enlisted personnel typically proceed to specialized training tailored to their specific job within a specialty (e.g., aircraft mechanic, infantry, nuclear electrician's mate) for several months or, in some cases, years. Once they complete this additional training, enlisted service members are sent to their first duty station. It should be noted that enlisted personnel typically join at a younger age (i.e., 18 or when they complete high school), though it is not uncommon for individuals to enter service later in life, spending time in other occupations or secondary education. Officers, on the other hand, have various routes to join: attending a service academy (e.g., the Naval Academy in Annapolis, Maryland, West Point), Reserve Officer Training Corps programs (ROTC), or by going to Officer Candidate School which is similar to the enlisted boot camp but with an emphasis on developing leadership skills. There are also several programs that allow enlisted service members to earn a commission and become officers. Depending on their job and specialty (e.g., infantry, surface, aviation), officers will also proceed to additional training before being sent to their first command. There are officer programs that allow senior enlisted to commission as Warrant Officers or Limited Duty Officers in fields that require a high degree of specialization.

The fundamental leadership structure of the military is the chain of command. This concept describes whom each member of the military reports to and takes orders from. An individual junior enlisted member is grouped with other junior personnel into a platoon, shop, division, etc. (the terms vary widely between each branch and even amongst different communities within each branch). Junior enlisted members are typically led by another enlisted service member with a few years of experience (noncommissioned officers, or NCOs, in the Army, Air Force and Marine

Corps; Petty Officers in the Navy and Coast Guard). Above them are Staff NCOs (Army, Air Force, Marines) and Chief Petty Officers (Navy, Coast Guard), who work with a junior officer (0–3 years of service) to run the platoon or division. Several platoons/divisions coalesce into companies/departments, which report to a Commanding Officer, aided by the Executive Officer (second in command), and Senior Enlisted Leader (works as an advisor and liaison between enlisted members and the Commanding Officer). *Although everyone has a supervisor to whom they report, all service members (even junior enlisted) are expected to look out for and support their lower ranking counterparts.*

The chain of command has much more responsibility and authority than would be typical of a civilian employer. In addition to acting as a work supervisor, they are responsible for the "care and feeding" of each of their service members, as well as their general well-being. Service members are encouraged to discuss personal issues with their chain of command (e.g., family illness, financial struggles), and commands have designated personnel to provide preliminary assistance (e.g., financial counseling, drug and alcohol programs advisor). Senior enlisted and junior officers are strongly encouraged to get to know their people, learn about the difficulties they face, and use command/military resources to help them face and overcome obstacles. This increased responsibility is also present in the military's disciplinary system. In stark contrast to the civilian world, the Commanding Officer is also delegated significant legal authorities, administering "nonjudicial punishment" (e.g., reprimand, reduction in rank, loss of pay, extra duty, and being placed on restriction) for lower violations of the Uniformed Code of Military Justice. The increased role the chain of command plays in a service member's life is thought to foster the semiconscious or unconscious notion that individuals have less control over events than is actually true. This external locus of control is thought to contribute to some posttraumatic symptoms and is described in more detail below.

The Pillars of Military Culture

> *[Armies] are institutions that create a world. [They] successfully engender the new member's respect, loyalty, love, affirmation, gratitude, and obedience.*
>
> Jonathan Shay, Achilles in Vietnam: Combat Trauma and the Undoing of Character [6]

With some background of military structure and organization in place, one can now begin to understand the three key pillars of military culture:

1. An external locus of control
2. Stoicism
3. Service to others above self

As described in detail above, the military is a highly structured organization. Because of this structure, it is paramount that the chain of command is observed, otherwise – as all service members are taught – the organization ceases to function. This mindset is repeatedly reinforced throughout one's military career to the point that it is ingrained in the psyche. It should also be noted that many aspects of a service member's life are controlled by their respective branch. For example, junior enlisted who are not married must live in military housing on base (called "barracks") or on board their ship. Furthermore, unlike the civilian sector, if a service member dislikes their job, they have no option to quit and must await the completion of their multi-year contract. Additionally, the maintenance that service member's perform on equipment is typically laid out in very specific checklists that must be followed sequentially. While many of their jobs still require a high degree of ingenuity to face complex problems in a dynamic environment, they are trained on reading and following detailed instructions. The military environment fosters the belief that the service member is not in control of the events in their lives. This culture has multiple important benefits such as increasing the reliability of the organization, preventing safety mishaps, and ensuring that service members can react quickly in times of duress to take complex action in service of their nation. When tragedies occur in spite of this training, preparation, and execution, or when a service member perceives they failed to take proper action to prevent the disaster, this sense of an external locus of control can lead to profound feelings of hopelessness or helplessness, traits which are frequently observed in combat veterans receiving trauma-focused treatment. This may also affect their readjustment to post-military life when they must take a more active role in making choices for their future.

Stoicism is a key trait that closely accompanies maintenance of the chain of command, because without either one of these, there is no hope for survival in times of war. Service members are taught to remain stoic in the face of adversity, and great generals and admirals are lauded for their ability to stay calm and collected during times of conflict. Despite recent campaigns to normalize seeking support for mental health conditions, the stigma still remains. Not only is emotionality felt to be detrimental to the mission, but it is also looked down upon, and the ones who show it are considered weak. As such, those who succeed in their military careers are the ones who "suck it up" and avoid succumbing to any emotional pitfalls.

Lastly, there is an increased focus on service and putting other unit members ahead of themselves. This is a culture that strives for cohesion of the unit, which can only be obtained by supporting others and the mission above oneself. If one member of the unit succeeds, the entire unit succeeds. The reverse is true as well, for if one member of the unit fails, the entire unit shoulders the consequences. As a result, service members are expected to support subordinates and their unit as a whole. Additionally, it is within the Commanding Officer's job description to ensure the command's service members' well-being (including housing, food, financial counseling, mandated time for fitness, etc.) at all times. It is because of this sense of duty to others that commands extend beyond a typical office environment and more closely resemble a family.

Combat and Its Effects

The experience of humans in war has been a cornerstone of storytelling for as long as we have been able to communicate. Although combat stress had been recognized as far back as ancient Greece, it was not until World War I (WWI) that the medical community began to identify the role of combat trauma in causing lasting psychological distress. During this time, physicians caring for soldiers that returned from combat described a number of patients with paralyzed limbs and other bizarre disorders of movement, blindness, hysteria, and mutism with seemingly no physical etiology. It was initially theorized that these symptoms were the direct result of nerve injury caused by exposure to repetitive gunshots and mortar explosions, leading to the concept of "shell shock." The term "shell shock" was first coined by Charles Myers, a psychiatrist well-known for his work with WWI soldiers in Britain. Dr. Myers described shell shock as mental shock which resulted from being "buried, lifted, or otherwise subjected to the physical effects of a bursting shell or other similar explosive" [7]. Both he and William Rivers, another British psychiatrist, were among the first to recognize that the suffering of these soldiers was genuine, and they advocated for more humane treatment. Though it was Major Arthur Hurst who revolutionized the conceptualization and treatment of shell shock.

Major Hurst, a general practitioner with no formal psychiatric expertise, shot the motion picture *War Neuroses* in 1917 as a means to further characterize the disorder. It was the first film of its kind and featured a number of patients whom he diagnosed with "war neuroses" (Hurst's preferred term to shell shock) [8, 9]. He characterized the syndrome of war neuroses as being comprised of a number of symptoms (which he identified as being neurologic in origin) to include poor appetite, tremor, paralysis, anxiety/hysteria, depression, dizziness, confusion, insomnia, nightmares, and blindness/deafness. In early 1918, Major Hurst opened a military hospital, Seale Hayne, dedicated to treating soldiers with war neuroses [10]. There, Hurst developed a treatment technique that closely resembles exposure therapy, focused on repeatedly reliving and reviewing the traumas of war until the images lost their power over the patient. Hurst even went so far as to recreate a battlefield for a final exercise he called "The Battle of Seale Hayne," which was designed to allow patients to relive the trauma of war in a controlled environment. Many former soldiers acted injured (to make the event seem more realistic) and were carried off the field by "medics." The technique was reportedly wildly successful with Major Hurst declaring, "We are now disappointed if complete recovery does not occur within 24 hours of commencing treatment, even in cases which may have been in other hospitals for over a year [10]."

Despite the increasing understanding that shell shock or war neuroses was a medical condition versus a disorder of constitution, there was little sympathy or understanding for these soldiers among the general public and even less so within the military. Many soldiers who later received diagnoses of shell shock or war neuroses were considered emotionally weak cowards. A large number of these soldiers were charged with desertion or insubordination and punished accordingly, with 306 soldiers in the British Army executed for cowardice in WWI [11, 12]. Consequently, the ideals of strength and heroism remained and were continually reinforced as critical internal and external barriers to seeking psychological care.

Combat Trauma in the Modern Day

Charles Myers, the first individual to use the term shell shock in a medical journal, soon realized the term was a misnomer, as many of the soldiers he treated had not been directly exposed to shelling [7]. While the term remained popular throughout WWI, mental health practitioners in World War II described soldiers with prolonged traumatic reactions as having "combat fatigue" or "battle fatigue." Military psychiatrists in Vietnam made an infamous claim that the rate of mental health casualties in the war was incredibly low, failing to predict or prepare for the increased recognition of chronic symptoms after traumatic experiences. It was this increased clinical and political focus on returning veterans with psychiatric difficulties that led to the description of "post-Vietnam syndrome." Researchers and patient advocacy groups recognized that these symptoms were not specific to combat experiences, and the term posttraumatic stress disorder (PTSD) was first included in the DSM-III in 1980.

Prolonged traumatic symptoms after exposure to combat are now represented in the DSM-5 as a number of trauma or stressor-related diagnoses. Current theories conceptualize traumatic stress reactions as existing on a continuum ranging from acute stress disorder (a stress reaction lasting between 3 days and 1 month following the traumatic event) to posttraumatic stress disorder (PTSD). The DSM-5 defines both acute stress disorder and PTSD as syndromes that occur after exposure to a traumatic incident either by way of directly experiencing it or by being repeatedly exposed to it (such as a medical professional caring for multiple patients with gunshot wounds), learning of a traumatic event occurring to someone close to them, or witnessing the traumatic event [5]. Symptoms of this disorder occur in four specific symptom clusters: avoidance (primarily of stimuli reminiscent of the trauma), negative emotions and cognitions, hyperarousal, and intrusive thoughts/memories of the trauma. This can be further delineated by the presence of dissociative symptoms, specifically depersonalization and derealization [5].

It is common for individuals to meet some, but not all, of these criteria, or for symptoms to exist with a range of occupational or interpersonal impairments. This is perhaps especially true of combat veterans in active service. Hypervigilance may be a strength for many military occupation specialties, and individuals who are constantly preparing for war and thinking about enemy threats are likely to perceive the world as inherently dangerous. Symptoms may, therefore, be difficult to recognize by both the clinician and the patient. As such, it is important to consider the individual's occupation and how it may mask or reinforce some of their symptoms.

Although much of the pathophysiology of PTSD has yet to be fully revealed, research in the area is rapidly expanding. Curiously, some imaging studies have described a number of notable structural differences in patients with PTSD to include decreased hippocampal volume, decreased left amygdala volume, and decreased volume of the anterior cingulate gyrus [13]. These findings are particularly interesting, given the known role of the amygdala and hippocampus in identifying and processing environmental threats. Other studies focusing on the neurochemical effects of PTSD have found evidence of increased norepinephrine levels centrally with seemingly downregulated adrenergic receptors, as well as upregulation of glucocorticoid receptors, but overall decreased glucocorticoid levels [14, 15]. One proposed mechanism is a chronically activated sympathetic nervous system that, in turn, leads to noradrenergic and glucocorticoid dysregulation, which may result in some of the structural changes described above.

When assessing patients for a trauma-related disorder, it is important to first understand the nature of the traumatic exposure. Particularly in military populations, the traumatic event may be atypical and is often not related to direct combat exposure. For example, consider the case of a 36-year-old enlisted male who presents with trauma-related symptoms. When queried about the trauma resulting in his symptoms, he reports reviewing drone footage of covert attacks for his job in the US Navy to document the details of each mission and maintain a written record of each assault. To assess whether this patient meets criteria for a trauma-related disorder, it would be important to understand if he has been exposed to actual or threatened death, serious injury, or sexual violence per the DSM-5 [5]. To do this, the nature of the films he reviewed must be clarified (e.g., do the videos contain images of individuals being killed vs. a nondescript building being bombed; how many of these videos does he watch; are the individuals in these videos enemy combatants, fellow service members, or innocent bystanders?). It should also be noted that there are a number of factors associated with increased risk of developing PTSD, which should be considered when assessing for trauma-related symptoms, including experiencing direct combat, severity of injury, childhood adversity, and lower military rank (and hence, likely a heightened sense of external locus of control) [16]. Additionally, it is important to determine if the reported symptoms are specifically associated with the traumatic event. As one may imagine, symptoms such as anxiety, depression, and insomnia are quite prevalent in military populations. It is important to distinguish the etiologies of the reported symptomology to ensure that the patient truly has a trauma-related disorder (e.g., insomnia secondary to nightmares about a traumatic event vs. insomnia secondary to obstructive sleep apnea).

Of course, there are a number of comorbidities which providers should be aware of when screening for posttraumatic stress disorder. Perhaps the most notable psychiatric comorbidities, particularly in the veteran population, are substance use disorders. One study reported that among veterans diagnosed with either or both an alcohol use disorder and drug use disorder, 55–75% also met criteria for a PTSD or depression diagnosis, and veterans with PTSD were 3–4.5 times more likely to be diagnosed with a substance use disorder [17]. Additionally, other psychiatric comorbidities such as independent depressive or anxiety disorders, as well as personality disorders (especially borderline personality disorder and antisocial personality disorder) are common among those diagnosed with PTSD. And, as with any psychiatric disorder, trauma-related disorders have a high comorbidity with sexual dysfunction, so a careful sexual history should be obtained to screen for this.

In addition to psychiatric comorbidities, there are also a number of nonpsychiatric medical comorbidities which providers should be aware of when treating this population. For combat veterans specifically, PTSD and traumatic brain injury (TBI) have very high rates of co-occurrence so careful screening for symptoms of a post-concussive syndrome is important [18–20]. Additionally, a number of studies have demonstrated that patients with PTSD are also at risk for a number of other medical issues including obesity, pain, musculoskeletal disorders, dyslipidemia, hypertension, autoimmune disease, and dementia; therefore a thorough medical examination is necessary for any patient presenting with symptoms consistent with PTSD [21–25]. As a brief aside, because of the hesitation to seek mental health treatment within the military, these patients are often better at expressing and seeking treatment for physical symptoms, as these may be perceived as more acceptable maladies. As such, medical providers treating patients within this population should have a low threshold to screen for psychiatric symptoms.

Defining the Problem

It is estimated that somewhere between 14% and 16% of US service members who have deployed to a combat zone return with trauma-related symptoms, with an estimated 11–20% of Iraq and Afghanistan veterans and nearly 30% of Vietnam veterans meeting DSM-5 criteria for posttraumatic stress disorder [26]. This is in comparison to 6.8% of the general population, as reported by the National Comorbidity Survey Replication [27]. However, as of 2014, only about 8% of the five million veterans receiving care through the VA system had been diagnosed with PTSD. Despite nearly three billion spent on PTSD treatment for veterans in 2012 and demand for mental healthcare in both the VA and Department of Defense (DoD) reaching an all-time high, likely hundreds of thousands of veterans meet criteria for PTSD but are not enrolled in any treatment.

The concept of transgenerational trauma is one which should also be considered when discussing the scope of combat-related posttraumatic stress disorder. Transgenerational trauma (also called intergenerational trauma) is a psychiatric concept which suggests that trauma can be transferred from one generation to the next. Although this phenomenon was originally observed among the children of Holocaust survivors, there has been an increasing body of research to support that children of service members with PTSD are far more likely than their peers to seek mental health treatment. Although there is no clearly defined mechanism, one can safely argue that the traumatized parent is not the only patient of the treating psychiatrist, and the physician should also screen for psychiatric conditions within the family unit.

Factors Impacting Care

It is also essential to briefly discuss the barriers to care both active duty members and veterans face in accessing and receiving mental health services. While active duty, there is significant stigma, not only because mental health care is perceived as a weakness, but also because it requires a service member to leave their unit for a period of time, which may be seen as placing oneself before the unit [28]. Additionally, some service members believe they are not "sick enough" to require care or, perhaps, that their symptoms are not secondary to a mental health condition at all (e.g., headaches, sexual dysfunction, poor sleep). Even if they do recognize that their symptoms may be secondary to a mental illness, concern that the mental health clinician might limit or remove them from duty also prevents them from coming forward. For example, a psychiatrist may recommend that a suicidal military policeman or woman not have access to firearms, which effectively removes them from their assigned job for an indefinite amount of time. It should be noted that military mental health providers face the unique additional challenge of having reporting responsibilities to the Commanding Officer about a patient's status and ability to complete his or her job in a safe manner [29]. Although active duty service members have most of the healthcare information protections that civilians do, an important caveat is the Commanding Officer must be informed when the service member's condition may interfere with the mission, or there is concern for risk of harm to self or others. Therefore, although mental health services are often made available, there are a number of reasons deterring service members from accessing care.

These barriers to care increase exponentially when a service member transitions to Veterans Affairs (VA) healthcare after completion of his or her time in service. This transition is particularly onerous due to the lack of a unified electronic medical record between DoD healthcare and VA healthcare, although there are increased efforts to improve the communication between these two systems. It can also be exceedingly difficult to gain access to prescriptions/medication management during this time, and case management/case coordination is notoriously limited. Once a veteran makes the transition, there is still a significant mistrust of the quality of care, particularly after a number of recent high-profile scandals [30]. Additionally, because of demand and limited resources, establishing care with VA mental health can be a months-long ordeal [31].

Upon transitioning out of the military, service members are evaluated for medical conditions which manifested while active duty (though they can request to be re-evaluated at any point through the VA system). Certain medical diagnoses, PTSD included, confer varying amounts of benefits which result in monthly disability payments, access to care, etc. While certainly not the norm, providers should consider secondary gain if a patient's symptoms are atypical for the diagnosis or if they appear disingenuous or overexaggerated.

Finally, though much of the medical literature and popular culture focuses on the negative effects of combat, it is important to recognize there are many positive experiences inherent in combat deployments. Previous generations, likely due to the higher proportion of citizens serving in the armed forces, appear to have appreciated this much more than we do today, and it is not uncommon for veterans to share bitter feelings toward the general public for not understanding this complex relationship. Studs Terkel writes in his book *The Good War*, that "if war were purely and absolutely bad in every single aspect and toxic in all its effects, it would probably not happen as often as it does. But in addition to all the destruction and loss of life, war also inspires the ancient human virtues of courage, loyalty, and selflessness that can be utterly intoxicating to the people who experience them [32]." In fact, this is one of the reasons that service members who previously deployed to a combat zone are more likely than their colleagues who have not, to sign on to do another tour. Consequently, one should not discount the sense of family and belongingness that comes from being entrenched in a unit exposed to the horrors of war with only each other to depend on. *Unlike treating victims of other types of trauma* (e.g., *abuse, assault, natural disaster*), *combat veterans will readily identify aspects of their experience that they wish to retain*. It is really these positive aspects of combat that can make successful treatment in this population so difficult to achieve.

Vignette

Mr. B is an actual patient. Some details have been omitted to preserve his confidentiality.

Mr. B enlisted in the US Navy at the age of 18 and was selected for the rate of builder (BU) in the Seabees. After completing basic and advanced training to gain technical expertise, he responded to a call for volunteers to join an elite unit within the Seabees to train to become an armed escort for military convoys. He attended several months of specialized weapon training and tactics before joining a unit that was deploying to Iraq (he would go on to deploy twice to Iraq and once to Afghanistan over the next 3 years).

Nearly every day during his deployments to Iraq and Afghanistan, his team would be tasked, usually at night, to escort a convoy of vehicles from one point to another in heavily armored vehicles called Mine-Resistant Ambush Protected vehicles or MRAPs. There were no easy or routine missions; ambushes and improvised explosive devices (IEDs) were an ever-present concern, though his unit grew accustomed to the tense realization that their lives were constantly in danger. On most missions, they encountered mortar attacks which were usually dismissed as less concerning due to their inaccuracy. Less frequent, but much more dangerous and feared, were the IEDs. They were typically strategically placed to destroy or immobilize the first vehicle, whereupon the enemy would open fire on the remainder of the convoy.

Mr. B reports being hit three times by an IED over the course of his deployments, all of which contributed in varying amounts to the painful memories he relates to combat. A close friend of his died in the first IED. In the second, he sustained a head injury and experienced loss of consciousness with a subsequent mild traumatic brain injury (TBI). Over the course of several sessions, however, it became apparent that the most distressing to him was the third, which occurred toward the end of his deployment to Afghanistan. He was traveling in the second vehicle when the first exploded into a ball of flames.

In our initial sessions, Mr. B was not entirely sure why the last incident was the most distressing, but this was a subject of frequent exploration as we continued working together. As we came to discover, one contributing factor was a powerful visual image of the explosion. He can still see this image very clearly, and when around flames, he has difficulty controlling the repetitive intrusion of this image.

In addition to the power of this image, the patient also described feeling as though he underwent a change over the course of his three deployments. Specifically, he became more aware of, and affected by, the events around him. He described himself in the first few years of service as being somewhat calloused and untouched by the ethical dilemmas inherent in combat, and he reflected relatively little on the people he was fighting. During those early years, the people attacking the convoys were simply evil, and it was his unit's job to defend themselves and their team. Gradually he became more aware of signs that this black and white conceptualization was missing something. He began to question the validity of the intelligence gathered to demonstrate that many of the IEDs were set by the property owners, as he noticed a number of signs indicating that the Taliban coerced and claimed that the Americans intended to cause them (noncombatants) harm. Additionally, he became more aware of the impact the war was having on the children in the country, and he noticed that these distressing thoughts increased in frequency and intensity once he had children of his own, several years after his last combat deployment.

Case Discussion

The experience of combat veterans has been a focus of the recorders of the human experience since the earliest forms of the written word. As our society places a greater emphasis on individual over community experiences and as our wars have become an event only experienced by a small minority of the population, we have become less comfortable listening to the experiences of modern warriors. The division between service members and civilians is frequently not only a reason for combat veterans seeking mental health care, but it is also one of the largest obstacles preventing them from seeking help. Clinicians must recognize the presence of this divide and learn skills to mitigate the impact of this obstacle. In the following paragraphs, we discuss the case above and highlight the knowledge and skills that may allow clinicians to bridge this divide. Before doing so, it is worth emphasizing that the advice that follows is not meant to replace the most important skill in communicating with patients: listening. Jonathan Shay, as the author of one of the most famous and certainly most useful pieces on communicating with veterans wrote, "Healing from trauma depends upon communalization of the trauma – being able to safely tell the story to someone who is listening and who can be trusted to retell it truthfully to others in the community. So before analyzing, before classifying, before thinking, before trying to *do* anything – we should *listen* [6]."

After the patient's name, the first information shared about him is the branch of service he joined. We emphasize this here to address a common and understandable mistake that people make in referring to all branches of the armed services as the Army, or all military service members as soldiers. There are many nations that have a single armed service, but in the United States, the various military branches (Army, Navy, Air Force, Marine Corps, and Coast Guard) each spend a great deal of their initial training of recruits instilling the unique history and customs of their respective branch. Calling a Marine a soldier may not cause a visible response, but it is likely to make it more challenging to build a therapeutic alliance, because in the minds of a service member, these are dramatically different experiences. And while it would not be reasonable to expect all clinicians to have an intricate knowledge of each service branch, it can be helpful for patients to know that the clinician is thoughtful about their line of work. This can be accomplished by demonstrating curiosity and asking questions about the patient's particular branch and what sets it apart from the others, laying the groundwork for establishing trust and respect in the relationship.

After Mr. B's name and branch of service, his rating, roughly equivalent to the term Military Occupation Specialty (MOS) in other branches, is reported identifying the service member's technical skill. Knowing about this term is helpful because it will provide information about the patient and convey thoughtfulness to the patient about their experience. We encourage and recommend that clinicians take the time to talk to their patient about the duties and requirements of their job and how they chose it. Clinicians will begin to appreciate the diverse roles that service members in each of the branches hold to support the overall mission.

It is worth being cautiously curious, however, as their rate/MOS may bear little similarity to the service member's actual job. Hearing the job title of "builder" does not automatically conjure an image of an armed escort ensuring the safe transport of people and materials within a war zone. It is also common for individuals to spend large portions of their time in service working outside of their rate/MOS, which was especially true during OEF (war in Afghanistan) and OIF (war in Iraq) where, for example, many sailors found themselves deployed to desert units working as armed guards for detainees. As such, it is always appropriate to ask whether or not the patient has spent time working outside of their rating.

The vignette described above discussed three separate traumatic incidents. The earlier sessions focused on the patient's first two IED experiences, both of which appeared more traumatic to the treating provider, as opposed to the third IED, due to his friend getting killed and the resultant TBI. However, while the patient endorsed some emotional distress stemming from these incidents, the third incident drove the majority of his trauma-related symptoms. By asking this patient to explore this discrepancy, a discussion was initiated regarding how his thinking about his role within the war changed and how he began to grapple with the ethical and moral aspects of his team's actions. The term "moral injury," used by Jonathan Shay to describe the long-lasting distress as a result of leadership failings, has become a term used to capture the emotional symptoms (other than fear) that can result from combat trauma such as anger, disgust, guilt, and shame. While the details of some traumas might appear more severe at the surface, it is important to consider the patient's perspective of which emotions and symptoms are most distressing to them, while acknowledging that these may not necessarily be fear or anxiety.

The information presented here was collected over several sessions. In the authors' experience, it is not unusual for combat veterans to reveal only a portion of their story in the initial session. There are a number of powerful psychological factors common in this community that prevent full disclosure of emotionally distressing symptoms (discussed in further detail in the "Factors Impacting Care" section of this chapter). Over the course of the last decade, impressive strides have been made to reduce the stigma associated with experiencing psychological symptoms and searching for or receiving psychological treatments, but this remains a barrier for many combat veterans. Addressing and understanding the shame, embarrassment, guilt, or other negative emotions which may conflict a patient about reaching out for care are an important first step in gathering a full history and developing a therapeutic alliance. As the clinician demonstrates a willingness to discuss the personal, painful, and embarrassing, rapport slowly builds, and other pertinent details are sure to present themselves.

Another obstacle to obtaining a complete history and building a therapeutic alliance is the fact that many veterans do not associate their symptoms with traumatic events, or if they do, focusing on a specific one is challenging. Allowing for space and time to explore multiple events is challenging but may be required in order to craft a comprehensive treatment plan. It can be helpful to create a timeline of events in order to structure the treatment and then address each event systematically.

A final obstacle that may present a barrier is the addition of positive emotions that the patient may associate with combat. Western literature is replete with examples of veterans struggling with fond memories of such a horrific time. Mr. B remains on active duty, having transferred to a position with greater upward mobility and stability, but remained deeply conflicted about leaving his unit. He missed the sense of community and felt that he may, in some way, have let them down. One of the most therapeutic actions he took was to search for ways to rekindle this sense of belonging and re-engage with the parts of his former job that brought him joy and purpose. The patient now frequently seeks out experiences at his current command to teach others about antiterrorism tactics and how to use/handle their weapons, even though this is far outside of his current job description. Mr. B describes feeling an improved sense of purpose and meaningfulness, and helping him to identify this sublimation and appreciate the conflict between both the positive and negative experiences of combat has been a powerful tool for healing.

Comments and Recommendations

Psychiatric disorders and particularly trauma and stressor-related disorders are among the leading causes of morbidity in the military. Below we discuss both the evidence-based treatments put forth for treating combat veterans, as well as provide a number of recommendations based solely on the authors' clinical experience with this population.

In 2017, the *VA/DoD Clinical Practice Guideline for the Management of Posttraumatic Stress Disorder and Acute Stress Disorder* (summarized in Table 4.1) was released with updated treatment recommendations [33]. In general, individual, manualized, trauma-focused therapy continues to be the recommended first-line treatment for all trauma-related disorders. This includes cognitive processing

Table 4.1 Summary of the 2017 VA/DoD clinical practice guidelines for treatment of trauma-related disorders [33]

Treatment type	Recommendation
Psychotherapy	
Exposure therapy (Prolonged exposure, PE)	Strongly recommend
Cognitive processing therapy (CPT)	Strongly recommend
Eye movement desensitization and reprocessing (EMDR)	Strongly recommend
Stress inoculation training (SIT), present-centered therapy (PCT), and interpersonal psychotherapy (IPT)	Weakly recommend
Dialectical behavior therapy (DBT), Skills training in affective and interpersonal regulation (STAIR), Acceptance and commitment therapy (ACT), Seeking safety, and supportive counseling	Insufficient evidence
Group therapy	Weakly recommend
Couples therapy (as a primary treatment)	Insufficient evidence
Pharmacotherapy-monotherapy	
Sertraline, paroxetine, fluoxetine, or venlafaxine	Strongly recommend
Nefazodone, imipramine, or phenelzine	Weakly recommend
Quetiapine, olanzapine, and other atypical antipsychotics (except for risperidone)	Weakly against
Divalproex, tiagabine, guanfacine, risperidone, benzodiazepines, ketamine, hydrocortisone, or D-cycloserine	Strongly against
Cannabis, cannabis derivatives	Strongly against
Escitalopram, bupropion, desipramine, doxepin, duloxetine, desvenlafaxine, fluvoxamine, mirtazapine, nortriptyline, trazodone, vilazodone, vortioxetine, and buspirone	Insufficient evidence
Prazosin (for nightmares)	Insufficient evidence
Pharmacotherapy-augmentation therapy	
Atypical antipsychotics, benzodiazepines, and divalproex	Strongly against
Topiramate, baclofen, or pregabalin	Weakly against
Prazosin (for nightmares)	Insufficient evidence
Non-pharmacological biologic therapy	
Repetitive transcranial magnetic stimulation (rTMS), Electroconvulsive therapy (ECT), Hyperbaric oxygen therapy (HBOT), Stellate ganglion block (SGB), or Vagal nerve stimulation (VNS)	Insufficient evidence

therapy (CPT), prolonged exposure (PE), and eye movement desensitization and reprocessing (EMDR), among others. Second-line treatments include non-trauma-focused psychotherapy and pharmacotherapy, which are summarized in the table below. Perhaps the most notable change in regard to pharmacologic interventions is for prazosin (Minipress). Although once thought to be a relatively successful intervention for trauma-based nightmares, prazosin is no longer recommended for or against nightmares due to increasing evidence that it may be less efficacious than previously believed. In general, selective serotonin reuptake inhibitors (SSRIs) are recommended for the depressive and anxiety symptoms due to PTSD with sertraline (Zoloft), paroxetine (Paxil), and fluoxetine (Prozac) having the strongest recommendations (in addition to venlafaxine [Effexor], a serotonin-norepinephrine reuptake inhibitor). It should also be noted that as cannabis and its derivatives (to include cannabidiols or CBD) become more readily available, clinicians are likely to receive more questions from patients regarding its efficaciousness. Currently, the guidelines strongly recommend against use of the agents as monotherapy, though no formal recommendations have been made regarding the use of these compounds in conjunction with other treatment modalities.

In addition to the above treatment recommendations, there are three key areas which these authors believe should be addressed during treatment: reintegration, children/family, and closure.

Reintegration is the principle of rediscovering purpose and intimacy. For a soldier, sailor, marine, or airman, the return from a deployment is psychologically complex. The media's typical portrayal of service members surprising exuberant family members upon their return fails to capture the weeks or months of adjusting back into a new routine for both the service member and their family. These brief, simplistic representations also set up the unrealistic expectation that a return home will be unequivocally positive. Working through traumatic experiences is part of this adjustment, and implementing a comprehensive strategy to identify and address these concerns can significantly improve the service members functioning and quality of life after deployment. One of the most difficult tasks for service members after returning from combat is readjusting to a day-to-day schedule that is dramatically less intense and regimented than when they were deployed. There is often significantly less group cohesion, and the sense of closeness and camaraderie felt within the unit is no longer present. If left unaddressed, this loss of a sense of belongingness (often identified as loneliness) can persist, even if it has been many years since the patient's combat experience. Providers should encourage a patient to look for ways to regain this connectedness. Some ideas include volunteer work, community involvement, or even looking for an occupation with a strong mentorship aspect (e.g., coach, teacher). As illustrated in the case of Mr. B, this can be particularly effective if the patient is able to recapture some of the positives of their military experience. Thus, mentoring or volunteering with young service members, or even teaching some of the skills involved in their military jobs, can be profoundly healing. Providers should also screen for sexual dysfunction and intimacy issues between the patient and his or her spouse or significant other, as this can be an intense barrier to reintegration for those suffering from a trauma-related disorder.

Providers should also remember that it is not just the patient who suffers after combat trauma. Therefore, it is important to integrate spouses and children into the treatment as well. Care should focus on providing safety, information, and assistance/referrals to community resources in order to facilitate a combat-injured family's recovery. Consideration should be given to individual therapy for family members, marital, and even family counseling in order to ensure that a family is able to relieve distress and communicate about the effects of combat trauma in a productive and effective way. It can also be helpful to connect the family to community resources (such as support groups) to help decrease the feeling of isolation or feeling as though nobody else can understand their circumstances. Further, this may have the secondary benefit of helping to facilitate reintegration. If the patient is still on active duty, consider referral to FOCUS (families overcoming under stress) [34] or FAP (family advocacy program) [35], which can be accessed on most military bases or online. The VA also has a number of programs and services which family members can access as well, though these vary by location [36].

Finally, it is important to allow the service member time to grieve. Oftentimes, in the midst of war, there is no time for a memorial service or a funeral. If loss is a prominent factor of a patient's trauma, consider encouraging the patient to participate in such an event. It can be formal or informal, religious, or otherwise, and it can be something they do alone or as part of a group (perhaps within their unit or command, if applicable). This ceremony can be adapted to allow for the opportunity to grieve the loss of a specific person or even a more abstract loss (e.g., loss of innocence, loss of "the way things were"). The ultimate goal of this event is to provide an opportunity for the patient to remember and show appreciation for that which was lost, allow time to grieve, and create hope for a new beginning [37, 38].

Summary of High-Yield Points

- While treating combat trauma can be quite difficult, particularly for providers with limited knowledge of the military and the unique cultural background it provides those who serve it, this work is becoming increasingly relevant as both awareness of the psychological effects of combat improves and operational tempo increases (i.e., an increase in the number of deployments, often in the context of war).
- Providers endeavoring in this work should, firstly, understand the power of and responsibility to the unit with whom our patients serve alongside. They should understand that not all combat experiences are negative and that frequently there are positive aspects which service members hold on to dearly. Successful treatment allows the patient to reconcile these opposing experiences.
- Additionally, many service members, while proud of their service, may feel as though only those who have served will understand their experiences and may be hesitant to open up to a civilian. In these cases, providers are encouraged to ask questions and do their own research in order to gain a better understanding of the patient's military and combat experience.
- Treatment should include an evidence-based, trauma-focused therapy, and special attention should be paid to recapturing the sense of community fostered in the military (whether that is through occupation, volunteering, or community involvement), while also allowing time to grieve any loss that may be a part of the patient's trauma.

- Providers may also consider incorporating some sort of ceremony into treatment in an effort to give the service member a venue to not only honor those lost, but also to provide a sense a closure which can frequently be overlooked during combat.
- Finally, providers would be wise to remember that service members and veterans do not exist in a vacuum; their spouses and children are also affected by combat trauma and treatment should address the family as a whole.
- Ultimately, if undertaken and approached with a sense of openness, curiosity, and willingness to share the burden of the traumatic experience, treatment of combat trauma can be an incredibly fulfilling and, quite literally, a life-saving intervention.

Acknowledgement LT Savannah Woodward and LCDR David Nissan are military service members and employees of the US government. This work was prepared as part of their official duties. Title 17U.S.C. 105 provides that copyright protection under this title is not available for any work of the US Government. Title 17U.S.C.101 defines a US Government work as work prepared by a military service member or employee of the US Government as part of that person's official duties.

References

1. Babylonian Talmud (Avodah Zarah 37b), citing Numbers 19:22: "And whatsoever the unclean person touches shall be unclean." The rabbis decreed that if a person defiled by the dead had touched another person, the person who had been touched is under a seven-day period of defilement, and cannot eat of Terumah or hallowed things until that period had expired (cf. BT Nazir 42b).
2. Junger S. Tribe: on homecoming and belonging. HarperColllins Publishers; 2016.
3. Schafer A. The Warrior Caste. https://slate.com/news-and-politics/2017/08/the-warrior-caste-of-military-families-that-fight-americas-wars.html. Accessed 16 May 2020.
4. Stern T, et al. Massachusetts general hospital psychiatry update & board preparation. 4th ed. MGH Psychiatry Academy; 2017.
5. American Psychiatric Association. Diagnostic and statistical manual of mental disorders. 5th ed., Text Revision. American Psychiatric Association; 2013.
6. Shay J. Achilles in Vietnam: combat trauma and the undoing of character. Scribner; 1994.
7. Myers CS. Autobiographical notes; F.C. Bartlett, BMFRS 5 (1948); idem, Am J Psychol. 50 (1937).
8. Hurst A. The man who filmed shell shock. Home Front, BBC. https://www.bbc.co.uk/programmes/articles/4VqPtrjsgcPKtgmYc2M5vXz/arthur-hurst-the-man-who-filmed-shell-shock. Accessed 2 May 2020.
9. Jones E. War neuroses and Arthur Hurts: a pioneering medical film about the treatment of psychiatric battle casualties. J Hist Med Allied Sci. 2016;67(3):245–373.
10. Shell Shock. Inside out. BBC. http://www.bbc.co.uk/insideout/extra/series-1/shell_shocked.shtml. Accessed 2 May 2020.
11. Trueman CN. World War One executions. The History Learning Site. historylearningsite.co.uk. Accessed 31 Mar 2015.
12. Shephard B. A war of nerves: soldiers and psychiatrists in the twentieth century. Harvard University Press; 2001.

13. Karl A, Schaefer M, Malta LS, et al. A meta-analysis of structural brain abnormalities in PTSD. Neurosci Biobehav Rev. 2006;30(7):1004–31.
14. Geracioti TD Jr, Baker DG, Ekhator NN, et al. CSF norepinephrine concentrations in post-traumatic stress disorder. Am J Psychiatr. 2001;158(8):1227–30.
15. Hendrickson RC, Rasking MA. Noradrenergic dysregulation in the pathophysiology of PTSD. Exp Neurol. 2016;284(B):181–95.
16. Jones M, Sundin J, Goodwin L, et al. What explains post-traumatic stress disorder (PTSD) in UK service personnel: deployment or something else? Psychol Med. 2013;43(8):1703–12.
17. Seal KH, Cohen G, Waldrop A, et al. Substance use disorders in Iraq and Afghanistan veterans in VA healthcare, 2001-2010: implications for screening, diagnosis, and treatment. Drug Alcohol Depend. 2011;116(1–3):93–101.
18. Halbauer JD, Ashford JW, Zeitzer JM, et al. Neuropsychiatric diagnosis and management of chronic sequelae of war-related mild to moderate traumatic brain injury. J Rehabil Res Dev. 2009;46(6):757–96.
19. Hoge CW, McGurk D, Thomas JL, et al. Mild traumatic brain injury in U.S. Soldiers returning from Iraq. N Engl J Med. 2008;351(1):13–22.
20. Walker WC, Franke LM, McDonald SD, et al. Prevalence of mental health conditions after military blast exposure, their co-occurrence, and their relation to mild traumatic brain injury. Brain Inj. 2015;29(13–14):1581–8.
21. Cohen BE, Marmar C, Ren L, et al. Association of cardiovascular risk factors with mental health diagnoses in Iraq and Afghanistan war veterans using VA health care. JAMA. 2009;302(5):489–92.
22. Howard JT, Sosnov JA, Janak JC, et al. Associations of initial injury severity and posttraumatic stress disorder diagnoses with long-term hypertension risk after combat injury. Hypertension. 2018;71(5):824–32.
23. O'Donovan A, Cohen BE, Seal KH, et al. Elevated risk for autoimmune disorders in Iraq and Afghanistan veterans with posttraumatic stress disorder. Biol Psychiatry. 2015;77(4):365–74.
24. Song H, Fang F, Tomasson G, et al. Association of stress-related disorders with subsequent autoimmune disease. JAMA. 2018;319(23):2388–400.
25. Spitzer C, Barnow S, Völzke H, et al. Trauma, posttraumatic stress disorder, and physical illness: findings from the general population. Psychosom Med. 2009;71(9):1012–7.
26. Study explores why Veterans seek-or don't seek-PTSD care. U.S. Department of Affairs. https://www.research.va.gov/currents/spring2014/spring2014-25.cfm. Accessed 3 May 2020.
27. Gradus JL. PTSD: National Center for PTSD. U.S. Department of Veteran Affairs. https://www.ptsd.va.gov/professional/treat/essentials/epidemiology.asp. Accessed 31 Aug 2019.
28. Langston V, Gould M, Greenberg N. Culture: what is its effect on stress in the military? Mil Med. 2007;172(9):931–5.
29. Kutz DL. Military psychiatry: a cross-cultural perspective. Mil Med. 1996;161(2:708):78–83.
30. Cheney AM, Koenig CJ, Miller CJ, et al. Veteran-centered barriers to VA mental healthcare services use. BMC Health Serv Res. 2018;18(1):591.
31. Whealin JM, Nelson D, Kawasaki MM, et al. Factors impacting rural Pacific Island veterans' access to care: a qualitative examination. Psychol Serv. 2017;14(3):279–88.
32. Terkel S. The good war: an oral history of World War Two. Pantheon Books; 1984.
33. VA/DoD Clinical Practice Guideline for the Management of Posttraumatic Stress Disorder and Acute Stress Disorder. Department of Veterans Affairs and Department of Defense. https://www.healthquality.va.gov/guidelines/MH/ptsd/VADoDPTSDCPGClinicianSummaryFinal.pdf. Accessed 31 Aug 2019.
34. The Focus Project. https://focusproject.org/. Accessed 30 May 20.
35. Military One Source. Department of Defense. https://www.militaryonesource.mil/family-relationships/family-life/preventing-abuse-neglect/the-family-advocacy-program. Accessed 30 May 2020.

36. Caregiver Tips – PTSD. U.S. Department of Veterans Affairs. https://www.caregiver.va.gov/Tips_by_Diagnosis/PTSD.asp. Accessed 30 May 2020.
37. Greenleaf AT, Roessger KM, Williams JM, et al. Effects of a rite of passage ceremony on veterans' Well-being. J Couns Dev. 2019;97(2):171–82.
38. Uniformed Services University: Funerals and Memorials A Part of Recovery. Center for the Study of Traumatic Stress. https://www.cstsonline.org/assets/media/documents/CSTS_FS_Leadership_Funeral%20and%20memorials_%20a%20part%20of%20recovery.pdf. Accessed 31 Aug 2020.

Part II

Special Populations

Co-occurring Disorders

5

Aaron Meyer, Gabriela G. Mejia, and Hilary M. Gould

Introduction

Co-occurring disorders, concurrent substance use and mental illness, often have synergistic effects that place an individual at increased risk of occupational, legal, and health hazards. These disorders affect those at the highest echelons of wealth and the most destitute. Addressing co-occurring disorders requires a multifaceted approach involving psychotherapy, support groups, and psychopharmacology. In this chapter, cultural aspects of co-occurring disorders are explored, including the role of public policy, healthcare organizations, and the legal system in combatting (and at times, perpetuating) the scourge of moralistic beliefs that have isolated this population from evidence-based interventions.

Substance use disorders are common in the United States and contribute to a large percentage of hospitalizations and mortality. There are about 20 million people with substance use disorders in the USA [1] . In 2010, 0.8% of global disability-adjusted life years were related to illicit substance use disorders [2]. Explanations for these rates are attributed to cardiovascular, digestive, respiratory, and endocrine diseases, cancers, suicide, overdoses, and injuries. In fact, of all hospitalized adult patients, 20% have a substance use disorder. These patients are three times more likely to leave the hospital against medical advice [3]. Consequences of leaving against medical advice are severe, with studies suggesting a doubling of 30-day mortality [4]. For patients with opioid use disorders, methadone induction has shown to reduce frequency of patients leaving against medical advice [3].

Mental health diagnoses often predate or co-occur with substance use disorders. In the USA in 2019, nearly half (49.2%) of patients with a substance use disorder were also diagnosed with a mental illness [1]. Concurrent diagnoses are especially common among patients with serious mental illness; patients with

A. Meyer (✉) · G. G. Mejia · H. M. Gould
Department of Psychiatry, University of California San Diego, San Diego, CA, USA
e-mail: aameyer@health.ucsd.edu; ggmejia@health.ucsd.edu; hgould@health.ucsd.edu

S. H. Koh et al. (eds.), *Diversity in Action*,
https://doi.org/10.1007/978-3-030-85401-0_5

schizophrenia have a 50% risk of developing a substance use disorder [5]. Disturbingly, a co-occurring disorder significantly increases the risk of psychiatric hospitalization, treatment nonadherence, and homelessness. Along with marketing, peer influence, and genetic predisposition, iatrogenic perpetuation of substance use disorders is a relevant issue. In a prospective analysis of 203 patients with co-occurring severe mental illness and substance use disorders, 43% were prescribed benzodiazepines. This group was twice as likely to abuse benzodiazepines than those who were not prescribed benzodiazepines [6]. The current opioid epidemic has been fueled in part by pharmaceutical advertising and physician prescribing.

Substance use disorders cost an estimated $700 billion a year, mostly related to lost productivity [7, 8]. Despite this high cost, there are significant structural barriers associated with care delivery. As Massachusetts' health expansion demonstrated, adding substance use disorder treatment to insurance coverage does not necessarily lead to increased utilization or care [9]. Lack of utilization is likely multifactorial and certainly not solely due to the insurer. Individuals decline to engage in treatment for a myriad of reasons including denial, fear of adverse impact on employment, and time constraints [9]. Unfortunately, the Mental Health Parity and Addiction Equity Act in 2008 does not require insurers to provide substance use disorder treatment. Instead, this law exclusively applied to businesses with 50 or more employees who were already providing insurance coverage for mental health and substance use treatment [10]. In 2014, the Affordable Care Act (ACA) required insurers to cover treatment for mental health and substance use disorders [10]. Even so, in 2017 17% of workers were exempt from these essential health benefit additions due to enrollment in older "grandfathered" plans [10]. Patients continue to face increased barriers utilizing substance use disorder treatment compared to other medical care. In one study of 11,732 privately insured participants, an underlying issue they identified was decreased individual awareness regarding whether their plan covered substance use disorder treatment [10]. Another study cites 24% of privately insured individuals did not receive treatment because of insurance difficulties, such as coverage or affordability. However, in the same study, 97% did not perceive a need for treatment which highlights the need of outreach initiatives to advertise the benefit and accessibility of substance use disorder treatment [9]. In recent years, mental health spending and coverage have been expanded, but substance use coverage has not followed suit. Private insurance, Medicare, and Medicaid total mental health share coverage increased from 44% (1986) to 68% (2014), while the share of spending for substance use disorder treatment abysmally went from 45% (1986) to 46% (2014) [11]. Between 1986 and 2014, mental health treatment shifted primarily from governments to insurance companies; yet, substance use disorder treatment continues to be financed primarily from government entities [11].

Currently, treatments authorized by insurance companies are not always aligned with best practices. Prior authorization requirements and nonquantitative limits on treatment and lifetime treatment limitations begs the question of whether there is true parity between physical and mental healthcare. Individuals with substance use disorders are often excluded from transplantation, acute care facilities, and outpatient parenteral antibiotic treatment [12]. A study through Health Resources and

Services Administration demonstrated that stigma was one of the most cited reasons for not participating in substance use treatment. Methadone treatment is often perceived as degrading and humiliating. Patients with co-occurring disorders are less likely to engage in treatment and are at increased risk for suicide [13]. Individuals are twice as likely to utilize services for mental health treatment rather than for management of a substance use disorder [14].

Background

Historical Significance

Humans have been abusing substances since the earliest historical records. Throughout history, there has been a spectrum of beliefs regarding the etiology of substance use disorders. In this chapter, four main substances are discussed: alcohol, opioids, stimulants, and tobacco. Although not covered in depth in this chapter, benzodiazepines, cannabis, inhalants, steroids, and other substances contribute to morbidity and mortality. Substances are rarely used in isolation and interactions can lead to unintended effects.

Alcohol

Alcohol has been consumed for at least the past 10,000 years. Some original inceptions include beer, without hops, and mead, an elixir made from honey. Christianity helped popularize wine through connecting its consumption with Jesus' last supper. Beneficial health effects of alcohol in treating snake bites have been cited by Cato the Elder. British physicians have considered alcohol's role in curing venereal disease [15]. There has also been a focus on alcohol's negative effects. For instance, slaves were banned from alcohol consumption due to perceived increased likelihood of upending social order. The English legal system began regulating alehouses in the fifteenth century. Alcohol increasingly became more accessible to working-class people during the Industrial Revolution, notably, with 25% of London households producing gin. As consumption of alcohol increased in the nineteenth century, a counter focus on the negative effects of alcohol arose through the "temperance movement." Physicians referred to alcohol as "a disease of the will." Homes for inebriates and asylums were established to treat alcohol use disorder during the Prohibition era.

Before Prohibition, there were no systematic efforts to quantify alcohol use [16]. In the USA, 1889 marked the founding of the Sociology Group, which investigated social problems. In 1893 they began addressing problems associated with alcohol consumption and rebranded to the Committee of Fifty [17]. Members of the Committee of Fifty were mainly upper-class business and financial elites. They drafted a volume titled *The Liquor Problem: A Summary of Investigations Conducted by the Committee of Fifty, 1893–1903*, which formed basis for further restrictions on alcohol use [16]. Congress passed Wartime Prohibition in 1917, and National Prohibition was passed in January 1920 (18th Amendment), until it was overturned in 1933 (21st Amendment) [16]. Despite doubling of enforcement budget between 1921 and 1930, efforts to curtail alcohol consumption were largely unsuccessful due to illegal manufacturing and trade. Additionally, there was increased support for alcohol consumption during Prohibition attributed to the romanticized thrill of danger. John Rockefeller and others founded the Research Council on Problems of Alcohol in 1937, in part to consider ramifications of repeal [18]. According to this group, "an alcoholic should be regarded as a sick person, just as one who is suffering from tuberculosis, cancer, heart disease, or other serious chronic disorder" [18].

Alcohol consumption, abuse, hospitalizations, and deaths have increased in the past two decades. A study examining alcohol-related deaths from US mortality data from the National Center for Health Statistics found that 2.6% of all deaths in 2017 involved alcohol [19]. Those at highest risk were men, middle-aged adults, and American Indians or Alaska Natives. Rate increases were highest among non-Hispanic white women, which is consistent with data on opioid use and other substance disorders.

Opioids

Opioid use disorder was originally considered a medical problem in the late 1800s. The Society for Promoting Legislation for Control and Cure of Habitual Drunkards (established in 1876) helped link substance dependence with medical treatment. Increasing use among lower socioeconomic groups in England led to concerns about "deviance" and increasingly punitive policies in the early 1900s [20]. The International Opium Convention of 1912 limited use of opiates and cocaine to medical use [21]. The Harrison Narcotic Act of 1914 required medical professionals to register with the Department of the Treasury and maintain prescribing records. In 1956, medical use of heroin was withdrawn in the USA (via the US Narcotic Drug Control Act), but any physician could still prescribe heroin to patients with opioid use disorder until 1968. Medication-assisted treatment emerged in the 1970s. Shifts in drug policy occurred in the 1980s, with the emergence of HIV/AIDS, leading to more favorable views of oral opioids such as methadone. In the 1990s, a number of pharmaceutical companies, physicians, and pain organizations began advocating for more aggressive use of opioids for chronic and nonmalignant pain conditions. During this time, opioid prescribing began to exponentially increase which led to dependence and growth in illegal marketplaces. Subsequently, other countries such as Australia and Switzerland renewed interest in heroin prescribing with the hopes of increasing access and interest in treatment and rehabilitation programs. A Geneva study investigated 46 patients randomized to receive heroin or methadone; at 6 months, the heroin group demonstrated reductions in illicit heroin use and legal infractions [22].

Concerningly, first-time heroin users have doubled to 169,000 between 2006 and 2013 [23]. Opioid use disorder is associated with significant cost, $51.2 billion in the USA related to productivity losses, drug costs, incarceration, and treatment for hepatitis C [23]. Overdose deaths have tripled since 2002 [23]. Harm reduction efforts, such as needle exchange programs, were banned due to concerns of facilitating substance use [24]. In 2015, Congress partially repealed this ban allowing federal funding for all aspects of needle exchange programs except clean needles [24].

Significant attention has been paid to geographical variance of overdose trends. Upper Appalachia is notorious for its high overdose fatality rates [25]. Native Americans are at the highest overdose risk and have the highest opioid overdose death rate, 8.4 deaths per 100,000 people [26]. Additionally, shifts in employment opportunities with decreased manufacturing and mining opportunities are associated with an increased overdose risk, particularly individuals without a college degree raised in a single-parent family. Sadly, for every 1% increase in unemployment, opioid fatalities increase by 3.6% [27]. In the 2010s, the increased heroin overdoses in urban areas were related to increased availability from drug trafficking organizations in Mexico and synthetic drug production from China. Soon after in 2013, the USA witnessed an exponential increase in fentanyl production and the overwhelming effects on overdose deaths [28]. By 2019, half of the drug overdose deaths in the USA involved synthetic opioids as they are both deliberately and inadvertently paired with other drugs [29]. These synthetics are significantly more potent than morphine (pure carfentanil is 10,000 times), and they continue to drive and expand the opioid epidemic [27].

Stimulants

Stimulant use via chewing coca leaves dates back 8,000 years ago in northern Peru. Throughout colonization, use was primarily endemic to South America because the coca leaf lost potency quickly. The active alkaloid, cocaine, was first isolated by German chemist, Friedrich Gaedcke, in 1855. By the 1880s, the medical community began recommending cocaine for treatment of depression and local anesthesia for ophthalmological procedures. Sigmund Freud touted it as miracle drug and partnered with pharmaceutical companies for sponsorship. Coca leaves were used in the soft drink Coca-Cola from 1886 to 1903. After several years, social and medical concerns surfaced, and the Harrison Act in 1914 banned all distribution of coca products (and opiates as described above).

Synthetic stimulants including amphetamine and methamphetamine were isolated in 1887 and 1919, respectively. By the 1950s and 1960s, methamphetamine was widely prescribed for obesity and depression [30]. In the early 1970s, Nixon declared a "war on drugs" to combat the sharp rise in cocaine abuse. The Controlled Substances Act of 1971 also led to a decline in prescribed amphetamines. The Reagan administration expanded these policies with emergence of the "Just Say No" movement, implementation of drug prevention programs in schools and signing the Anti-Drug Abuse Act in 1986. This law established mandatory prison penalties for specific drug offenses and led to a massive surge in incarcerations. By the 1990s there was a resurgence of methamphetamine popularity, originally isolated to "meth labs" in California but later spreading nationwide.

Current estimates for stimulant misuse are on the rise with 5.5 million Americans using cocaine and 1.9 million using methamphetamine in 2018 [31]. In some parts of the country, stimulant use exceeds opioid use. Amphetamine-related hospital costs reached 2.17 billion in 2015 [32]. Overdoses involving psychostimulants have increased in the past two decades, in part due to synthetic opioids being mixed into stimulants often without user awareness. In 2018, greater than 50% of psychostimulant-related overdose deaths involved opioids [28].

Tobacco

Archaeological evidence reveals tobacco use many millennia ago in ancient indigenous communities in Mesoamerica and South America. Tobacco was a heavily traded commodity and use increased nearly exponentially from the 1800s to mid-1960s, especially with the invention of cigarettes [33]. Since the identification of harmful health consequences and publication of the Surgeon General's report in 1964, rates in the USA have declined. Statewide campaigns, such as the California Tobacco Control Program, have been instrumental in decreasing tobacco use via policy measures (e.g., taxes, reducing secondhand smoke, regulation of tobacco industry, providing cessation services) targeted to create social norm and cultural changes.

Currently, tobacco use has remained relatively stable, in part due to increased consumption of e-cigarettes and related products. It continues to remain the most common substance use disorder and leading source of preventable disease, disability, and death in the USA [34]. In 2019, 14.0% of adults (34.1 million) smoked cigarettes. More than 480,000 deaths every year are attributed to cigarette smoking, and data suggests that 16 million Americans live with a smoking-related disease [34]. Annual costs are approximately $300 billion, including direct medical care and lost productivity due to premature death and secondhand smoke [34]. Importantly, tobacco use disorders remain undertreated, even among individuals attending substance use programs. Less than half (47%) of all substance use treatment facilities offer tobacco cessation services with only one-quarter offering nicotine replacement therapy [35]. Moreover, while tobacco use rates are declining nationally, subgroup rates are disproportionate. Individuals who smoke menthol cigarettes, live in rural environments, have low socioeconomic status, identify as LGBTQ, and/or have serious mental illness are more likely to have continued use [34].

Cultural Considerations

Cultural factors are important to consider when discussing co-occurring disorders. Defining the terms "culture," "ethnicity," and "race" is necessary to facilitate dialogue. Cultural factors may either stigmatize or protect certain groups of people within larger systems of law enforcement, legal, and healthcare services.

Culture is the characteristics and knowledge of a particular group of people, which may involve ethnic and racial characteristics [36]. It is dynamic and changes over time. It can also involve age, class, and power dynamics. Culture can be used to distance or reinforce stigma. For instance, whiteness has been defined as a hegemonic system of domination to maintain power and influence in mainstream society. Core principles of whiteness are that it is invisible, socially constructed, and grants unearned privileges to members of the culture it represents [37].

White privilege is seemingly a worldwide phenomenon, with roots stemming from European colonialism. In the field of psychiatry, DSM diagnostic categories and criteria are presumed "culture-free" despite originating from Europe and Northern America [36]. Reinforcing the dominant invisibility, highlighting specific "culture-bound" disorders, shields whiteness from a similar psychopathological focus. European and North American psychiatrists have presumptively assumed authority to ascribe diagnoses to not only North American and European culture but other cultures as well. Along with highlighting cultural "otherness," cultural richness has been further subjugated by a reductionist appeal to neurobiology. Culture in medical settings often distances the clinician from the patient (e.g., cultural differences may be viewed as an impediment to shared understanding) [36]. Poor attention to the importance of culturally competent care in psychiatry often leads to lower utilization of outpatient mental health services [36].

Racialization of substance use disorders has been repeatedly utilized throughout time and regions. Examples in the USA include the use of phrases such as "cocaine-crazed Negroes" and "Chinese opium dens," despite the reality that narcotic use was highest among whites. The 1986 Anti-Drug Abuse Act enforced similar sentencing for possession of crack cocaine (perceived as a Black drug) at 1/100th the amount of powder cocaine (perceived as a white drug). This led to targeting of communities of color with increased spending on incarceration in these neighborhoods. Similarly within healthcare systems, buprenorphine was marketed to general medicine clinics as an option for "stable," "suburban" populations (implicitly linked to whiteness). Contrastingly, methadone clinics are often located in minority neighborhoods despite a stated preference for buprenorphine [8]. While individuals in developed countries and wealthier environments are more likely to use substances, people who are socially and economically disadvantaged are more likely to develop substance use disorders [38]. The intersection of public policy, healthcare organizations, and the legal system impact the context in which patients receive care.

Vignette

Malachi is a 46-year-old homeless male with opioid use disorder admitted to hospital medicine for management of bacteremia. This is not his first hospitalization at this hospital as he has been admitted previously for the treatment of cellulitis to both lower extremities. His bed was positioned in the emergency department (ED) hallway where he avoided eye contact with people he did not know. While in the ED, his nurses complained of difficulty obtaining intravenous line access. He endured loud sighs as ultrasound-guided placement of his intravenous line was finally successful. Malachi declined his dinner that evening (two half-slices of white bread with deli turkey) due to nausea from opiate withdrawal. His attempts to obtain treatment for withdrawal symptoms were unsuccessful, and he suffered the humiliation of defecating in his bed due to diarrhea. Despite his protests, his bedsheets were not changed for 3 hours. The ED nurse informed him that he would be admitted.

After he showered and changed into ill-fitting hospital-donated clothes, he decided to go outside and smoke a cigarette. Upon returning, he was sternly reminded by the unit clerk, "next time, you better sign out." He replied that he was unaware of the unit expectations and would remember to sign out next time. Two hours later, he wanted to smoke another cigarette. The binder to sign out was nowhere to be found and attempts to locate it were unsuccessful. A hospital staff member informed him that he was allowed to smoke a cigarette. Upon return, he found two security officers and a medicine intern in his room. They asked about his whereabouts and suspiciously questioned his time off the unit. The young male intern informed him that he will need a urine drug screen. Malachi was then presented with a behavioral contract. He was enraged when he read "I will be discharged if I leave the unit" and "I am to remain on the unit at all times."

Malachi angrily crumpled up the piece of paper and tossed it at the intern. Immediately turning bright red, the intern sputtered, "the hospital is not a place for drug users. It's a place for people who want to get better." The security officers then proceeded to demand access to his personal belongings and confiscated two lighters from his backpack. They quickly followed the intern out of the room, making eye contact with Malachi saying, "we have our eyes on you." Malachi went to bed feeling angry and upset that he was accused but also increasingly uncomfortable and ashamed about his craving for heroin.

The next morning, Malachi awoke to the sound of a large cylindrical structure being wheeled into his room by hospital staff. He was informed that this was a "video-monitoring unit" to discourage "funny business." This device would provide 24/7 surveillance, essentially leaving him devoid of privacy. Due to ongoing opiate withdrawal, Malachi had to make several trips to the bathroom. At each use, hospital staff made a point to knock loudly on his bathroom door, often saying "everything all right in there?" He did not know why the nurses would wake him up in the middle of the night by jostling the arm with his intravenous line.

On Hospital Day 3, Malachi had made up his mind to leave the hospital. His withdrawal symptoms had escalated considerably. He was too uncomfortable to discuss his rationale with the physician and did not know what the intern meant when he said, "you don't have the capacity to leave." He soon found out, however, when the same two security guards firmly instructed him to lay back down on the bed. Arguing that he has "had it with this hospital," he was aggressively situated in bed while physical restraints were applied to both wrists and ankles. Crying out loudly "get me out of here," he eventually fell asleep after intramuscular medications were administered.

Although his bacterial infection was clearing, the physician informed him that there were no accepting inpatient rehabilitation facilities because of his drug history and insurance coverage. Malachi pleaded with the intern to come back daily to the ED, but the intern scoffed "you think we would let you out of here with an IV? Give me a break." That night, Malachi left the hospital. His absence was noticed 3 hours later. He was not there to hear the nurse complain, "shit, he left with his IV."

Discussion

Patients like Malachi present difficult challenges to healthcare systems, both in terms of treatment and policy recommendations. Multifactorial etiologies (medical, psychiatric, substance) combined with multidisciplinary involvement (physician, nurse, clinical care partner, hospital security, hospital administration) and systemic factors (fee for service versus value-based payments, available outpatient treatment options) require a comprehensive, coordinated approach that is challenging to organize and influence.

Malachi has chronic bacteremia that has not been successfully treated despite numerous hospitalizations and ED visits. His irritable impulsivity is likely related to opioid withdrawal but could be a sign of an underlying psychiatric disorder, such as bipolar disorder. Verbalizing a desire to leave against medical advice will prompt considerations of capacity. Determining a patient's understanding of the rationale for hospitalization and risks/benefits of leaving against medical advice is necessary. Patients must be able to articulate a greater understanding of their current condition and risks of discharging against medical advice in accordance with the severity of their condition. There are several tools available to assist clinicians in these decisions.

Recognizing nonspecific behavioral manifestations of substance use disorders should lead to consultation with an inpatient psychiatrist for diagnostic clarification and treatment recommendations. Prompt consideration of medication-assisted treatment to decrease the discomfort of withdrawal will help decrease the likelihood of patients leaving against medical advice. Physicians and staff developing an awareness of organizational stigma surrounding substance use disorder and the impact on the medical care available to these individuals, for both related and unrelated issues, is critical for equitable care delivery. Examples include outpatient parenteral antibiotic therapy guidelines excluding patients with intravenous substance use disorders, behavioral agreements that restrictively confine patients to their hospital room, and lack of substance use navigators within hospital settings. All these practices are common problem areas that isolate patients with substance use disorders from medical care. Reducing stigma among healthcare providers is challenging in environments that lack resources to address the problem. Rather than retreating to cynicism, civic engagement with local behavioral health leaders may help reduce the sense of helplessness and futility many healthcare workers face when treating patients presenting to emergency departments. Advocating for increased resources, such as substance use navigators who can assist patients engage with a complex, Rube Goldbergian, health system may be useful.

In Malachi's case, several modifications are required to provide optimal clinical care. First and foremost, treating patients with respect should be the default, not diagnosis dependent. Demeaning comments reinforce stigma and isolate the patient from beneficent care. His substance use and withdrawal symptoms should have been more thoroughly assessed. This would have increased the opportunity for his provider to offer nicotine replacement therapy or medication to manage discomfort associated with opiate withdrawal. A consult to psychiatry may have been useful to help clarify psychiatric history and diagnoses, manage his substance use while in the hospital, and offer recommendations for his behavioral disturbances. To prevent the miscommunications that occurred, upon admittance, the hospital staff should have provided Malachi with clear instructions and expectations regarding leaving his room. Several members of the team including the medicine intern, nurse, and security guard should have been more mindful of their biases and language. Malachi's decision to leave against medical advice perpetuated the pattern of untreated medical, psychiatric, and substance use problems.

Culturally Competent Care in Co-occurring Disorders

To provide culturally competent care for patients with co-occurring disorders, mental healthcare providers must recognize the role of the environment they are seeking care in, obtain personal and familial history, assess for social risk factors, and identify personal values and motivations. Examination of specific populations demonstrates the need for targeted and adapated interventions. Communication should be effective, attending to native language and nuanced interactions. Awareness of personal and systemic limitations, gaps, and biases should be recognized, and steps should be taken to reduce misunderstandings and barriers to care.

Social Risk Factors

Isolation

Social identity and social supports impact the development of substance use disorders, particularly during formative adolescent years. Nearly all adults who go on to develop substance use disorders begin using during adolescence. For those that develop a substance use disorders in adolescence, nearly 60% also have a concurrent mental illness [39]. Using substances may be associated with an increased or decreased number of social support sources, which are perceived as an "identity gain" or "identity loss," respectively [40]. Social connection is vital for humans, and poor social support and isolation are risk factors for developing both mental health and substance use disorders. Attending to the social network and potential loss of social connections during recovery is an important part of the treatment process and sustaining change.

Isolation can be grouped into three subtypes: (1) being unliked (not receiving social ties), (2) disengaged (not sending ties to others), and (3) outside-oriented (having out-of-network ties) [41]. Individuals with fewer social supports and more isolative behaviors are at greater risk for adverse health outcomes, including antisocial acts, mood disturbances, and suicide [42]. Laboratory research has also demonstrated the deleterious effects of depriving rats from social engagement, including increased cocaine abuse [43]. While social isolation and rejection can increase risk of using substances, many also turn to substances to ameliorate feelings of loneliness [44] which perpetuates the disorder.

Stigma

Given the importance of social supports, community, and connection, it is not surprising that stigma, or marked disapproval of an individual, is associated with less access and utilization of care and worse mental health outcomes [45]. Substance use disorders are one of the most stigmatized health conditions in the world. They are often understood as extrinsic, environmental problems rather than biological or genetic ones. Therefore, if an individual is unable to control their substance use, the individual is to blame. Additionally, there is a moral aspect that further reinforces stigma, which is closely linked with the emotion of shame. Individuals with substance use disorders are often thought to be "weak and incompetent, more responsible for their disorder, and less pitiable and worthy of help" [45]. Similar stigmatizing language is also used against individuals with mental illness; use of the terms "maniac," "lunatic," and "psycho" perpetuate beliefs that individuals with mental illness are violent. Individuals with both substance use and psychiatric diagnoses are likely to be subject to more stigma than either one alone.

Stigma can affect an individual in three different ways: (1) experienced stigma, including acts of discrimination; (2) perceived stigma, how one believes society views them; and (3) self-stigma, or internalization of public perception [7]. Stigma related to substance use disorders is related to social stereotypes, internalization of these stereotypes, and reinforcement through societal shaming behaviors. Use of the term "addict" is often linked to a moral judgment or internalization as a "bad person" [7].

Unfortunately, physicians are also exposed to a system of blame, shame, and stigma for substance use disorders. Studies have documented that physicians may view individuals with substance use disorders as having lower importance and more likely to commit violence and manipulate others [7]. Surprisingly, these views do not always change with more training and education. In a study of psychiatry residents, negative attitudes toward patients with substance use disorder increased throughout training. Addiction psychiatrists and community psychiatrists had more negative attitudes toward patients with a co-occurring mental health and substance use disorder than patients with either diagnosis alone [7]. Negative beliefs about patients with substance use disorders are partly related to the perception that this population places an undue burden on our healthcare system. Additionally, despite understanding that substance use disorders create reward circuitry dysfunction, moralistic oversimplification attitudes (e.g., "this guy should just shape up") remain prevalent among healthcare workers. There is also a bias in hospital settings toward primarily interacting with individuals who have severe untreated substance use disorders rather than treating individuals who are in recovery. Unfortunately, trainee exposure to the "hidden curriculum" may foster negative attitudes rather than positive mentorship that contextualizes substance use disorders within a medical framework indicating a need for larger systemic change. Notably, physicians experience substance use disorder rates similar to the general population, but the formal treatment they are offered through physician health programs is thought to be attributed to their significantly smaller relapse rate from the general population.

Addressing public stigma can alleviate the severity of self-stigma. One way to address public stigma is through decriminalization, as laws are seen as a codification of social norms []. The swinging pendulum from criminal to medical interventions for substance use disorders can be viewed across time as described above in the "Historical Significance" section. Additionally, treatment for substance use disorders typically includes both psychoeducation and support groups for patients and family members that can help connect them to a supportive social group, overcome shame and blamed based thinking, and realize they are not alone.

Special Populations

Pregnancy, Postpartum, and Motherhood

From 1999 to 2015, prescription opioid fatalities increased by 471% for women compared to 218% for men [46]. Similar increases in misuse and mortality for women have been observed in alcohol and other substances [19]. Despite the growing rates of substance abuse concerns in women, they are less likely to receive treatment. It is hypothesized that this is related to increased stigma, higher burden of caregiving responsibilities, and treatment approaches that have been designed based on research conducted primarily on male populations. Substance use in the context of pregnancy and motherhood may be particularly challenging. The postpartum period is a critical time where many mothers may start using substances again after pausing during pregnancy and is associated with postpartum depression. The American College of Obstetricians and Gynecologists assert that women with an opioid use disorder should not face criminal or civil penalties including loss of custody [47]. Loss of custody is associated with substance relapse and increased risk for depression. Fear of child separation is one reason women opt to avoid substance use disorder treatment. Black and Latinx women with opioid use disorders are more likely than white women with opioid use disorders to be incarcerated and separated from their children. Twenty-three states classify substance use in pregnancy as child abuse, and three states classify substance use as grounds for civil commitment.

Women with substance use disorders have higher rates of mental health diagnoses than men, which may be attributed to a combination of adverse childhood experiences, lifetime trauma, and low self-esteem []. The Substance Use and Mental Health Services Administration (SAMHSA) notes that "trauma is an almost universal experience" for women with co-occurring disorders [48]. Whereas men with substance use disorders are more likely to exhibit externalizing behaviors (e.g., aggression), women are more likely to internalize (e.g., self-criticism). These externalizing behaviors decrease with age in men, but internalizing behaviors increase with age in women.

Physical and Cognitive Disabilities

Individuals with disabilities are at higher risk for developing co-occurring mental illness and substance use disorders. They are also less likely to engage in treatment [49] and are more likely to be heavy users compared to individuals without disabilities [50]. Disabilities may be physical (e.g., deaf and hard of hearing) and/or cognitive (e.g., traumatic brain injury). Increased risk for developing substance use disorders appears to be related to social isolation, limited access to services, poor health literacy, unemployment, and level of disability acceptance [51]. Treatment services are critical. One study found that suicidal behavior is increased in deaf individuals with co-occurring disorders compared to deaf individuals with a mental health diagnosis alone [49]. While access to care remains challenging, efforts to increase access via environmental modifications (e.g., wheelchair ramps) and resource materials (e.g., Braille, sign language interpretation) are being made in support programs.

Incarcerated Populations

Incarcerated populations face significant challenges and limited resources. These limitations, coupled with a multitude of factors, place them at increased risk for both substance use disorders and mental illness [52]. Prisoners reported increased use of cannabis (40%), cocaine (21.4%), methamphetamine (12.2%), and heroin (8.2%) compared to the general population. Symptoms of mental illness are also significantly higher, specifically mania (43.2% versus 2%), depression (23.5% versus 7%), and psychosis (15.4% versus 3%). Forty-one percent of incarcerated individuals have a co-occurring disorder. Incarceration alone increases the risk for suicide attempt (2.3% versus 0.4%) and completion compared to the general population [53]. Mood disorders in an incarcerated person increase the individual's suicide risk to 13%. Placement in maximum security settings increase the risk of suicide attempts [54].

Rates of co-occurring serious mental illness and substance use disorders are high in incarcerated populations (4–6x in jail, 3–4x in prison compared to national averages) [54]. Elevated rates of substance use disorders are related to federal and state drug policies (in 2015, >50% of federal prison population were related to drug offenses), homelessness, and higher rates of criminal behaviors [55]. An increased focus on community services (e.g., drug courts, mental health courts, assertive community treatment programs) for incarcerated individuals with co-occurring disorders has led to decreased rates of incarceration.

Treatment of substance use disorders in jail and prison settings is often rudimentary and limited, with only 11% of individuals receiving any treatment at all [7]. Perceived social support for prisoners was negatively correlated with number of substance use disorders [7]. In 2015, the US population was 13% Black, but the US prison population was 38% Black [7]. Evidence suggests that the general public assigns greater blame to Black individuals with substance use disorders than their white counterparts [7]. White inmates are also more likely than Black inmates to receive substance use treatment [7].

Additionally, there is inadequate access to medication-assisted treatments. If these treatments are provided, inmates are typically charged extra for this service. As of August 2018, only Rhode Island provides all three forms (methadone, buprenorphine, naltrexone) of medication-assisted treatment, and 28 states do not prescribe any form of medication-assisted treatment [7]. Paltry medication formularies often lead to psychiatric decompensation due to reduced access to nonformulary medications and challenges related to restrictions on dosage and use. Logistical factors such as clinicians having a Drug Enforcement Administration waiver may also affect access to pharmacological treatments. Medication cessation can lead to behavioral dysregulation and increased risk for placement in administrative segregation (solitary confinement) [54]. Lack of reentry programs can lead to further destabilization.

Military Service Members and Veterans

Active duty and veteran service members suffer from higher than average prevalence rates of both mental health disorders and substance use disorders, which places them at increased risk of developing co-occurring disorders. Higher rates of substance abuse, particularly alcohol misuse, are observed in those that have deployed [55, 56]. This is likely due to a combination of factors including the culture, setting, and experiences, such as exposure to combat. Prescriptions for pain medications also increased exponentially in the early 2000s among military physicians [56], increasing concerns for opioid use disorders. Service members are likely to have co-occurring substance and mental health disorders, such as posttraumatic stress disorder, depression, and anxiety. Those with co-occurring disorders are at increased risk for suicide. The suicide rate for service members exceeded suicides in the general population, and more than 1,100 military members died by suicide between 2005 and 2009 [55]. Efforts have been made to address these growing concerns including reducing access to alcohol on military sites and reinforcing underage laws, reducing stigma to accessing treatment, and offering more confidential and intensive services to treat substance use and co-occurring disorders [56].

Indigenous Populations

Indigenous populations have a high prevalence of substance use and co-occurring disorders. Historically, American Indians and Alaska Natives have had the highest rates of alcohol, marijuana, cocaine, hallucinogen, and methamphetamine use disorders [1, 57]. Rates for psychosocial stressors, adverse childhood experiences, and poverty are also elevated. Substance use disorders in this population affect not only individuals and families but communities on a larger scale. In addition to increased risk due to disparities in social determinants of health, these populations often have limited access to treatment across rural and urban settings. Access to treatment is challenging due to transportation issues, limited insurance coverage, low socioeconomic status, stigma, and shortage of treatment programs (particularly interventions that have culturally informed adaptations) [57]. Encouragingly, access to medication-assisted treatments continues to increase every year and the expansion of telemedicine services is likely to benefit rural populations [1].

Treatment for Co-occurring Disorders

Traditionally, treatments for substance use disorders were sequestered from general and mental health care services. Services provided were also limited, often reduced to urgent or emergency care rather than treatment and recovery services. The benefits of treating substance and mental health disorders concurrently are evident. Integrated treatment approaches including psychosocial interventions, case management (e.g., housing, finances, education/vocation), peer supports (e.g., 12-step groups, recovery support specialists), and family services (e.g., psychoeducation, support groups) are recommended. These approaches are not just beneficial for patient outcomes but also valuable for larger systems of care, such as reducing unnecessary expensive hospital visits. Table 5.1 outlines unique and shared treatment approaches across alcohol, opioid, stimulant, and tobacco use disorders. Despite information about the effectiveness of comprehensive and integrated treatments, the majority of patients with co-occurring disorders receive treatment for only one disorder or no treatment at all [1]. Additional work is needed to inform public policy, address stigma, and shift the perspective of substance use disorders as a social or criminal problem rather than a public health need.

Alcohol

Six percent of all deaths globally and 3% of deaths in the USA are related to alcohol use [18, 19]. Prolonged cessation from alcohol abuse without support is successful for 20% of population suffering from alcohol use disorder [18]. However, only 8.3% of 15 million adults struggling with alcohol use disorder received treatment in 2015 [58]. Twelve-step programs started with Alcoholics Anonymous (AA), founded in 1934 after the repeal of Prohibition [18]. Importantly, while other groups were focused on societal problems associated with alcohol use, AA focused on the individual's consumption of alcohol. AA chose to avoid other aspects of alcohol use disorder, such as underlying etiology (genetic, societal, medical, personal). The group emphasized the need for spirituality conversion as central to recovery. Members of AA found solace in descriptions of alcohol as an "allergy" and "obsession," advocating abstinence in order for individuals to address spiritual maladies. Central to AA is "identity diffusion," where individuals listen to personal stories from other members, allowing them to connect to shared experiences in the group [59]. After completion of residential treatment, rates of abstinence double with participation in AA compared to no participation [60]. Similarly, increased participation in AA is associated with increased periods of sobriety [60]. A Cochrane review demonstrated equal levels of effectiveness of 12-step programs compared to other interventions such as self-help groups [61].

For individuals who require more intensive structure than recovery meetings, residential treatment is often sought. Residential treatment is a 24-hour nonhospital level of care setting with intensive substance abuse programming. People with co-occurring disorders often are treated in residential facilities because of their more

Table 5.1 Treatment recommendations for substance use and co-occurring disorders

	Pharmacotherapy/ medication-assisted treatment	Other treatments	Experimental treatments requiring more research
Alcohol	Disulfiram Naltrexone Injectable naltrexone Acamprosate	Modified therapeutic communities (inpatient, residential, or recovery treatment) Peer supports (e.g., 12-step programs, recovery support specialists) Motivational interviewing and enhancement Behavioral couples therapy	Transcranial magnetic stimulation Buprenorphine Varenicline Intranasal oxytocin Gabapentin Prazosin Topiramate Buspirone
Opioids	Methadone Buprenorphine Naltrexone	Needle exchange programs Modified therapeutic communities Peer supports Motivational interviewing and enhancement	Ketamine Heroin-assisted treatment Transcranial magnetic stimulation Buspirone
Stimulants	N/A	Contingency management therapy Community reinforcement approach Modified therapeutic communities Peer supports Motivational interviewing and enhancement	Dexamphetamine Methylphenidate Topiramate Disulfiram Buprenorphine Naltrexone Bupropion N-acetylcysteine Mirtazapine Valproic acid Transcranial magnetic stimulation Cognitive behavioral therapy
Tobacco	Nicotine replacement therapy Bupropion Varenicline	Motivational interviewing and enhancement Telephone support and quit lines Cognitive-behavioral therapy and mindfulness interventions	Nortriptyline N-acetylcysteine Transcranial magnetic stimulation

complex treatment needs, and evidence suggests that residential treatment settings are effective in reducing substance use and promoting higher quality of life. As untreated depression or posttraumatic stress disorder hastens alcohol craving and relapse, integrated residential care settings are important for those with co-occurring disorders [63]. Notably, duration of residential treatment differs by country; Swiss residential treatment duration is about five times (122 days) that of the USA (25 days) [64]. Although depressive symptoms at admission to residential treatment were associated with alcohol use at 1 year after residential treatment discharge, improvements in depressive scores were not associated with subsequent alcohol use at 1 year [64]. Co-management, including pharmacologically, for alcohol use disorder and major depression leads to decreased relapse rates and increased sobriety [65].

Unfortunately, prescription rates for treatment of alcohol use disorders are woefully low; from 2002 to 2007, one study indicated that only 9% of individuals received one of the four medications (i.e., disulfiram, naltrexone, injectable naltrexone, acamprosate) the Federal Drug Administration (FDA) has approved for alcohol use disorder [58]. Medications that have been used to treat other substance use disorders may also aid the treatment of alcohol use disorder. Specifically, high doses of buprenorphine has shown decreased alcohol consumption, theoretically by blocking reward circuitry [62]. Similarly, varenicline decreased the number of heavy drinking days [62]. Decreasing glutamate through topiramate has also demonstrated a concomitant decrease in stress-related alcohol consumption [62]. Tracking serum glutamate levels are of importance as individuals with higher serum glutamate levels were more likely to respond to acamprosate (returning to normal serum glutamate levels) than those with lower baseline glutamate levels. Intranasal oxytocin is associated with decreased alcohol cravings, likely through stress-mediated pathways [62]. Data suggests that gabapentin is efficacious in reducing withdrawal symptoms and increasing duration of sobriety [65].

In addition to psychosocial and pharmacologic treatments, neuromodulation is a potential avenue to address alcohol use disorder. Due to compulsive behavior associated with alcohol use and positive results using transcranial magnetic stimulation (TMS) in patients with obsessive-compulsive disorder, TMS has also been posited as a possible treatment for alcohol use disorder [66]. By targeting dorsolateral prefrontal cortex and medial prefrontal cortex, investigators hope to disrupt pathways implicated in alcohol abuse [67]. In early studies, repetitive transcranial magnetic stimulation directed to dorsolateral prefrontal cortex and medial prefrontal cortex resulted in decreased alcohol craving compared to placebo [67]. Similar results have been demonstrated with transcranial direct current stimulation [67]. This has implications for future indications of transcranial magnetic stimulation.

Opioids

Rates of opioid misuse rose exponentially in the past few decades, resulting in high disability, infectious disease burden, and overdose deaths. First line recommended and FDA-approved treatment is medication-assisted treatment including buprenorphine, methadone, and extended-release naltrexone. Pharmacotherapy should be combined with behavioral counseling. Studies have demonstrated support for decreased opioid-related deaths and infectious disease transmission, increased engagement in treatment and functioning, and improved neonatal outcomes once medication-assisted therapies have been introduced [47, 68, 69]. However, access to these treatments remains sparse with nearly all US states having insufficient treatment options. On average, only 11% of patients with opioid use disorder receive medication-assisted treatment [70].

In addition to currently approved medications, researchers are investigating alternative methods of treating opioid use disorder. One potential option is ketamine [71]. In one promising study, abstinence rates were 85% at 1 month and 24% at

1 year for high-dose ketamine (2 mg/kg) versus 6% for low-dose ketamine (0.2 mg/kg). This study was limited by lack of a placebo group [72]. Noninvasive brain stimulation including TMS, transcranial direct current stimulation, and auricular vagus nerve stimulation may have therapeutic benefits as an augmentation strategy, particularly during withdrawal and cravings [73]. Research is still preliminary and ongoing studies with larger samples, placebo groups, and generalizable findings are needed.

Supervised injectable heroin treatment was started during the 1990s. This intervention is used when first-line options (methadone, buprenorphine, residential treatment) are unsuccessful. Patients inject about 200 mg of heroin with direct supervision [21]. Introduction of supervised injection sites has led to a decrease in illicit heroin use along with use of cocaine and alcohol. Social functioning including housing, drug-free contacts, employment, and incarceration rates have improved [21]. Patients are prohibited from leaving the site with any heroin. Negative connotations associated with substance use disorders have infected public policy and hospital practices. While heroin-assisted treatment is utilized in some European countries, its use is banned in the USA.

Six countries (i.e., Canada, Germany, Spain, Switzerland, the Netherlands and the UK) have studied heroin-assisted treatment (HAT) to determine if this option is superior to the standard of care, especially when other options have failed. The most common reasons for prescribing heroin among English psychiatrists was continued illicit heroin use by injection, methadone refusal, crime reduction (e.g., purchasing heroin through sex work), and previous treatment failure [21]. In Germany, HAT led to health system net savings of ~$6,000 per patient per year compared to a net cost of ~$2,000 per patient per year with methadone maintenance. Also, HAT programs maintained higher retention rates [21]. Broadening treatment required legislative changes to Germany's federal narcotics control law. Similarly, a multicenter study in the Netherlands demonstrated therapeutic benefit (i.e., physical health, mental health, and social functioning) of HAT compared to methadone [21]. Political opposition has proven the rate-limiting step in many of these countries [75].

Stimulants

Methamphetamine intoxication is associated with psychosis. Its effects can be explained by dopamine binding and sympathetic stimulation by monoamine release. Frequent, prolonged methamphetamine use can lead to mood disturbances, impulsivity, and cognitive deficits [76]. Depression and anxiety are common comorbidities among patients with methamphetamine use. Over half of the women in one study reported a history of sexual assault [77]. In a study of 16 patients with methamphetamine use disorder, 53% experienced psychiatric disorders (i.e., unipolar depression, attention-deficit/hyperactivity disorder, substance-induced psychosis) [77]. It is unknown whether cognitive deficits related to methamphetamine use are completely reversible; however, attentional problems improve with sustained sobriety [76]. Patients who inject methamphetamine, versus inhale, demonstrated an increased risk for suicidal ideation and attempts as well as violent behavior [77].

The global market for stimulants is expanding. Use of cocaine and methamphetamine has been increasing for the past decade, reaching a high in 2018 of 19 million cocaine users (primarily in North America/Western Europe) and 27 million amphetamine users (primarily in Southeast Asia) [38]. Seizures from amphetamine use quadrupled between 2009 and 2018 [38]. Treatment for stimulant use disorder is particularly challenging as no medications have FDA approval or demonstrated consistent efficacy. Psychosocial interventions, such as contingency management, have demonstrated support in reducing stimulant use and improving functioning and treatment engagement. Additionally, there is some evidence that prescription psychostimulants may promote sustained drug abstinence. Trials with dexamphetamine have demonstrated prolonged methamphetamine cessation and decreased craving [78]. Once daily dosing was used with maximum dose of 110 mg/day. Buprenorphine showed greater decrease in craving compared to methadone [79], and naltrexone may be helpful regarding cravings in laboratory and clinical studies [80]. Bupropion and N-acetylcysteine are helpful at reducing methamphetamine withdrawal symptoms. Research findings for modafinil are mixed and limited. One study supported adding mirtazapine to cognitive behavioral therapy/motivational interviewing to decrease methamphetamine use [81]. Ongoing research is needed, and individuals with stimulant use disorders are considerably undertreated.

Tobacco

Smoking is the leading cause of preventable disease, disability, and death in the USA [34]. Although many smokers express interest in quitting smoking or smokeless tobacco, much fewer are successful in doing so. On average, individuals undergo 30 quit attempts before successful discontinuation [82]. First-line treatment for smoking cessation includes a combination of medication (bupropion and varenicline) and nicotine replacement therapy (NRT; transdermal, lozenges, gum). Combining short- and long-acting NRT can be more effective than using one form only. Patients may also benefit from additional counseling via quit hotlines, phone apps, individual, and/or group therapies. Strategies that have demonstrated efficacy include setting a quit date, recognizing behavioral and environmental triggers, and having identified reasons for quitting. Similar to other substance use disorders, early studies indicate TMS may be helpful on craving and intake [83].

Individuals with schizophrenia have the highest rates of tobacco use (70–80%) compared to those with other mental health diagnoses [5]. Data suggests that treatment with first-generation antipsychotics may worsen substance use disorders, particularly tobacco use disorders [5]. Increased tobacco use is attributed to extrapyramidal side effects associated with first-generation antipsychotics. Smoking cessation interventions may be more effective with atypical antipsychotics, but larger studies are necessary to support these studies with small sample sizes [5]. Additional research is needed to inform best practice prescribing patterns in psychotic patients with a known tobacco use disorder.

Conclusion

Co-occurring disorders are common but undertreated due to a combination of factors related to addiction and systemic barriers to care including stigma, discrimination, limited resources, and lack of access to appropriate treatments. Even among healthcare professionals, negative attitudes toward individuals with a substance use disorder are extremely prevalent. Although increased training is not always effective at reducing stigma, hospitals are encouraged to utilize substance use navigators to better guide treatment and advocate for patients. Evidence-based treatments are underutilized, especially in custodial and hospital settings. Inadequate recognition and treatment of co-occurring disorders often have deleterious consequences. Efforts to address substance use disorders as diagnoses, rather than moral failings, will improve patient care.

Summary of High-Yield Points

- Mental health diagnoses often predate or co-occur with substance use disorders.
- Individuals with co-occurring disorders are at increased risk for suicide, poor treatment adherence, and homelessness.
- Social isolation is a common risk factor for developing a substance use disorder.
- Patients are more likely to have their mental health diagnosis treated than their substance use disorder.
- Clinician attitudes toward patients with co-occurring disorders affect utilization of healthcare services.
- Even when substance use disorder treatment is covered by insurance providers, patients face increased barriers and are often unaware that this resource is available to them.
- In addition to 12-step programs and FDA-approved medications, transcranial magnetic stimulation has been posited as possible treatment for alcohol use disorder and other substance use disorders.
- Treatment for stimulant use disorder is particularly challenging as no medications have FDA approval or demonstrated consistent efficacy.
- Heroin-assisted treatment is utilized in other countries for patients who are difficult to engage with medication-assisted treatment or fail to respond to the standard of care.

References

1. U.S. Department of Health and Human Services, Substance Abuse and Mental Health Services Administration, Center for Behavioral Health Statistics and Quality. Key substance use and mental health indicators in the United States: results from the 2019 National Survey on Drug Use and Health. 2019.
2. Degenhardt L, Whiteford HA, Ferrari AJ, Baxter AJ, Charlson FJ, Hall WD, Freedman G, Burstein R, Johns N, Engell RE, Flaxman A. Global burden of disease attributable to illicit drug use and dependence: findings from the Global Burden of Disease Study 2010. Lancet. 2013;382(9904):1564–74.
3. Ti L, Ti L. Leaving the hospital against medical advice among people who use illicit drugs: a systematic review. Am J Public Health. 2015;105(12):2587.
4. Tan SY, Feng JY, Joyce C, Fisher J, Mostaghimi A. Association of hospital discharge against medical advice with readmission and in-hospital mortality. JAMA Netw Open. 2020;3(6):e206009.
5. Green AI, Drake RE, Brunette MF, Noordsy DL. Schizophrenia and co-occurring substance use disorder. Am J Psychiatry. 2007;164(3):402–8. https://doi.org/10.1176/ajp.2007.164.3.402. PMID: 17329463
6. Brunette MF, Noordsy DL, Xie H, Drake RE. Benzodiazepine use and abuse among patients with severe mental illness and co-occurring substance use disorders. Psychiatr Serv. 2003;54(10):1395–401. https://doi.org/10.1176/appi.ps.54.10.1395. PMID: 14557527
7. Avery JD, Avery JJ, editors. The stigma of addiction: an essential guide. Springer; 2019.
8. National Institute on Drug Abuse. Trends & Statistics. 2017.
9. Ali MM, Teich JL, Mutter R. The role of perceived need and health insurance in substance use treatment: implications for the Affordable Care Act. J Subst Abus Treat. 2015;54:14–20.
10. Mojtabai R, Mauro C, Wall MM, Barry CL, Olfson M. Private health insurance coverage of drug use disorder treatment: 2005–2018. PLoS One. 2020;15(10):e0240298.
11. Mark TL, Yee T, Levit KR, Camacho-Cook J, Cutler E, Carroll CD. Insurance financing increased for mental health conditions but not for substance use disorders, 1986–2014. Health Aff. 2016;35(6):958–65.
12. Tsai AC, Kiang MV, Barnett ML, Beletsky L, Keyes KM, McGinty EE, Smith LR, Strathdee SA, Wakeman SE, Venkataramani AS. Stigma as a fundamental hindrance to the United States opioid overdose crisis response. PLoS Med. 2019;16(11):e1002969.
13. Yates K, Lång U, Cederlöf M, Boland F, Taylor P, Cannon M, McNicholas F, DeVylder J, Kelleher I. Association of psychotic experiences with subsequent risk of suicidal ideation, suicide attempts, and suicide deaths: a systematic review and meta-analysis of longitudinal population studies. JAMA Psychiat. 2019;76(2):180–9.
14. Hatzenbuehler ML, Keyes KM, Narrow WE, Grant BF, Hasin DS. Racial/ethnic disparities in service utilization for individuals with co-occurring mental health and substance use disorders in the general population. J Clin Psychiatry. 2008;69(7):1112.
15. Anderson P, Baumberg B. Alcohol in Europe, vol. 2. London: Institute of Alcohol Studies; 2006. p. 73–5.
16. Miron JA, Zwiebel J. Alcohol consumption during prohibition. National Bureau of Economic Research; 1991.
17. Levine HG. The Committee of Fifty and the origins of alcohol control. J Drug Issues. 1983;13(1):95–116.
18. Kurtz E. Alcoholics anonymous and the disease concept of alcoholism. Alcohol Treat Q. 2002;20(3–4):5–39.
19. White AM, Castle IJP, Hingson RW, Powell PA. Using death certificates to explore changes in alcohol-related mortality in the United States, 1999 to 2017. Alcohol Clin Exp Res. 2020;44(1):178–87.
20. Metrebian N. Influences on the prescribing of heroin for the treatment of opiate dependence in the United Kingdom. London: University of London; 2005.

21. Strang J, Groshkova T, Metrebian N. European Monitoring Centre for Drugs and Drug Addiction. New heroin-assisted treatment: recent evidence and current practices of supervised injectable heroin treatment in Europe and beyond. Luxembourg: Publications Office of the European Union; 2012.
22. Perneger T, Giner F, del Rio M, Mino A. Randomized trial of heroin maintenance programme for addicts who fail in conventional drug treatment. BMJ. 1998;317(7150):13–8.
23. Jiang R, Lee I, Lee TA, Pickard AS. The societal cost of heroin use disorder in the United States. PLoS One. 2017;12(5):e0177323.
24. Weinmeyer R. Needle exchange programs' status in US politics. AMA J Ethics. 2016;18(3):252–7.
25. Cohen A. How white users made heroin a public-health problem. The Atlantic. 2015.
26. Mack KA, Jones CM, Ballesteros MF. Illicit drug use, illicit drug use disorders, and drug overdose deaths in metropolitan and nonmetropolitan areas—United States. Am J Transplant. 2017;17(12):3241–52.
27. Peters DJ, Monnat SM, Hochstetler AL, Berg MT. The opioid hydra: understanding overdose mortality epidemics and syndemics across the rural-urban continuum. Rural Sociol. 2020;85(3):589–622.
28. Jones CM, Bekheet F, Park JN, Alexander GC. The evolving overdose epidemic: synthetic opioids and rising stimulant-related harms. Epidemiol Rev. 2020;42(1):154–66. https://doi.org/10.1093/epirev/mxaa011.
29. Mattson CL, Tanz LJ, Quinn K, Kariisa M, Patel P, Davis NL. Trends and geographic patterns in drug and synthetic opioid overdose deaths — United States, 2013–2019. MMWR Morb Mortal Wkly Rep. 2021;70:202–7. https://doi.org/10.15585/mmwr.mm7006a4.
30. Anderson AL, Li SH, Biswas K, McSherry F, Holmes T, Iturriaga E, Kahn R, Chiang N, Beresford T, Campbell J, Haning W. Modafinil for the treatment of methamphetamine dependence. Drug Alcohol Depend. 2012;120(1–3):135–41.
31. Substance Abuse and Mental Health Services Administration: Center for Behavioral Health Statistics and Quality. Key substance use and mental health indicators in the United States: results from the 2018 National Survey on Drug Use and Health (HHS Publication No. PEP19–5068, NSDUH series H-54). Rockville: Substance Abuse and Mental Health Services Administration; 2019.
32. Winkelman TN, Admon LK, Jennings L, Shippee ND, Richardson CR, Bart G. Evaluation of amphetamine related hospitalizations and associated clinical outcomes and costs in the United States. JAMA. 2018;1(6):e183758.
33. United States. Public Health Service. Office of the Surgeon General, National Center for Chronic Disease Prevention, & Health Promotion (US). Office on Smoking. Preventing tobacco use among young people: a report of the surgeon general, vol. Vol. 10. US Department of Health and Human Services, Public Health Service, Centers for Disease Control and Prevention, National Center for Chronic Disease Prevention and Health Promotion, Office on Smoking and Health; 1994.
34. US Department of Health and Human Services. The health consequences of smoking—50 years of progress: a report of the surgeon general. Rockville: U.S. Department of Health and Human Services; 2014.
35. Substance Abuse and Mental Health Services Administration, National Mental Health Services Survey (N-MHSS): 2017. Data on Mental Health Treatment Facilities. BHSIS Series S-98, HHS Publication No. (SMA) 17-5049. Rockville, MD: Substance Abuse and Mental Health Services Administration, 2018.
36. Maharajh HD, Abdool PS. Cultural aspects of suicide. TheScientificWorldJOURNAL. 2005;1:5.
37. Schmitt T. Stuff White People Like... To Keep: re-appropriation and whiteness in America. Augsburg Honors Rev. 2012;5(1):4.
38. United Nations Office on Drugs and Crime. World drug report 2020. 25 June 2020. https://wdr.unodc.org/wdr2020/index.html.
39. Hser YI, Grella CE, Hubbard RL, et al. An evaluation of drug treatments for adolescents in 4 US cities. Arch Gen Psychiatry. 2001;58(7):689–695.

40. Dingle GA, Cruwys T, Frings D. Social identities as pathways into and out of addiction. Front Psychol. 2015.
41. Hussong AM, Ennett ST, McNeish D, Rothenberg WA, Cole V, Gottfredson NC, Faris RW. Teen social networks and depressive symptoms-substance use associations: developmental and demographic variation. J Stud Alcohol Drugs. 2018;79(5):770–80.
42. Copeland M, Fisher JC, Moody J, Feinberg ME. Different kinds of lonely: dimensions of isolation and substance use in adolescence. J Youth Adolesc. 2018;47(8):1755–70.
43. Fosnocht AQ, Lucerne KE, Ellis AS, Olimpo NA, Briand LA. Adolescent social isolation increases cocaine seeking in male and female mice. Behav Brain Res. 2019;359:589–96.
44. Rapier R, McKernan S, Stauffer CS. An inverse relationship between perceived social support and substance use frequency in socially stigmatized populations. Addict Behav Rep. 2019;10:100188.
45. Wilkens C, Foote J. "Bad Parents,""Codependents," and other stigmatizing myths about substance use disorder in the family. In: The stigma of addiction. Springer; 2019. p. 33–53.
46. U.S. Department of Health and Human Services Final report: opioid use, misuse, and overdose in women. 2017.
47. American College of Obstetricians and Gynecologists (ACOG), American Society of Addiction Medicine (ASAM). Committee opinion: opioid abuse, dependence, and addiction in pregnancy, vol. 524. Committee on Health Care for Underserved Women and the American Society of Addiction Medicine; 2012. p. 1–7.
48. Substance Abuse and Mental Health Services Administration. SAMHSA's Concept of Trauma and guidance for a traumainformed approach. 2014. https://store.samhsa.gov/system/files/sma14-4884.pdf
49. Embree JA. Prevalence of suicide attempts in a deaf population with co-occurring substance use disorder. JADARA. 2019;45(2):1–15.
50. Anderson ML, Chang BH, Kini N. Alcohol and drug use among deaf and hard-of-hearing individuals: a secondary analysis of NHANES 2013–2014. Subst Abus. 2018;39(3):390–7.
51. Moore D, Li L. Prevalence and risk factors of illicit drug use by people with disabilities. Am J Addict. 1998;7(2):93–102.
52. Peters RH, Bartoi MG, Sherman PB. Screening and assessment of co-occurring disorders in the justice system. Delmar: GAINS Center; 1997.
53. Gates ML, Turney A, Ferguson E, Walker V, Staples-Horne M. Associations among substance use, mental health disorders, and self-harm in a prison population: examining group risk for suicide attempt. Int J Environ Res Public Health. 2017;14(3):317.
54. Peters RH, Wexler HK, Lurigio AJ. Co-occurring substance use and mental disorders in the criminal justice system: a new frontier of clinical practice and research. Psychiatr Rehabil J. 2015;38:1–6.
55. Maguen S, Metzler TJ, Bosch J, Marmar CR, Knight SJ, Neylan TC. Killing in combat may be independently associated with suicidal ideation. Depress Anxiety. 2012;29(11):918–23.
56. Institute of Medicine. Substance use disorders in the US armed forces. Washington, DC: National Academies Press; 2013. https://www.nap.edu/catalog/13441/substance-use-disorders-in-the-us-armed-forces.
57. Dickerson DL, Spear S, Marinelli-Casey P, Rawson R, Li L, Hser YI. American Indians/Alaska natives and substance abuse treatment outcomes: positive signs and continuing challenges. J Addict Dis. 2010;30(1):63–74.
58. Kranzler HR, Soyka M. Diagnosis and pharmacotherapy of alcohol use disorder: a review. JAMA. 2018;320(8):815–24.
59. Cain C. Personal stories: identity acquisition and self-understanding in alcoholics anonymous. Ethos. 1991;19(2):210–53.
60. Kaskutas LA. Alcoholics anonymous effectiveness: faith meets science. J Addict Dis. 2009;28(2):145–57.

61. Ferri M, Amato L, Davoli M. Alcoholics anonymous and other 12-step programmes for alcohol dependence. Cochrane Database Syst Rev. 2006;(3):CD005032.
62. Litten RZ, Wilford BB, Falk DE, Ryan ML, Fertig JB. Potential medications for the treatment of alcohol use disorder: an evaluation of clinical efficacy and safety. Subst Abus. 2016;37(2):286–98.
63. Reif S, George P, Braude L, Dougherty RH, Daniels AS, Ghose SS, Delphin-Rittmon ME. Residential treatment for individuals with substance use disorders: assessing the evidence. Psychiatr Serv. 2014;65(3):301–12.
64. Suter M, Strik W, Moggi F. Depressive symptoms as a predictor of alcohol relapse after residential treatment programs for alcohol use disorder. J Subst Abus Treat. 2011;41(3):225–32.
65. Mason BJ. Emerging pharmacotherapies for alcohol use disorder. Neuropharmacology. 2017;122:244–53.
66. Burchi E, Makris N, Lee MR, Pallanti S, Hollander E. Compulsivity in alcohol use disorder and obsessive compulsive disorder: implications for neuromodulation. Front Behav Neurosci. 2019;13:70.
67. Philip NS, Sorensen DO, McCalley DM, Hanlon CA. Non-invasive brain stimulation for alcohol use disorders: state of the art and future directions. Neurotherapeutics. 2020;17(1):116–26.
68. Fullerton CA, Kim M, Thomas CP, Lyman DR, Montejano LB, Dougherty RH, et al. Medication-assisted treatment with methadone: assessing the evidence. Psychiatr Serv. 2014;65(2):146–57.
69. Maglione MA, Raaen L, Chen C, Azhar G, Shahidinia N, Shen M, et al. Effects of medication assisted treatment (MAT) for opioid use disorder on functional outcomes: a systematic review. J Subst Abus Treat. 2018;89:28–51.
70. Oesterle TS, Thusius NJ, Rummans TA, Gold MS. Medication-assisted treatment for opioid-use disorder. Mayo Clin Proc. 2019;94:2072–86. https://doi.org/10.1016/j.mayocp.2019.03.029.
71. Jones JL, Mateus CF, Malcolm RJ, Brady KT, Back SE. Efficacy of ketamine in the treatment of substance use disorders: a systematic review. Front Psych. 2018;9:277.
72. Ezquerra-Romano II, Lawn W, Krupitsky E, Morgan CJ. Ketamine for the treatment of addiction: evidence and potential mechanisms. Neuropharmacology. 2018;142:72–82.
73. Young JR, Smani SA, Mischel NA, Kritzer MD, Appelbaum LG, Patkar AA. Non-invasive brain stimulation modalities for the treatment and prevention of opioid use disorder: a systematic review of the literature. J Addict Dis. 2020;38(2):186–99.
74. Sawynok J. The therapeutic use of heroin: a review of the pharmacological literature. Can J Physiol Pharmacol. 1986;64(1):1–6. https://doi.org/10.1139/y86-001. PMID: 2420426
75. Fischer B, Oviedo-Joekes E, Blanken P, Haasen C, Rehm J, Schechter MT, Strang J, van den Brink W. Heroin-assisted treatment (HAT) a decade later: a brief update on science and politics. J Urban Health. 2007;84(4):552–62.
76. Bernhardt N, Petzold J, Groß C, Scheck A, Pooseh S, Mayer-Pelinski R, Zimmermann US, Smolka MN, Pilhatsch M. Neurocognitive dysfunctions and their therapeutic modulation in patients with methamphetamine dependence: a pilot study. Front Psych. 2020;11:581.
77. Zweben JE, Cohen JB, Christian D, Galloway GP, Salinardi M, Parent D, Iguchi M. Psychiatric symptoms in methamphetamine users. Am J Addict. 2004;13(2):181–90.
78. Longo M, Wickes W, Smout M, Harrison S, Cahill S, White JM. Randomized controlled trial of dexamphetamine maintenance for the treatment of methamphetamine dependence. Addiction. 2010;105(1):146–54.
79. Clark M, Featherstone R. Management of acute withdrawal and detoxification for adults who misuse methamphetamine: a review of the clinical evidence and guidelines. Ottawa: Canadian Agency for Drugs and Technologies in Health; 2019.
80. Morley KC, Cornish JL, Faingold A, Wood K, Haber PS. Pharmacotherapeutic agents in the treatment of methamphetamine dependence. Expert Opin Investig Drugs. 2017;26(5):563–78.

81. Colfax GN, Santos GM, Das M, Santos DM, Matheson T, Gasper J, Shoptaw S, Vittinghoff E. Mirtazapine to reduce methamphetamine use: a randomized controlled trial. Arch Gen Psychiatry. 2011;68:1168–75.
82. Chaiton M, Diemert L, Cohen JE, Bondy SJ, Selby P, Philipneri A, Schwartz R. Estimating the number of quit attempts it takes to quit smoking successfully in a longitudinal cohort of smokers. BMJ Open. 2016;6(6):e011045.
83. Antonelli M, Fattore L, Sestito L, Di Giuda D, Diana M, Addolorato G. Transcranial magnetic stimulation: a review about its efficacy in the treatment of alcohol, tobacco and cocaine addiction. Addict Behav. 2021;114:106760.

Telepsychiatry to Rural Populations

6

Gregory Evangelatos, G. Andrew Valasquez, Christine Le, Juan Sosa, Jessica Thackaberry, and Donald M. Hilty

Vignette 1

Theme: The interface of depression, psychosis, culture, and telemental health (TMH) in a rural emergency department.

HPI: A.Q. is a 29-year-old English-speaking Hispanic American male who presented in the emergency department of a rural community (population 4000) hospital due to depression, hopelessness, and auditory hallucinations (AH) telling him to kill himself. After being admitted to the medical floor of the hospital – as there was also unstable diabetic control – the patient denied experiencing auditory hallucinations or thoughts of self-harm. His provider was relieved but wary as his new "good" mood did not correspond with his restricted and flat affect.

G. Evangelatos · C. Le · J. Sosa
Department of Psychiatry, Kaweah Delta Medical Center, Visalia, CA, USA
e-mail: gevang@kdhcd.org; jsosa@kdhcd.org

G. A. Valasquez
Department of Psychiatry, Kaweah Delta Medical Center, Visalia, CA, USA

American University of Antigua College of Medicine, Osbourn, Antigua and Barbuda

J. Thackaberry
Department of Psychiatry, University of California San Diego, San Diego, CA, USA
e-mail: jthackaberry@health.ucsd.edu

D. M. Hilty (✉)
Mental Health Service, Northern California Veterans Administration Health Care System, Mather, CA, USA

Department of Psychiatry & Behavioral Sciences, University of California Davis, Sacramento, CA, USA
e-mail: donald.hilty@va.gov

S. H. Koh et al. (eds.), *Diversity in Action*,
https://doi.org/10.1007/978-3-030-85401-0_6

TMH consultation: The telepsychiatrist started with routine questions but shifted to social questions after noting supposed disinterest and some resistance to discuss the symptoms. Using the Diagnostic and Statistical Manual (DSM) Cultural Formulation Interview format [1], questions emphasized the patient's culture, heritage, interpretation of his experiences, and expectations for help. He was born in Mexico, and the family immigrated to the USA at age 3, so he grew up in California and became the first of his family to go to college. He had past periods of depression – that term was acceptable – but "We never much talked about it." He was encouraged to "move on," go to church, and keep busy.

MSE: The patient was withdrawn and anxious at first but warmed up over the first 15 minutes of the interview. His speech was notable for initial terse comments and then used more demonstrative descriptions; English appeared to be very well spoken. Mood was "depressed" and affect quite restricted. Thoughts were linear, and the content included worry, hopelessness, and disbelief about the AH. His insight/judgment was fair, despite his initial hesitance to talk or share. He reported suicidal ideation due to the intensity of AH, but not a preference to die, no homicidal ideation. Cognition was intact.

PE/Lab/Imaging: Stabilizing glucose; no head imaging was completed.

A/P: A.Q. met the criteria for a recurrent major depression, severe with psychotic features. He was agreeable to continue antidepressant sertraline 50 mg AM and to start an antipsychotic olanzapine 5 mg HS, as he also had some insomnia. The telepsychiatrist had the PCP attend the last 5 minutes to discuss the plan, the medications, and maintaining privacy. It was suggested that depression (only) be used without going into AH with family. A.Q. was discharged home in 2 days with family. When inquired about his opinion over conducting interviews over telehealth, he stated he hardly noticed a difference and also remarked "It's pretty cool, I guess…we could really talk." The patient also stated he had a preference to retaining his telehealth provider instead of seeing a new provider in-person, if given the option.

Summary

1. TMH increased access to care with a specialist trained in cultural issues.
2. TMH may offer a wide range of services and may require augmentation with interpreters and/or cultural consultants, depending on the case.

Introduction

Healthcare systems in the USA and abroad struggle to provide timely, evidence-based care, particularly for culturally diverse patients in rural areas with behavioral disorders. Telepsychiatry, telebehavioral health, and telemental health are terms used interchangeably throughout the literature and defined as mental health care delivered at a distance. For the purposes of this chapter, the term "TMH" will be used to describe any provision of mental health care via telemedicine. The challenge to deliver culturally appropriate rural behavioral health (BH) care has attracted national and global attention [2, 3]. The Hispanic population in rural and frontier America is the most rapidly growing segment of the population in nonmetropolitan counties since 2005, according to US Department of Agriculture [4]. Rural depressed patients have three times more hospitalizations, a 70% likelihood of an inadequate trial of antidepressant per national guidelines, and higher reported rates of suicide attempts [5, 6]. Rural primary care providers (PCPs) are often the target of interventions, since they typically report having inadequate skills to manage behavioral health issues [7, 8]. Administrators, staff, and other team members must also face and overcome obstacles to care, cultural elements, and reimbursement for sustainability.

Culture itself and its components can include race, ethnicity, spirituality, religion, sexual preference, gender identity, geography (i.e., urban, rural, global), special populations (e.g., incarcerated), age, language, socioeconomics, education, and other parameters [9]. Culture has a central role in facilitating patient-centered care (PCC) [10]. Care is defined as patient-centered when the following occur: (1) patients are asked to explain their illness/suffering, (2) why they think it is occurring, (3) how their social group understands/explains it, (4) standard/alternative approaches to care, and (5) how their culture affects the doctor-patient relationship [10]. Lack of available interpreter services may contribute to poor healthcare access and utilization for limited English proficiency (LEP) patients, which further limits access to psychiatric services [11].

Academic health centers (AHCs), statewide/county networks, and interstate telemental health programs are often linked with rural primary care offices. A variety of clinical and educational models have been employed for implementation [12]. A developmental approach to rural TMH addresses stages of needs identification, infrastructure survey, partnership organization, structural configuration, and pilot implementation [13]. Systems of care and their leaders are moving fast now with traditional video/synchronous telepsychiatry (STP), novel (e.g., asynchronous, social media), and emerging (e.g., web- and mobile–/wireless-based) models.

There are many challenges to providing culturally competent care by TMH – it requires a starting point of "good" clinical skills and additional skills related to culture and technology in providers, clinical staff, and technology/administrative support. Cultural and language differences were initially believed to be more challenging for TMH compared to in-person consultations [14], but TMH has been shown to be effective in many culturally diverse populations including Hispanics/Latinos, Asians, Native American, Eastern Europeans, and special populations (e.g., individuals using sign language) [15]. Systems face funding, logistics, sustainability, training, and administrative adjustments prior to adoption. In Vignette 1, A.Q was resistant to express his suffering, may have needed a specialist, and divulged much more after cultural issues were addressed through TMH. This is a powerful demonstration of mental health, cultural, psychiatric consultation to primary care, and TMH – particularly memorable to healthcare providers in very remote and isolated communities.

This chapter will help inform the reader(s)' approach to (1) understand the need for culturally competent BH service in rural communities and provide an outline to move forward; (2) develop reasonable, meaningful outcomes for clinical, cultural, and training initiatives and select appropriate model(s) of care; and (3) identify, manage, and evaluate obstacles related to culture/stigma, funding, logistics, and technology.

What Is Culturally Competent Care and How Can TMH Help in Rural Settings?

Approaches to Provide Culturally Competent Care

The Outline for Cultural Formulation, Cultural Formulation Interview, and the CFI Supplementary Modules in the DSM-5 [1] help clinicians learn how to ask about, and more broadly, gain perspective on the cultural issues. The bio-psycho-socio-cultural (BPSC) model has been suggested as an expansion of the biopsychosocial model by Engel [16] to specifically define and delineate culture and diversity components implied in the social component [17–19]. The BPSC model includes, but is not limited to symptoms, presentation, meaning, causation, family factors, coping styles, treatment seeking, mistrust, stigma, immigration, and overall health status; additionally, the culture of the clinician affects the interaction, particularly the inability to speak the patient's language [20, 21]. Table 6.1 outlines historical shifts in care, training, and policy moving forward with major milestones from 1969 to 2016.

The social and cultural elements in the BPSC are separated out because the boundaries of normality and pathology vary across cultures for specific types of behavior. Thresholds of tolerance for specific symptoms vary across cultures, social settings, and families. A judgment of a behavior is affected by internalized norms, and mistaken interpretations can contribute to vulnerability, suffering, and missed opportunities for care. Cultural or familial beliefs and traditions can affect course and outcome of illness including instillation of maladaptive or adaptive coping strategies, access to care, and engagement of alternative care practices. Furthermore, differences between the clinician and patient have implications for accuracy, mutual understanding, and acceptance of illness, treatment planning, and prognosis.

Stories are well-described across cultures in their role in healing, conveying abstract meaning (e.g., myths), moving people to change (e.g., politics), and applying knowledge and teaching skills [36]. Stories are sometimes the only way to understand a patient's perspective and path. They constitute a less hierarchical approach by facilitating a patient to tell their story in their own words. Since the ability to communicate with patients is essential in clinical care, it is a common practice to use interpreters on-site for LEP patients; however, when resources are limited, sometimes family members or untrained interpreters are used. There are significant and often detrimental consequences to this, including miscommunicating medical complaints [37] or de-emphasizing critical information [38].

Table 6.1 Milestones in the cross-cultural behavioral health, psychiatry, cultural competence and training

Year	Event	Comment
1969	Transcultural or cross-cultural psychiatry recognized by the American Psychiatric Association (APA)	[22]
1964	Title VI Civil Rights Act of 1964 (Civil Rights Law)	Forbade discrimination on the basis of sex and race in hiring, promoting, and firing [23]
1989	Cultural competence defined	[24]
1990	The Americans with Disabilities (ADA) Act	Prohibits private employers, state and local governments, employment agencies, and labor unions from discriminating [25]
1993	State of California began a process that became known as the California Cultural Competence Plan	Counties asked to assess language and provide services to 3000 non-English-speaking or 5% or the Medi-Cal population
1994	APA Outline for Cultural Formulation in Diagnostic and Statistical Manual (DSM)-IV	
1997	New York State Cultural and Linguistic Competency Standards	[26]
1992	American Counseling Association	Cross-Cultural Competencies and Objectives [27]
2000	SAMHSA Cultural Competence Standards in Managed Care Mental Health Services	Four underserved/underrepresented Racial/ethnic groups [28]
2000	United States Center for Mental Health Services	Cultural competence standards in managed care mental health services [28]
2000	Association of American Medical Colleges (AAMC)	Cultural Competence in Medical Education [29]
2001	Surgeon General's Report on Mental Health, Culture, Race, and Ethnicity	[30]
2001	The National Association of Social Workers	Standards for Cultural Competence [31]
2003	The American Psychological Association Guidelines	Multicultural education, training, research, practice, and organizational change [32]
2006	Agency for Health Care Research and Quality (AHQR) published the National Health Care Disparities Report	Disparities based on race, ethnicity, and socioeconomic status continue to exist and have a devastating personal and societal cost [33]
2007	Accreditation Council of Graduate Medical Education (ACGME) Residency Review Committee	Cultural competence requirements into its Guidelines for Psychiatry Residencies [34]
2013	DSM-5 Cultural Formulation Interview and Supplementary Modules	16-item interview and accompanying questions [1]
2014	Health Services Research Administration (HRSA)	Culture, Language, and Health Literacy Resources
2014	Liaison Committee of Medical Education (LCME)	Specific competencies for 2015 in culture and diversity for medical education [35]
2016	Biopsychosociocultural Model, Psychology, and Cognitive Sciences	Concept paper [10]

Vignette 2

Theme: The impact of culture on immigrant families and the need for "wrap-around" case management in a community.

HPI: E.S. was a 28-year-old patient with diagnosis of schizophrenia, living in a rural community of 40,000, who was taken to the emergency department by local police department for bizarre behavior. The patient had been walking on the street. Upon evaluation the patient was disorganized and complained of command-type auditory hallucinations. The patient had multiple previous psychiatric hospitalizations and had failed trials of antipsychotic monotherapy. After adding adjunctive treatment to his antipsychotic, his psychotic behavior improved.

MSE: The patient was initially withdrawn, as if absent, and at times did not move. Over time, he became more active: speech was fluent, mood was "okay," and a range of affect appeared. These thoughts became less disorganized and, eventually, he discussed his hobbies of reading books, taking walks, and playing with games on the cell phone.

A/P: For a patient with schizophrenia who struggled with the negative symptoms for many years, the ability to converse about his hobbies was a marker of improvement. Use of a depot antipsychotic paliperidone monthly enhanced the likelihood of medication adherence. The patient was discharged to a step-down facility. However, shortly thereafter he wandered away, and it was unclear for a period where he was. He did not have his own cell phone. He did not go to a follow-up appointment at the clinic. Unfortunately, E.S. was hit by a vehicle and died from the injuries sustained.

The emotional adjustments for his family were endless, including a void left by the loss of E.S. His immigrant mother from Mexico only spoke Spanish and thus a cultural and language barrier needed to be addressed as to deliver the proper message. In this situation, a certified Spanish-speaking interpreter was used for a meeting with the mother and the rural MH treating team. The mother became tearful when the condolences were delivered, as one would expect with the loss of a child. Her subtle, emotional responses would have been difficult to elicit, engage, and comprehend had an interpreter not been used. Even though some staff shared the same culture, there were language nuances for the family, and though E.S.' mother had lost a piece of her happiness, she was thankful the condolence was delivered in a way she could digest.

Summary

1. Review of the case did not indicate suicidal intentions, but implementing wrap-around services in the community in addition to his residence may have been indicated.
2. Another suggestion was equipping him with a cell phone, which would allow him to check in (e.g., send a text), be reached, and/or even allow family to track

his movements. Its linkage with an enjoyed hobby was a good "hook." More broadly, if privacy and security could be arranged, brief teleconferences with providers may have helped support him better.

One hurdle regarding BH disorders in minority populations is that they are often difficult to recognize and diagnose due to complex beliefs, differences in help-seeking, and stigmatization. All of these factors affect access and/or treatment initiation/completion, and if there is a lack of access to culturally sensitive treatment, these matters are amplified. Therefore, some cultural outcome targets would be to reduce the level of stigma through increased awareness at the community level and to increase access to culturally sensitive treatment options through enhanced training to providers and patient engagement about preferences with treatment modalities including telepsychiatry (TP).

A recent study of illness beliefs among Chinese Americans showed that many patients with depression were reluctant to refer to their illness as psychiatric in nature due to fear of being stigmatized [39]. Therefore, one way to address stigma of BH disorders would be to increase awareness within specific minority communities through public awareness campaigns in the appropriate language, health fairs/outreach, and engagement with local PCPs. Another cultural outcome target could be to increase access to culturally sensitive psychiatric treatment in common non-English languages. In the primary care setting, this requires a broad administrative approach to "format" the clinic (e.g., entry, forms, and work flow), train PCPs and staff, and manage other complexities.

Setting Goals with Patients

Outcome targets for culturally diverse patients with BH disorders via TP are similar to those of in-person care, involving measures with qualitative and quantitative dimensions. These should be founded on training, supervisory, and feedback practices that are evidence-based. Shared decision-making equalizes the information and power symmetry between doctors and patients, allowing both parties to share information and develop consensus in a decision [40]. It is important to provide adequate education and translation for patients with limited English proficiency (LEP) by those with formal training to ensure this information is conveyed and understood by both parties (clinician and patient/family).

There are innumerable target outcomes one would seek in patient care, but two important clinical outcomes are (1) increased rate of engagement in and adherence with treatment and (2) reduced utilization of high-intensity services (e.g., emergency departments, inpatient hospitalizations). Adherence – rather than compliance – embodies this philosophy and is an important measurement of a patient's commitment to treatment (i.e., weekly TP sessions, medication). PCC facilitates engagement and places the patient as the driver of care, rather than a passenger of care. Indeed, in the broadest sense, many treatment "failures" can be traced back to inadequate therapeutic alliance and shared decision-making for the participants.

One example of such a "treatment failure" is medication and appointment non-adherence, which is seen very often in both primary care and psychiatric settings. It is often attributed to factors such as medication side effects and cost/access, but misunderstandings between a clinician and the patient can result in nonadherence, and furthermore, treatment plans with rare appointments often result in appointment no-shows. A randomized study highlighted the positive effects of tele-monitoring of medication adherence in patients with schizophrenia, resulting in fewer emergency room visits and fewer reported day-to-day symptoms. Therefore, increasing access to culturally competent telemedicine technologies and TP services may be an effective way to mitigate adherence issues and reduce the rate of hospitalizations.

TMH and Its Use in Cultural Populations

Evaluation of TP/TMH has gone through three phases [15]. First, the review of TMH's effectiveness considered it effective in terms of increasing access to care, being well accepted, and having good educational outcomes. Second, a validity and reliability of clinical care compared to in-person services [41, 42], including building of rapport based on nonverbal cues. Comparison (or "as good as") studies and TP outcomes are not inferior to in-person care [15, 43]. Third, frameworks are needed to organize the administrative approach to evaluation and costs/economic assessments [15, 41, 42, 44].

Some TMH models of care have specifically been studied regarding culturally diverse populations, including direct care and consultation-liaison services; there were initial concerns as to whether a cultural difference between a patient and provider might be an obstacle [14]. Initial studies of culturally competent TP consultation to rural primary care were first done about 20 years ago [45], and others furthered the effort [46]. Now, many descriptive studies have reported positive outcomes [47], and TP's effectiveness appears to be accepted across cultures [15], including Hispanics/Latinos, Asians, Native American, Eastern Europeans, and other populations (e.g., individuals using sign language). Nonetheless, the evidence base could be improved with randomized studies and measurable outcomes.

How Do We Provide Culturally Competent Care Via TMH?

Assess Needs for Cultural and Language "Fit" Between Patients and Providers

Studies have assessed the capacity of TMH to serve culturally diverse populations with regard to the cultural and language interface between patients and providers [3], both for in-person primary care [48] and specific to telemedicine services [47]. In one study, PCPs and staff rated the importance of valuing cultural differences and being able to speak (or use an interpreter) in the patient's primary language at 5.4 on a Likert scale from 1 to 7 (not important to very important) [3]. Ratings of the importance of quality of care were at 4.9, access to care better with TP at 4.5 and availability of competent trained interpreter at 4.4 [3]. Subanalysis of PCP versus staff ratings did not differ. Those surveyed did not think providers and patients must share the same ethnicity, culture, or language, but they thought more interpreters were needed. This work is more specific but is consistent with that of others in primary care [48] and specific to telemedicine services [47].

Attend to Language and Culture over Distance

Many rural sites face challenges in meeting the specific needs of Hispanics and Asians using TMH [47, 49–51]. Specific challenges include difficulty understanding and using technology and working with providers who are not fluent in the patient's native language or with the patient's culture. These cultural differences can vary and include generally being averse to pharmacotherapy and/or avoidant of psychiatric services altogether.

Studies with Native Americans [14, 52], Eastern Europeans [53], and other populations (e.g., individuals using sign language) [54] show that patients prefer to use their primary language for expression.

Untrained interpreters' errors [37, 38] have led to a call for credentialing of interpreters [55]. For example, nurses fare better with concrete medical complaints of patients but struggle in capturing the narrative or cultural metaphors [12, 56], which is potentially very significant in psychiatric care [3]. Using interpreters at an academic center to join or "three-party" conference by phone may be more costly and is not the same as in-person service but enhances services. Federally qualified health centers (FQHCs) and rural health clinics (RHCs) often have ample interpreters, but TP to these sites has limited reimbursement as the consultant is seen as "outside" the clinics' walls.

Training Approaches to Telehealth and Culture

Competency-based medical education (CBME) focuses on skill development more than knowledge acquisition [57, 58]. In medicine, the most common frameworks used for organizing competencies are from the CanMEDS [59], the American Association of Medical Colleges [60], and the Accreditation Council of Graduate Medical Education [61]. The evidence-based CanMEDS competency framework describes the knowledge, skills, and abilities that specialist physicians need for better patient outcomes, based on the seven roles that all physicians play: (1) medical expert, (2) communicator, (3) collaborator, (4) manager, (5) health advocate, (6) scholar, and (7) professional [59, 62]. Similarly, the AAMC for medical students' outcomes are evidence-based, including the domains of medical knowledge, patient care skills and attitudes, interpersonal and communication skills and attitudes, ethical judgment, professionalism, lifelong learning and experience-based improvement, and community and systems-based practice [60].

Table 6.2 outlines competencies for clinicians/faculty, trainees, and other providers available for TP [63], social media [64], mobile health/psych apps [65], and telemedicine competencies across specialties [19]. A few of the TP competencies are based on in-person, collaborative, and integrated care services [63, 66, 67]. Three areas of skill development for residents using TP are technical, administrative, and collaborative care skills [68]. Regarding teaching and learning methods, relational, communication, interprofessional, medicolegal, community psychiatry, cultural, and health system skills are suggested [69].

Training for technology and cultural competency starts at the level of residency training, and a key question is how to do this. Residents already have a large amount of required competencies and educational demands, but training in telehealth is crucial to prepare residents for an evolving technological landscape. Residents also are expected to have basic competencies in cultural psychiatry, and combining both cultural and telehealth competencies could be an effective strategy, with many programs requiring neither formal training in cultural nor TP. Utilizing the Cultural Formulation Interview, mentioned previously, basic competencies in cultural mental health can be established. Training curricula need to set goals and align teaching and evaluation toward clinical skills, and those of TP can be included in this outcome measure.

Several large healthcare systems serving rural populations have adopted culturally competent telehealth care models. For example, the University of Hawaii child and adolescent psychiatry fellows attended trainings to provide more culturally effective care to rural communities utilizing telehealth [70]. Another example is the Alaskan healthcare system, which piloted a small study creating not only telehealth competencies for teleconference interviews but also cultural competencies with training from content experts in the regional culture, including Alaska Native elders and university professors. Rural residency programs have incorporated utilizing culturally based competencies into their TP education [71].

A review of the TMH evidenced-based literature across psychiatry/medicine, psychology, social work, counseling, marriage/family, behavioral analysis, and other behavioral sciences found no common TMH competencies across disciplines [72]. There are several challenges to achieving consensus across disciplines due to varying scopes of practice, training differences, distinct case conceptualizations, and diverse faculty development priorities. Disciplines and organizations involved with TMH may consider certification/accreditation to ensure quality care. Interdisciplinary competencies have been proposed, including those for psychology, social work, marriage/family therapy, psychiatry, and telemedicine in general. These include competencies in patient care, communication, systems-based practice, professionalism, knowledge, and technology [73].

Models of Care: Enhancing Access, Providing Flexibility, and Leveraging Resources

Models of TP care may be organized into low, moderate, or high intensity levels of care based on intensity of care intervention, technology complexity, specialist time, patient acuity, and use of other resources as depicted by Table 6.3 [74]. Services,

Table 6.2 A framework for telebehavioral health competencies for clinicians and trainees based on telepsychiatric competencies

Area/topic	Novice/advanced beginner (e.g., advanced medical student, early resident, other trainees)	Competent/proficient (e.g., advanced resident/graduating resident/ faculty/attending/interdisciplinary team member)	Expert (e.g., advanced faculty/attending/ interdisciplinary team member)
Patient care			
History-taking	Standard history	Informed consent for telehealth (check state to see if form needed; option not to do telehealth is discussed) Contextualized history (e.g., aware of geographic and cultural specificity)	Informed consent problems (e.g., lacks capacity, just like in-person care) In-depth, well-paced, and concise interview
Engagement and interpersonal skills	Establishes therapeutic alliance Builds trust and rapport	Identify and manage problem(s) with alliance/trust/rapport Adjust interview to technological and patient needs/preferences	Determine best appropriate assessment adjustments based on the setting (in-person vs. TP)
Assessment and physical examination	Stratify risk and protective factors based on epidemiology (e.g., suicide, homicide risk) Administer tools (e.g., MMSE) from a distance[CM] Ascertain need for literal PE	Assess risks for suicide/harm to others and develop follow-up plan Ensure identification of significant exam findings (e.g., movement disorders; intoxication/withdrawal) Examine and administer tools with adjustments (e.g., use staff to complete or do part of PE)	Synthesize information (including risk vs. protective factors and collateral information) Administer tools contextually (e.g., substitute score item for non-reproducible task at distance) Teach staff/others how to do parts of PE and troubleshoot PE problems far end

(continued)

Table 6.2 (continued)

Area/topic	Novice/advanced beginner (e.g., advanced medical student, early resident, other trainees)	Competent/proficient (e.g., advanced resident/graduating resident/faculty/attending/interdisciplinary team member)	Expert (e.g., advanced faculty/attending/interdisciplinary team member)
Management and treatment planning	Biopsychosociocultural (BPSC) outline Participates in providing summary and recommendations Medical decision-making on safety, need for treatment and other interventions Follow-up with PCP or TP by note Follow-up with necessary others	BPSC outline with depth and identification of safety and risk factors Able to provide summary and recommendations to patient and interprofessional team Awareness of treatment continuum (levels of care) Follows in-person medication recommendations (i.e., reviews options, side effects, and alternatives if applicable, provides specific instructions for PCP to initiate, titrate, and augment) Formulate plan for calls, Rx and such Follow-up with PCP by TP or phone	BPSC outline with prioritization, with emergency plan execution, and obstacles anticipated Tailors recommendations to available resources, cultural specificity, and patient preference Engages patient, referring doctor or other providers succinctly Select "best" mode: e-mail, telephone, or other (and if it changes the process); terminate video if too problematic For medication recommendations: considers safety and adherence factors; plan for follow-up and monitoring; aware of legal and jurisdictional issues related to prescribing
Documentation	Draft TP note hard copy or rudimentary EHR	Initial/revised draft primary or other specialty care modification for consultation Complex EHR (e.g., Cerner, Epic)	Provide sufficient detail to allow implementation of plan over time and within local context/resources Phone, e-mail, and asynchronous notes
Billing	Learn why billing is important and how it is configured	Identify diagnoses for billing	Final time spent, diagnosis and codes Consideration of health advocacy issues related to billing; access to care
Privacy and confidentiality (medicolegal issues[CM])	Learn in-person basic regulations	Be aware of regulations and learn translation of principles to video and adjunct regulations, if applicable Be aware that technologies are encrypted differently	Practice within in-person and telemedicine standards Be aware of pitfalls with technologies (e.g., cellular phones are not private; Gmail is not HIPAA compliant)

Communication[MS]			
Cultural, diversity, and social determinants of health	Consider diversity of patients, families, and communities: language fluency, customs Consider one's culture, values, behaviors, and preferences[CM] Learn how social determinants affect in-person care[CM]	Adjust in consideration of patient culture and preference Language fluency: double check/confirm Ways to elicit cultural meaning of illness/wellness Be aware that social determinants may affect interest in, using of, and experience with telemedicine	Follow cultural formulation frameworks Ask if culture affects using TP (general exploration) or explanation of illness Consider patient-doctor relationship in context of culture, values, behaviors, and preferences Adjust interview, assessment, and treatment per social determinants; consider in-person care if critical need
Language/interpreter ability	Use the interpreter	Time management and preferred types (e.g., professional > family)	Verbal and nonverbal dimensions
Communication	Clear communication with patient, family, and healthcare professionals	Clarify and amplify communication	Troubleshoot communication difficulties
Systems-based practice [MS]			
Outreach to community	Participates and engages	Visit community in-person before TP Identifies relevant resources and needs within community	Establishes and maintains relationships with communities Thoughtful integration of in-person and TP care, if applicable
Interprofessional education (IPE) and team work	Participates and experiences different roles; works effectively	Work with interprofessional team and familiar with IPE Begins to teach within IPE	Supports interdisciplinary team care (e.g., care coordinators – MA-RN-PA/PCP/NP – therapists)
Collaborative primary care	Considers consult from perspective of referring provider's perspectives/needs	Understands the referring provider's needs and adapts consult and note appropriately	Engages providers with unclear needs Uses individual consult as an opportunity for building ongoing relationship Integrates indirect care (e.g., case or chart review) into practice

(continued)

Table 6.2 (continued)

Area/topic	Novice/advanced beginner (e.g., advanced medical student, early resident, other trainees)	Competent/proficient (e.g., advanced resident/graduating resident/ faculty/attending/interdisciplinary team member)	Expert (e.g., advanced faculty/attending/ interdisciplinary team member)
Rural health	Learns about rural access, epidemiology, cost, and other	Learns rural health basics	Practices and role models
Special populations	Learns differences (e.g., veterans, child/adolescent/parent/family, geriatric)	Recognizes differences and adapts assessment and management approaches accordingly	Practices and role models
Safety	Learns systematic assessment	Identifies problems and stratifies risk	Adjusts risk and its management to TP system practice
Care models	Learns what in-person, TP care, and consulting TP care are	Facility with traditional referral to psychiatry, consultation care, and TP Begins to learn collaborative care	Has facility with models of consultation, integrated, stepped and hybrid care; practices with one that fits context
Licensure regulations as applied to telemedicine care model (medicolegal issues[CM])	Learn in-person regulations and that there are differences between states	Be aware that in-person and telemedicine regulations may/not differ	Practice within telemedicine regulations state to state or within unique system (e.g., veterans affairs)
Professionalism [MS]			
Attitude	Learn and be open to technology	Interprofessional clinical practice and teaching/learning	Leadership in groups/teams
Integrity and ethical behavior	Demonstrates behavior consistent with integrity	Role models	Role models and gives feedback
Scope	Becomes aware of scope issues of in-person, TP care, and TP consultation	Practices within scope(s)	Provides feedback on scope and boundary issues; troubleshoots problems
Practice-based learning [MS]			
Administration	Learn basics of in-person care	Be aware that in-person and telemedicine care have differences	Practice with adjustments to telemedicine care
QI	Learns how to participate in QI	Applies QI information to cases and system	Analyzes QI options, selects, and evaluates
Teaching and learning	Participates and contributes	Organizes and furthers	Provides context and next steps
Knowledge			

Knowledge	Relevance History	Relevance History Evidence base	History Evidence base Clinical guidelines
Technology			
Adapt to technology	Identify differences between TP and in-person care Tries to project self 15% more (voice/animation) Realize some nonverbal limitations (e.g., offering a tissue, handshake)	Takes steps to engage and put patient at ease Expect and plan for differences Identify barriers à replacement behavior Adding in third part by phone	Uses humor, self-deprecatory remarks, or "top moments" to ease Analyze what actually happened and make adjustments for next time Additional ways to express empathy
Remote site design	Observe	Identify problems and possible solutions to try Modification: toys for a child to play with and furniture	Pre-planning: continuous, iterative improvement Modification: use professional staff for remote play therapy)
Technology operation^{CM}	Familiarity with microphone, camera and prn second camera Observe how multiple technologies (e.g., primary and secondary camera) are used simultaneously	Operate hardware, software, and accessories Basic troubleshooting (e.g., re-boot system; call for assistance) Operate use of multiple technologies	Optimize hardware, software, and accessories based on context (for enhancement and avoiding distraction) Manage all troubleshooting operations on near end and advice on far end prn Optimize use of multiple technologies

Adapted from: Hilty et al. [63]

Abbreviations:

1. CM = based on submission for CanMEDS TP competencies
2. MS = US Milestones; consistent with non-TP, regular competencies of the Accreditation Council of Graduate Medical Education (ACGME)
3. PE = physical examination
4. PCP = primary care provider
5. QI = quality improvement

models, and outcomes can be stratified by the designation of primary service provider (e.g., PCP) and secondary consultant (e.g., psychiatrist). Ultimately the objective is to match the needs of the patient and PCP to a specialist that can optimize flexibility and maximize value.

Low-intensity interventions include tele-education, formal case review, and doctor-to-doctor "curbside" consultations either in-person, by telephone, through e-mail, or through the electronic medical record [12]. Mid-intensity programs may offer consultations with continuing medical education to help PCPs with medication dosing and decision-making [12] or asynchronous telepsychiatry for English- and Spanish-speaking patients in primary care [75]. High-intensity care involves fully integrated programs and collaborative care and requires resources and extensive time, as evidenced by randomized controlled trials and extensive collaborative care work [12, 76, 77].

Prior to the onset of TP services, patients with BH disorders could go months to years before gaining access to a BH professional for various reasons, including geographic distances (rural community) or physical limitations. A 2014 study found that Latinx in rural areas are the fastest growing subpopulation but have the largest discrepancy in utilization and access to culturally competent healthcare services [78]. As TP services become more available and utilized, it can be expected that many disparities such as limited access to providers and transportation costs will be mitigated. The same study above compared two groups, one who received telepsychiatry neurocognitive testing and the other group who received in-person neurocognitive testing [78]. The conclusion of the study showed no significant difference between cognitive scores TP or in-person modalities, thus supporting the growing evidence that TP services in rural areas are applicable and feasible.

Asynchronous telepsychiatry is feasible, valid, reliable, and cost-effective for English and Spanish-speaking patients in primary care [75]. Similar asynchronous methods are used in other medical specialties including radiology, dermatology, ophthalmology, cardiology, and pathology. One example of an asynchronous TP model uses a basic questionnaire for screening by the provider of the patient, video capture of that interview, and uploaded patient history for a remote psychiatrist to review in a HIPAA-adherent manner [41, 42]. Following the consultation, the remote psychiatrist may develop a treatment plan for the PCP to implement a brief psychotherapy (e.g., problem-solving therapy) and/or to prescribe a psychotropic medication. In most instances, the PCP has the option of e-mail or phone follow-up consultations.

Refugees and Disaster Victims and TMH

Through the course of history, world events have driven the migration of mass populations to different areas of the world. Many of these people have had family members killed by war, or they themselves have witnessed atrocities against humanity or become victims of hate crimes. Due to trauma, refugees and disaster victims find themselves vulnerable and require culturally sensitive care [79]. Interestingly, TMH with the patient and provider using a common language – even if it is not the primary one for patient – was preferred over seeing a provider from their own culture due to ambiguity of the latter's political views. In addition, the use of TP rather than an in-person translator as some patients saw the TP one as less intrusive to the patient-physician interaction [53]. These findings are different from the majority of studies, which show that TP facilitates cultural "fit" in the patient-provider relationship.

What Are the Dos and Don'ts of Addressing Barriers, Problems and Sustainability Issues

Implementation of a TMH program requires a strong administrative program that should attend to process, procedures, and policy. Flexible basic or advanced approaches to culturally competent care, TMH, and program administration are suggested – importantly, all should include ongoing evaluation and outcome measurements. The fundamentals of evaluation are necessary for clinical managers, clinicians, and designated TMH experts because the approach and processes that guide "good" evaluation and outcome targets may require a "fundamental shift in philosophy—from seeing what happens with planned services – to advanced planning of outcome targets, and then subsequent design of the services" [19].

Successful implementation is enhanced when there is strong foundational support from all levels of the organization and an interdisciplinary team that shares responsibilities and overlapping roles. The administrative approach should consider change (e.g., "good" idea vs. formal hypothesis), amount of preparation/depth of work (e.g., adding a little something to pre-existing clinical programs vs. marked improvement of one), degree of proactivity (e.g., a user-friendly, partially proactive approach versus a systematic, proactive approach), and scope of investigation (i.e., limited but systematic cross-sectional evaluation versus a large, longitudinal, outcome one). A summary of administrative successes and failures may guide new and current programs (Table 6.4).

Successful implementation of telemedicine and TP is largely dependent on continued outcome targets and evaluation. Acceptance by providers and other team members are required for an effective system to deliver the product [80]. Research of the cost-benefit ratio suggests TMH at higher volumes (i.e., numbers of consultations) is less costly compared with face-to-face care [81]. Many current TP programs are grant-funded and depend on continued applications and support for sustainability, thus making widespread implementation across institutions difficult [80]. Therefore, from a logistical standpoint, programs have to balance start-up, demand, and supply costs.

Table 6.3 Continuum of in-person and telepsychiatric models for psychiatry and primary care based on clinical outcomes, team member roles, and resource allocation

Intensity	Model method	Model examples and features
High	TP collaborative care (synchronous video)	Versus in-person care in terms of diagnosis and treatment of depression in children and adolescents
		Medication use for depression in children/adolescents and adults
		Adults with PTSD
		Children/adolescents with ADHD
		Federally qualified health center for pharmacotherapy and psychotherapy for depression
	RCT hybrid care: TP with other methods (synchronous in-person and video)	STP and asynchronous TP for children with ADHD, with parents and teachers, with screening using a checklist, a diagnostic assessment instrument, rating scales for inattention, hyperactivity, role performance, and other impairments
	RCT disease management for depression (synchronous video and telephone)	Improved TP and usual care outcomes over 12 months; the latter group benefitted from the Hawthorne effect and providers' application of skills from the intervention group[10]
	Non-RCT, informal stepped care	Grant-funded e-MH service with a priori outcome evaluation with (1) two-tiered triaging of patients with depression based on MH screening and TP consultation to (2) therapy on site and/or initiation/change of antidepressant by PCP and (3) ongoing telepsychiatric consultation (by telephone, e-mail, or video) and (4) continuing medical education and (5) staff retraining
Mid	Initial +/− follow-up TP consultation (synchronous video and telephone)	The consultation care or consultation-liaison (CL) model increases capacity of MH services with diagnostic assessment and medication changes in 91% and 57% of cases, respectively, leading to clinical improvements in 56% of cases
		PCP knowledge, skills, and complexity of questions improve over time,[7] particularly in rural PCPs
	Adding a geriatric nurse practitioner (GNP) (synchronous in-person/video and asynchronous to supervisor	Adding a geriatric nurse practitioner (GNP) to an outpatient diagnostic multidisciplinary facility for patients with cognitive disorders may improve the providers' concordance rate of the advice from the diagnostic facility and reduce subjective burden of the informal caregiver[49]
	Veterans affairs TP (synchronous video)	Geographically dispersed population; in 2012, VA MH providers conducted 340,842 interactive video encounters
	Non-RCT child and adolescent program to boost MH services	Contract for child and adolescent MH screening, therapy on site, telepsychiatric consultation (phone, e-mail or video), continuing medical education and staff training improved patient outcomes and site-based staff skills
	Asynchronous telepsychiatry	This involves the PCP interviews a patient with video recording and sends the video with historical information for review by a distant psychiatrist; feasible, valid, reliable, and cost-effective in English- and Spanish-speaking patients in primary care
	Asynchronous e-consultation	Specialists, using e-mail, text, and/or documented notes. This requires a system within electronic health record, training, and monitoring

Low	In-person and telephone doctor-to-doctor "curbside" consultations	Meet approximately 33% of informational PCPs' needs "in-time" Part of collaborative care Purposeful and timely
	Telephone or e-mail doctor-to-doctor "curbside" consultations	A multispecialty phone and e-mail consultation system to PCPs for the care of adults and children across specialties with developmental disabilities Adults awaiting TP consultation as part of a disease management, as a way to accelerate care; a third did not need the TP Align PCPs' diagnoses and medication treatments Improve PCPs' knowledge and skills Improve nursing home TP care for depression or dementia, by making evaluation easier and more efficiently using consultant time. Part of TP collaborative care and integrated care
	Oversight of PCP for PCMH (synchronous video and telephone)	Improve patient care and health desk-mounted video systems offer great convenience for therapy to cancer patients to avoid travel, but the cost used to be prohibitive for most consumers
	Case review with PCPs (synchronous video and telephone)	Case review of diagnosis and follow-up after a discussion helps change treatment plans and improves knowledge Videoconference "virtual grand rounds" are led by a team of MH specialists to review and discuss cases, by Specialty Care Access Network-Extension of Community Healthcare Outcomes (SCAN-ECHO) model at the University of New Mexico
	One-time cultural consultation (synchronous video and telephone, if necessary)	Cultural consultation to rural primary in order to match patients and specialists by culture, ethnicity, and language
	Distance neurocognitive assessment (synchronous video)	Neurocognitive assessment via TP using a Spanish language battery was comparable to in-person (IP) testing for rural Latino patients
	E-mail	Primary care team member and behavioral health clinician

Adapted from: Hilty et al. [74]
Abbreviations: *BH* mental/behavioral health, *app* application, *STP (video)* synchronous telepsychiatry, *ATP* Asynchronous TP, *PCP* primary care provider, *PTSD* post-traumatic stress disorder, *ADHD* attention-deficit hyper/activity disorder, *RCT* randomized controlled trial

Barriers in Patient/Provider Culture and Access to Technology

Barriers to BH (and TMH) care exist at the level of patients, clinicians, clinics/hospitals, and systems of care. Some barriers are easily modifiable, while others are not. Clinical patient barriers include stigmatization, low awareness of a "problem," and limited sharing/denial of BH symptoms. Systems are increasingly seeing TP/TMH as an opportunity to leverage BH expertise across sites in a way that increases efficiency – the basic idea is no different than using national interpreter system for distributing interpreters. These efforts will not improve access and efficient care for all cultures if patients do not seek help at medical clinics, regardless of the reason. Additionally, some patients may shun away from healthcare if staff and providers do not have any overlap in diversity factors. This may contribute to preference for alternative approaches (e.g., shaman, natural remedies, traditions).

Demographic factors can affect accessing care and technology across several levels including income, education, race, and geographic location. Patients living in poverty often have difficulty receiving culturally appropriate psychiatric care, both in person and by telecommunication. Furthermore, rural ethnic minority groups report nearly double the poverty rate of the white rural populations [75]. Poverty can limit access to technology, either by inadequate accessibility or by access with only antiquated systems [75].

Physician and Workflow Barriers

Physicians have been slow to adopt TMH services. Barriers are typically classified into three categories: (1) personal barriers (e.g., attitude), (2) clinical workflow and technology barriers, and (3) licensure, credentialing, and reimbursement barriers [37]. Personal physician barriers include concerns about difficulty establishing rapport or therapeutic relationship and limitations to assessing nonverbal signs of psychiatric illness (e.g., initial greeting, poor hygiene, alcohol on breath, social skills). These barriers can be easily overcome by technology trainings, experience, and shadowing other physicians that utilize TMH. Characteristics of the physician may also affect interest and skill in adopting TMH, with some differences emerging across generations.

Addressing clinical workflow and technology barriers are critical in implementation. This includes additional time to plan and organize operations for a TMH visit, which are not needed for an in-person encounter (e.g., room preparation, equipment availability, up-to-date software). An instrumental step is the development of a workplace culture in which in-person and TMH care are part of workflow. BH clinics function well in this capacity due to the regular patient appointment schedule (e.g., 15-, 30-, or 45-minute visits), timeliness of the therapeutic "hour," and generalizable care across private, clinic, and AHC practices. Workflow barriers of TMH include orienting patients to it, staff flexibility and dependability, and provider-distant site coordination – in the initial phases of establishing a program, TMH has more demands than in-person care. If TMH is combined with in-person visits for other patients and/or additional technologies, the transitions take coordination.

Table 6.4 Top 10 reasons for program failures and dos to ensure quality

Top Ten Reasons for the Failure of a Telemedicine Program

1. Inadequate needs assessment in the region that the program is planning to serve.
2. Inadequate overall and financial support of the program from senior leadership of the organization.
3. Telemedicine and outreach are not consistent with overall mission of the organization.
4. Unreliable or inconsistent service from specialists providing the consultations.
5. Lack of a physician champion.
6. Inadequate technical support or unreliable telecommunications.
7. Inadequate time to develop the program (e.g., time to develop financial stability after start-up funds).
8. Inadequate attention up-front to the appropriate policy and procedures (e.g., consent process).
9. Beginning with too complex of cases; in other words, doing cases that fail at the beginning, so that you lose your referring physician support.
10. Failing to build in adequate resources and procedures to document benefits of the program for both the service area and the provider organization (may be key for grant or organizational support).

Steps for Delivering Quality Services

1. Use clinically proven technology.
2. For each consult, be certain that the technical quality equipment is appropriately matched to the service and needs of the patient and their condition.
3. Evaluate options, implementation, and maintenance of telepsychiatry with a team of clinicians, technicians, and administrators in both the hub and the spoke sites.
4. Adequately train the hub site coordinator and spoke site coordinator in the technical and procedural aspects of the service.
5. Provide adequate training for the telepsychiatrist with the technology, work with them to adapt clinical practice to fit its use, and be certain that they are aware of its limitations.
6. Ensure the telepsychiatrist has general and specific expertise (e.g., consultation-liaison for consults to primary care, geriatric psychiatry for a geriatric patient).
7. Develop referral and/or consultation guidelines, as well as adequate procedures forgetting the key component(s) of the record to the consulting physician.
8. Ensure satisfactory telecommunication by regular technical maintenance and prompt troubleshooting.
9. Coordinate timing of consults (i.e., patients are there at the right time, telepsychiatrist has adequate time, and/or referring physicians or staff stop in if desired).
10. Adequately evaluate satisfaction and outcomes for each consultation (patient, referring physician, and consulting physician) and the program (coordinator, technical staff, and administration). Have adequate feedback mechanisms of this information to telemedicine staff and providers.

Some of this may be better managed through the integration of care within the electronic health record (EHR), but the two juxtaposed and the addition of the more technologies require time to coordinate the components. The exception is use of patient questionnaires and other data (e.g., mobile health apps) which may reduce interview, decision-making time, and documentation. Generally, though, it takes time and practice to develop fluency and efficiency with these modalities.

Licensing and credentialing may be significant barriers, but with planning these can partially be overcome. Licenses are required in states where patients are located, unless it is a one-time assessment or consultation. Licensing can be both complex and expensive if planning to provide care across many states and additional exploration of state/federal laws may be necessary. Credentialing is easier for providers with TP training or experience, there are existing TP proctors (who may teach/train at the same time), and there is reciprocity between health systems (e.g., rural hospital accepts an AHC's credentialing).

Reimbursement barriers still exist. For many years, telemedicine and TP were not billable services, but instead covered by grants or out-of-pocket payments [80]. Although many grants are available for TP research, funding is limited and requires reapplication. Often times when the funding ends, so does the program. There is a substantial difference in reimbursement rates between states. Insurance payers generally reimburse, but not always; education may be needed to facilitate this. TP can help the underserved, but it is seen as "outside" the FQHC and RHC walls, TP is not a financially viable option for the providers (i.e., providers get the regular Medicaid rate and not the higher rate as if they were on site). TP reimbursement to urban FQHCs is not consistently covered, as Medicare restrictions on geographic location require that in order for the TP to be reimbursed, the patient be located in a designated health professional shortage area (HPSA) [82].

A case study by Whitten and Adams [83] found that issues of reimbursement had a strong negative impact on sustainability, primarily due to a fixed process of reimbursement for telemedicine services not yet properly established. Health policymakers have made efforts to address this issue, and currently 46 states now have some type of Medicare or Medicaid reimbursement for behavioral health care provided via videoconferencing. Although this has improved the accessibility of TP, many restrictions on its use still exist [80]. Members of congress understand TP's ability to increase access, but education is required to help them understand its effectiveness and efficiency for consultation, emergencies/crises, and direct care.

Funding and Cost Analysis

In order to best assess cost outcomes of each individual TP program, it may be beneficial to involve a health economist with specialized expertise. To help reduce costs, programs may consider consulting with experts beforehand to come up with a feasible and sustainable program. In cases where expert help is unavailable or too costly, there is benefit to understanding and delineating between differing types of cost analyses [84]. Programs may utilize a variety of methods, including: cost-offset, break-even, cost-effectiveness, and cost-benefit analyses. No one framework is likely adequate for a given program; rather the types of analyses are meant to vary by the relevant questions related to particular metrics or measures. A lexicon of assessment and outcome measures has been developed by the American Telemedicine Association (ATA) [44] that identifies the lack of standardized metrics and definitions required to operationalize cost frameworks.

Several costs and benefit factors may be worth tracking to aid in program evaluation. Cost assessments and value assessments overlap [44], and both should be evaluated in context of a program's pre-established goals. Each program will vary in what they value and calculate in terms of cost. For example, large academic institutions may choose to operate specific TP programs at a (comparative) loss to meet some larger clinical or training mandate (such as reduction in no-shows, improvement in patient satisfaction, or reduction of wait times), while smaller programs, or individual practices, may be utilizing TP modalities specifically to increase efficiency and revenue streams.

The most significant and necessary paradigm shift in the US model of healthcare for increased utilization of TP is in reimbursement. There are trends toward greater TP and limited telephone care (e.g., hematology and thromboembolic diseases) reimbursement with private payers, and some pressure in governance to allow Center for Medicare and Medicaid Service (CMS) to reimburse more widely. Veterans Affairs and other capitated or managed care organizations see the utility and efficiency of low-end technology use, as they do not necessarily depend on specific code-based reimbursement. However, technology is not a high priority of value-based care and accountable care organizations that are driven by CMS and the Affordable Care Act [85]. These organizations are more dependent on specific income-generating RVUs for income and also require broader system changes to allow for expansion into more fluid payment structures and reimbursement modalities. Physicians are a crucial leverage point in these systems, as their work is the prominent mode of reimbursement, and they are complemented by interdisciplinary teams and stepped care models [12]. The shift to allow increases in reimbursement and rethinking of models of reimbursement also requires allowance of faculty development for teaching, supervision, and evaluation [86–89], especially in AHCs.

Evaluation

There is literature describing specifics with regard to evaluation of outcomes in TMH, focusing on operationalization, models of care, and various populations/settings of provision of TMH [12]. The most important takeaway being the need for TMH programs to utilize a lexicon in evaluating their programs that will allow for comparison and improvement based on the existing programs and literature. This is more difficult than it seems, with so many different programs throughout the world implementing TMH, and the wide variety of uses for the technology, as well as the wide variety of payers and systems providing the care. The ATA has developed a lexicon for outcome measures to be used to communicate between programs, focusing on clinical and administrative outcomes, special populations, and cost and economic outcomes [12]. It is their hope that this lexicon can be utilized across programs to evaluate and improve the field of TMH as a whole. Table 6.5 outlines these specific recommendations. Additionally, other evaluation techniques include a method for prioritizing, making decisions, and implementing program change based on iterative feedback [18] and adjusting TMH outcomes for different populations and settings [15],

TMH Administration and Models of Care

Successful intervention models and modules in telemedicine for primary care have some common denominators, according to work in the USA, Australia, Canada, and England: (1) mutual incentive for primary care and specialty partners (e.g., improved quality of care); (2) commitment from physicians, staff, and administration to pursue telemedicine and alternate modes of consultation; (3) systematic or multiple interventions that meet the needs of the site; (4) a system approach for the primary care system to monitor the flow of patients and measure outcomes; and (5) consultants who are able to bridge the differing philosophies that may be unique to rural primary care and urban academic settings and to specific cultural groups [90].

The choice to employ a consultation model has historically been seen as well-advised, since other models (e.g., direct patient care) are understandably more time intensive for the psychiatrist and are less apt to develop skills for the PCP [91, 92]. Overall, telemedicine in a consultative model may reduce provider isolation, provide case-based learning [93], and aide decision support [94]. These interventions have been shown to help patients with depression who are managed by PCPs receive adequate doses of antidepressants and recover from depression [90, 95]; they have relied on TP consultations more for triage, new treatment plans, and changes in treatment plans than for diagnosis compared to suburban providers [90], allowing more provision of care in the medical clinic without delay of waiting for a psychiatric intake appointment [96] and accelerating the service delivery [74]. Without interventions by PCPs, patients may not receive treatment or have substantial delay in treatment due to wait times to see psychiatrists in the community [97].

Discussion

Perhaps the most significant changes in approach to culturally competent care over the past three decades are: (1) shifting from knowledge to skills as central to provider training and patient outcomes, (2) moving away from a specialized clinician based on a single culture (e.g., matching his/her own to training that provides flexibility/versatility to help many diverse populations), and (3) team-based collaboration, shaped by many disciplines including cultural anthropology, psychology, social work, and other BH/social sciences.

The gold standard for clinical care is linguistic, cultural, *and* racial concordance. The concordance facilitates patient and provider satisfaction, as well as patient adherence to treatment [98–101]. Overall, clinical outcomes appear to be excellent with cultural competency training [102]. The use of a non-primary, shared language (e.g., a third language shared by both patient and clinician when neither's primary language can be used), is advocated in some parts of the world to provide more culturally competent care, such as in Europe; however, this is not often available in developing countries [103].

Table 6.5 Baseline assessments help to identify and manage cost outcomes

Value proposition	Comparison of clinical and other health service outcomes by overall resources allocated Standardized and reported taxonomy of resources allocated and outcomes measured There is no consensus yet on the best determinations for economic evaluations in TMH
Travel direct	Direct cost associated with provider and/or patient travel to care site(s) All direct costs should be identified, operationalized, and reported for comparison Should be included within the broad category of costs. Precise definition may not be possible given differing perspectives, but all components should be identified, operationalized, and reported
Travel indirect	Indirect costs associated with provider and/or patient travel to care site All indirect costs should be identified, operationalized, and reported for comparison Should be conceptualized as comparison to normal care, e.g., loss of work productivity is comparable given 1 hour away regardless of mode of delivery. Indirect costs are both inputs to a cost model as well as potential positive outcomes of telehealth (reduction). Evaluators should determine and report up-front whether indirect costs are inputs to a cost model or expected outcomes
Technology direct	Direct patient and provider costs associated with the technology utilized to deliver telehealth services All direct costs should be identified, operationalized, and reported for comparison Need to determine upfront whether costs are calculated as a whole, or divided between providers and patients. Inputs to consider include hardware and depreciation, software and licensing, infrastructure, network, and maintenance costs
Technology indirect	Indirect patient and provider costs associated with the technology utilized to deliver telehealth services Indirect costs include expenses incurred as a result of technology downtimes, specialized licenses, and administration There is crossover between direct and indirect technology costs. Direct costs should focus on tangible assets, while indirect costs are often intangible resources allocated based on the need for tangible assets
Public vs. private	Payer perspective Whether a project, program, or system utilizes public or private funding. This is not an outcome measure but rather a perspective. Outcome measures should be evaluated based upon the financial perspective under which a program operates
Cost avoidance	Current or future direct costs avoided due to a specific intervention or program There are currently no industry standards for cost avoidance measures Consideration should be given to measuring items such as hospitalizations, visits, and other costs. These should be operationalized and reported as possible

(continued)

Table 6.5 (continued)

Missed obligations	Indirect cost: missed obligations Should be measured as part of overall indirect costs Where possible a baseline assessment should be conducted against care as usual. As an outcome measure, the assumption is that TMH impacts indirect costs/burden, thus requiring a comparison Burden on social network Societal resources associated with either the provision of or inadequate access to TMH services Burden on social network should include direct burden to support resources and broad burden to societal infrastructure. When conducting research a positive or negative directional association should be identified a priori
Personnel (administrative, provider, provider extender, presenter)	Personnel costs associated with the provision of TMH services
Supplies	Direct cost of auxiliary supplies required for TMH services

Policy/Advocacy

National organizations are also making changes, and this progress is building on many historical movements (see Table 6.1). The Institute of Medicine (IOM) has outlined the steps toward cultural competence including self-assessment, humility, valuing diversity, vigilance (toward power dynamics), and responsiveness to cultural differences. The Liaison Committee of Medical Education (LCME), Committee on the Accreditation of Canadian Medical Schools (CACMS), American Association of Medical Colleges (AAMC), and others (e.g., Health Services Research Association [HRSA]) are moving forward in these steps as well. The IOM has recommended that medical school programs "integrate cross-cultural education into the training of all current and future health professionals" and the Liaison Committee on Medical Education updated competencies: 3.3 (Diversity/Pipeline Programs and Partnerships), 7.5 (Societal Problems), and 7.6 (Cultural Competence and Health Care Disparities) [104–106], to improve cultural competence.

The movement to *skills* from *knowledge* – consistent with the competency-based medical education movement – will shape culturally competent care, its implementation, and attempts to overcome barriers for in-person and TMH care. Interdisciplinary collaboration – enlisting educators into partnering with cultural leaders, researchers, and clinicians – will make this movement stronger. There is a rich history in the USA from training movements since the 1960s [107] that can be drawn from. The first set of telecompetencies – TP in 2015 – provides a replicable framework with (1) novice/advanced beginner, competent/proficient, and expert levels; (2) domains of patient care, communications, systems-based practice, professionalism, practice-based improvement, knowledge, and technology know-how; and (3) andragogic methods to teach and evaluate skills (see Table 6.2) [63].

Psychology's strength in identifying and assessing practice competencies during graduate training [108, 109] is welcomed.

Limitations of this work include a relatively thin evidence base, aside from individual studies cited. Many topics and themes have been adapted from in-person care, but primary research may be needed to verify if patients are open to care by TMH and if the TMH process has any difference in outcomes from those of in-person care. Second, while this work is based on the literature, it is not based on a consensus process by experts (e.g., Delphi). Third, further discussion, input, and analysis by an interdisciplinary process are suggested to flush out nuances. While there is established literature on BH and ethnic groups, and how to deliver competent care to these diverse groups, additional research and evidence is needed on culturally competent TP (e.g., the ability of clinicians to engage patients across diversity factors) and specifically language-related factors (e.g., individuals using sign language; effect of interpreters).

Conclusion

Rural healthcare systems are challenged to provide timely, evidence-based care, particularly for culturally diverse patients with behavioral disorders. TP and TMH improve access to care for underserved populations and leverage scarce resources like specialty expertise and language interpreters. Principles and approaches exist to provide culturally competent care in-person and via TP. Administrative efforts help to overcome barriers, limitations, and other threats to sustainability. Education and training of an interdisciplinary team, selection of the best care model(s) of consultation, and efficiency with reimbursement help PCPs deliver quality care. More structured, in-depth research is required to ascertain to what these healthcare participants go through, which care models fit best, and the pros/cons of different system interventions.

Summary of High-Yield Points

- Patient-centered care (PCC) requires carefully planned systems using a bio-psycho-social-cultural model and providers who are well versed in the patient's cultural background and curious to learn from the patient. This can feasibly be done via telemedicine with synchronous video conference or asynchronous store-and-forward consultations to allow a more diverse range of patients to be seen by highly skilled providers.
- Some cultures inherently include stigma surrounding mental illness and require increased effort on the part of the provider and the system in order to reach members of these cultures to provide excellent mental health care. This stigma can extend itself to the telemedicine utilized to reach these patients geographically.
- Culturally competent care can be provided in many ways, most frequently involving a team model where the mental health specialist works with the

primary care provider and their team to improve general knowledge of mental health issues and expand access to specialty care.

- Efforts are being made to develop core competencies for telemental health looking at interdisciplinary teams and their uses of technologies to treat patients. These competencies can then be translated into outcomes and goals for teaching new providers to do this work in the future.
- Constant evaluation of programs both fiscally and with regard to clinical outcomes is necessary to sustain a telemental health program provided in a culturally competent manner.

References

1. American Psychiatric Association, Cultural Formulation Interview Supplementary Modules; 2013. Website: http://www.multiculturalmentalhealth.ca/wp-content/uploads/2013/10/2013_CFI_supplementarymodules.pdf. Accessed 30 July 2020.
2. Hilty DM, Feliberti J, Evangelatos G, et al. Competent cultural telebehavioral healthcare to diverse populations: administration, evaluation, and financing. J Tech Behav Sci. 2018;4(3):186–200.
3. Hilty DM, Lim RF, Nasatir-Hilty SE, Koike AK, et al. Planning for telepsychiatric consultation: a needs assessment for cultural and language services at rural sites in California. J Rur Ment Health. 2015;39(3–4):153–61. https://doi.org/10.1037/rmh0000035.
4. U.S. Department of Agriculture. What is Rural? 2015. Retrieved from http://ric.nal.usda.gov/what-is-rural/.
5. Rost K, Williams C, Wherry J, et al. The process and outcomes of care for major depression in rural family practice settings. J Rur Health. 1995;11:114–8.
6. Rost K, Zhang M, Fortney J, et al. Rural-urban differences in depression treatment and suicidality. Med Care. 1998;36:1098–107.
7. Geller JM. Rural primary care providers' perceptions of their roles in the provision of mental health services: voices from the plains. J Rur Health. 1999;15(3):326–34.
8. Geller JM, Muus KJ. The role of rural primary care physicians in the provision of mental health services: letter to the field,# 5. Frontier Mental Health Services Resources Network; 2002.
9. Lim R, Lu F. Culture and psychiatric education. Acad Psychiat. 2008;32(4):269–71.
10. Hilty DM. Advancing science, clinical care and education: shall we update Engel's biopsychosocial model to a bio-psycho-socio-cultural model? Psychol Cogn Sci Open J. 2016;1(1):e1–6. https://doi.org/10.17140/PCSOJ-1-e001.
11. Kim G, Aguado Loi CX, Chiriboga DA, et al. Limited English proficiency as a barrier to mental health service use: a study of Latino and Asian immigrants with psychiatric disorders. J Psychiat Resear. 2010;45(1):104–10. https://doi.org/10.1016/j.jpsychires.2010.04.031.
12. Hilty DM, Yellowlees PM, Parish MB, et al. Telepsychiatry: effective, evidence-based and at a tipping point in healthcare delivery. Psych Clin N Am. 2015;38(3):559–92. https://doi.org/10.1016/j.psc.2015.05.006.
13. Shore JH, Manson SM. A developmental model for rural telepsychiatry. Psychiatr Serv. 2005;56(8):976–80.
14. Shore JH, Brooks E, Savin D, Orton H, Grigsby J, Manson SM. Acceptability of telepsychiatry in American Indians. Telemed J e-Health. 2008;14(5):461–6.
15. Hilty DM, Ferrer D, Parish MB, et al. The effectiveness of telemental health: a 2013 review. Telemed J E-Health. 2013;19(6):444–54. https://doi.org/10.1089/tmj.2013.007.
16. Engel G. The need for a new medical model: a challenge for biomedicine. Sci. 1977;196(4286):129–36.

17. Hilty DM, Evangelatos G, Valasquez A, et al. Telebehavioral health for rural culturally diverse populations: approaches for clinical services, competencies and administration. J Tech Behav Sci. 2018;2(3):206–20.
18. Hilty DM, Yellowlees PM, Nasatir SEH, et al. Program evaluation and practical: supporting pragmatic data-driven clinical videoconferencing CV services. In: Behavioral telehealth, Clinical video conferencing: program development and practice, vol. 1. New York: Springer Press; 2014. p. 105–34.
19. Hilty DM, Doarn C, Armstrong A et al. A framework for telemedicine training and e-health: competency-based education, evaluation and implications. Short Course, American Telemedicine Association, Minneapolis, MN; 2016.
20. Berger JT. Culture and ethnicity in clinical care. Arch Intern Med. 1998;158(19):2085–90.
21. Office of the Surgeon General Center for Mental Health Services and National Institute of Mental Health. Mental Health: Culture, Race, and Ethnicity: A Supplement to Mental Health: A Report of the Surgeon General; 2001, Rockville. http://www.ncbi.nlm.nih.gov/books/NBK44242/. Accessed 30 July 2020.
22. American Psychiatric Association. Position statement on the delineation of transcultural psychiatry as a specialized field of study. Am J Psychiatry. 1969;126:453–5.
23. Civil Rights Act of 1964, Public Law 88-352.
24. Cross TL, Bazron BJ, Dennis KW, et al. Towards a culturally competent system of care, vol. 1. Washington, DC: CASSP Technical Assistance Center, Georgetown University Child Development Center; 1989.
25. Americans with Disabilities Act, 1990, Public Law 101-336; 1990.
26. New York State Office of Mental Health. Cultural and Linguistic Competency Standards. New York: Office of Mental Health; 1997.
27. American Counseling Association: Cross-Cultural Competencies and Objectives; 1992. Retrieved from http://www.counseling.org/Publications/
28. United States Center for Mental Health Services. Cultural competence standards in managed care mental health services: four underserved/underrepresented racial/ethnic groups (Publication No. SMA00–3457). Washington, DC: Substance Abuse and Mental Health Services Administration; 2000. Retrieved from http://mentalhealth.samhsa.gov/publications/allpubs/sma00–3457/default.asp
29. Association of American Medical Colleges. The AAMC Initiative for Cultural Competence in Medical Education; 2000. Retrieved from http://www.aamc.org/meded/tacct/culturalcomped.pdf.
30. US Department of Health and Human Services. Mental Health: Culture, Race, and Ethnicity. A Supplement to Mental Health: A Report of the Surgeon General. Rockville, MD, DHHS, 2001.
31. National Association of Social Workers: Standards for Cultural Competence in Social Work Practice; 2001. Retrieved from http://www.socialworkers.org/sections/credentials/cultural_comp.asp
32. American Psychological Association. Guidelines on multicultural education, training, research, practice, and organizational change for psychologists. Am Psychol. 2003;58:377–402.
33. Agency for Healthcare Research and Quality: National Healthcare Disparities Report, 2006. Rockville, MD, Agency for Healthcare Research and Quality; 2006. Retrieved from http://www.ahrq.gov/qual/nhdr06/nhdr06.htm
34. Accreditation Council for Graduate Medical Education: Residency Review Committee, Guidelines for Psychiatric Residencies; 2007. Available at www.acgme.org/acWebsite/downloads/RRC_progReq/400pr07012007.pdf
35. LCME accreditation standards. Washington, DC: Liaison Committee on Medical Education, March 12, 2003. Retrieved from www.lcme.org. Accessed 30 July 2020.
36. Greenburg M, Shergill S, Szmukler G, et al. Narratives in psychiatry. London: Jessica Kingsley Publishing; 2002.

37. Brooks TR. Pitfalls in communication with Hispanic and African-American patients: do translators help or harm? J Nat Med Assoc. 1992;84(11):941–7.
38. Brua C. Role-blurring and ethical grey zones associated with lay interpreters: three case studies. Comm Med. 2008;5(1):73–9.
39. Yeung A, Chang D, Gresham R. Illness beliefs of depressed Chinese American patients in primary care. J Nerv Ment Dis. 2004;192(4):324–7.
40. Hamann J, Leucht S, Kissling W. Shared decision making in psychiatry. Acta Psychiat Scand. 2003;107(6):403–9.
41. Yellowlees PM, Odor A, Parish MB, et al. A feasibility study of asynchronous telepsychiatry for psychiatric consultations. Psych Serv. 2010;61(8):838–40. https://doi.org/10.1176/ps.2010.61.8.838.
42. Yellowlees PM, Shore JH, Roberts L, et al. Practice guidelines for videoconferencing-based telemental health. Telemed J e-Health. 2010;16(10):1074–89.
43. Richardson L, McCauley E, Katon W. Collaborative care for adolescent depression: a pilot study. Gen Hosp Psychiat. 2009;31:36–45.
44. Shore JH, Mishkind MC, Bernard J, et al. A lexicon of assessment and outcome measures for telemental health. Tel e-Health. 2013;20(3):282–92. https://doi.org/10.1089/tmj.2013.0357.
45. Cerda GM, Hilty DM, Hales RE, Nesbitt TS. Use of telemedicine with ethnic groups. Psychiatr Serv. 1999;50(10):1364. https://doi.org/10.1176/ps.50.10.1364.
46. Yellowlees PM, Marks SL, Hilty DM, et al. Using e-health to enable culturally appropriate mental health care in rural areas. Telemed J eHealth. 2008;14(5):486–92.
47. Moreno FA, Chong J, Dumbauld J, et al. Use of standard webcam and Internet equipment for telepsychiatry treatment of depression among underserved Hispanics. Psychiatr Serv. 2012;63(12):1213–7. https://doi.org/10.1176/appi.ps.201100274.
48. Beach MC, Price EG, Gary TL, et al. Cultural competence: a systematic review of health care provider educational interventions. Med Care. 2005;43(4):356–73.
49. Chong J, Moreno F. Feasibility and acceptability of clinic-based telepsychiatry for low-income Hispanic primary care patients. Telemed e-Health. 2012;18(4):297–304. https://doi.org/10.1089/tmj.2011.0126.
50. Nieves JE, Stack KM. Hispanics and telepsychiatry; 2007.
51. Ye J, Shim R, Lukaszewski T, et al. Telepsychiatry services for Korean immigrants. Telemed J eHealth. 2012;18(10):797–802. https://doi.org/10.1089/tmj.2012.0041.
52. Weiner MF, Rossetti HC, Harrah K. Videoconference diagnosis and management of Choctaw Indian dementia patients. Alzheim Dem. 2011;7(6):562–6. https://doi.org/10.1016/j.jalz.2011.02.006.
53. Mucic D. Transcultural telepsychiatry and its impact on patient satisfaction. J Telemed Telecare. 2010;16(5):237–42. https://doi.org/10.1258/jtt.2009.090811.
54. Lopez AM, Cruz M, Lazarus S, Webster P, Jones EG, Weinstein RS. Case report: use of American sign language in telepsychiatry consultation. Telemed J e-Health. 2004;10(3):389–91.
55. Carlson J. Breaking down language barriers. Hospital interpreters get credentialed with new certification programs. Mod Healthcare. 2010;40(46):32–4.
56. Elderkin-Thompson V, Silver RC, Waitzkin H. When nurses double as interpreters: a study of Spanish-speaking patients in a US primary care setting. Soc Sci Med. 2001;52(9):1343–58. https://doi.org/10.1016/S0277-9536(00)00234-3.
57. Frank JR, Mungroo R, Ahmad Y, et al. Toward a definition of competency-based education in medicine: a systematic review of published definitions. Med Teach. 2010;32(8):631–7. https://doi.org/10.3109/0142159X.2010.500898.
58. Accreditation of Medical Education Programs Leading to the MD Degree, 2014. At https://www.lcme.org/publications/2015-16-functions-and-structure-with-appendix.pdf.
59. Royal College of Physicians and Surgeons, CanMEDS Framework; 2005. Retrieved from http://www.royalcollege.ca/portal/page/portal/rc/canmeds/framework. Accessed 30 July 2020.
60. American Association of Medical Colleges, Core Medical Student Competencies; 2015. Retrieved from https://www.aamc.org. Accessed 30 July 2020.

61. Accreditation Council on Graduate Medical Education. Common program requirements; 2013. Retrieved from https://www.acgme.org/acgmeweb/Portals/0/PFAssets/ProgramRequirements/CPRs2013.pdf. Accessed 30 July 2020.
62. Frank JR. The CanMEDS 2005 physician competency framework; 2005. Retrieved from http://rcpsc.medical.org/canmeds/CanMEDS2005/CanMEDS2005_e.pdf. Accessed 30 July 2020.
63. Hilty DM, Crawford A, Teshima J, et al. A framework for telepsychiatric training and e-health: competency-based education, evaluation and implications. Int Rev Psychiat. 2015;27(6):569–92. https://doi.org/10.3109/09540261.2015.1091292.
64. Hilty DM, Zalpuri I, Stubbe D, et al. Social media/networking as part of e-behavioral health and psychiatric education: Competencies, teaching methods, and implications. J Tech Behav Sci. 2018;3(4):268–93.
65. Hilty DM, Chan S, Torous J, et al. A framework for competencies for the use of mobile technologies in psychiatry and medicine. JMIR Uhealth Mob Health. 2020;8(2). http://mhealth.jmir.org/2020/2/e12229/
66. Cowley D, Dunaway K, Forstein M, Frosch E, Han J, Joseph R, Unutzer J. Teaching psychiatry residents to work at the interface of mental health and primary care. Acad Psychiatry. 2014;38:398–404.
67. Ratzliff A, Norfleet K, Chan YF, Raney L, Unützer J. Perceived educational needs of the integrated care psychiatric consultant. Acad Psychiatry. 2015;39(4):448–56.
68. Sunderji N, Crawford C, Jovanovic M. Telepsychiatry in graduate medical education: a narrative review. Acad Psychiat. 2015;39(1):55–62. https://doi.org/10.1007/s40596-014-0176-x.
69. Crawford A, Sunderji N, López J, Soklaridis S. Defining competencies for the practice of telepsychiatry through an assessment of resident learning needs. BMC Med Educ. 2016;16(1):28.
70. Alicata D, Schroepfer A, Unten T, Agoha R, Helm S, Fukuda M, et al. Telemental health training, team building, and workforce development in cultural context: the Hawaii experience. J Child Adolesc Psychopharmacol. 2016;26(3):260–5.
71. Gifford V, Niles B, Rivkin I, et al. Continuing education training focused on the development of behavioral telehealth competencies in behavioral healthcare providers. Rur Remot Health. 2012;12:2108.
72. Hilty DM, Maheu M, Drude K, et al. Telebehavioral health, telemental health, e-therapy and e-health competencies: the need for an interdisciplinary framework. J Tech Behav Sci. 2017;2(3–4):171–89.
73. Maheu M, Drude K, Hertlein K, et al. Telemental health, e-therapy and e- health competencies: an interdisciplinary framework. J Technol Behav Sci. 2018;3(2):108–40; correction 3(2): 107.
74. Hilty DM, Rabinowitz T, McCarron RM, Katzelnick DJ, Chang T, Bauer AM, Fortney J. An update on telepsychiatry and how it can leverage collaborative, stepped, and integrated services to primary care. Psychosomatics. 2018;59(3):227–50.
75. Yellowlees PM, Odor A, Losif AM, et al. Transcultural psychiatry made simple—asynchronous telepsychiatry as an approach to providing culturally relevant care. Telemed J e-Health. 2013;19(4):1–6. https://doi.org/10.1089/tmj.2012.0077.
76. Fortney JC, Pyne JM, Mouden SP, et al. Practice-based versus telemedicine-based collaborative care for depression in rural federally qualified health centers: a pragmatic randomized comparative effectiveness trial. Am J Psychiat. 2013;170(4):414–25. https://doi.org/10.1176/appi.ajp.2012.12050696.
77. Fortney JC, Pyne JM, Turner E, et al. Telemedicine integration of mental health into rural primary care settings. Int Rev Psychiat. 2015;27(6):525–39. https://doi.org/10.3109/09540261.2015.1085838.
78. López-Cevallos DF, Harvey SM, Warren JT. Medical mistrust, perceived discrimination, and satisfaction with health care among young-adult rural Latinos. J Rur Health. 2014;30(4):344–51.
79. Mucic D, Hilty DM. Key issues in e-mental health. New York: Springer Publishing; 2015.

80. Lauckner C, Whitten PJ. The state and sustainability of telepsychiatry programs. Behav Health Serv Res. 2016;43(2):305–18. https://doi.org/10.1007/s11414-015-9461-z.
81. Hyler SE, Gangure DP. A review of the costs of telepsychiatry. Psychiatr Serv. 2003;54(7):976–80. https://doi.org/10.1176/appi.ps.54.7.976.
82. Health Resources and Services Administration. Shortage designation: health professional shortage areas & medically underserved areas/populations [Internet]. US Department of Health and Human Services: Rockville, MD; 2019. Retrieved from http://www.hrsa.gov/shortage/. Accessed 30 July 2020.
83. Whitten P, Adams I. Success and failure: a case study of two rural telemedicine projects. J Telemed Telecare. 2003;9(3):125–9. https://doi.org/10.1258/135763303767149906.
84. Weinstein MC, Stason WB. Foundations of cost-effectiveness analysis for health and medical practices. N Engl J Med. 1977;296:716–21.
85. Hilty DM, Hwang T, Turvey C. Staying abreast of information in the information age: digital continuing education and levering technology to stay current for clinical psychiatric practice. Curr Psychiatry Rep. 2018;20(3):15. https://doi.org/10.1007/s11920-018-0878-y.
86. Litzelman DK, Stratos GA, Marriott DJ, et al. Factorial validation of a widely disseminated educational framework for evaluating clinical teachers. Acad Med. 1998;73(8):688–95.
87. McLean M, Cilliers F, Van Wyk JM. Faculty development: yesterday, today and tomorrow. Med Teach. 2008;30:555–84. https://doi.org/10.1080/01421590802109834.
88. Skeff KM, Stratos GA, Mount JFS. Faculty development in medicine: a field in evolution. Teach Teach Educ. 2007;23:280–5. https://doi.org/10.1016/j.tate.2006.12.019.
89. Srinivasan M, Li ST, Meyers FJ, et al. Teaching as a competency for medical educators: competencies for medical educators. Acad Med. 2011;86(10):1211–20. https://doi.org/10.1097/ACM.0b013e31822c5b9a.
90. Hilty DM, Nesbitt TS, Kuenneth TA, et al. Rural versus suburban primary care needs, utilization, and satisfaction with telepsychiatric consultation. J Rural Health. 2007;23(2):163–5. https://doi.org/10.1111/j.1748-0361.2007.00084.x.
91. Katon W, Von Korff M, Lin E, et al. Collaborative management to achieve treatment guidelines. JAMA. 1995;273(13):1026–31.
92. Strathdee G. Primary care-psychiatry interaction: a British perspective. Gen Hospit Psychiat. 1987;9:102–10.
93. Greenberg WE, Paulsen RH. Moving into the neighborhood: preparing residents to participate in a primary care environment. Harvard Rev Psychiat. 1996;4(2):107–9.
94. Armstrong IJ, Haston WS. Medical decision support for remote general practitioners using telemedicine. J Telemed Telecare. 1997;3(1):27–34. https://doi.org/10.1258/1357633971930166.
95. Simon GE, VonKorff M, Rutter C, et al. Randomised trial of monitoring, feedback, and management of care by telephone to improve treatment of depression in primary care. BMJ. 2000;320:550–4.
96. Hilty DM, Yellowlees PM, Nesbitt TS. Evolution of telepsychiatry to rural sites: change over time in types of referral and PCP knowledge, skill, and satisfaction. Gen Hosp Psychiat. 2006;28(5):367–73. https://doi.org/10.1016/j.genhosppsych.2006.05.009.
97. Marcin JP, Nesbitt TS, Struve S, et al. Financial benefits of a pediatric intensive care unit-based telemedicine program to a rural adult intensive care unit: impact of keeping acutely ill and injured children in their local community. Telemed J e-Health. 2004;10 Suppl 2:S1–5.
98. Freeman GK, Rai H, Walker JJ, et al. Non-English speakers consulting with the GP in their own language: a cross-sectional survey. Br J Gen Pract. 2002;52(474):36–8.
99. Perez-Stable EJ. Language access and Latino health care disparities. Med Care. 2007;45(11):1009–11.
100. Pöchhacker F. Language barriers in Vienna hospitals. Ethn Health. 2000;5:113–9.
101. Saha S, Komaromy M, Koepsell TD, et al. Patient-physician racial concordance and the perceived quality and use of health care. Arch Intern Med. 1999;159(9):997–1004.
102. Ton H, Koike A, Hales RE, et al. A qualitative needs assessment for development of a cultural consultation service. Transcult Psychiatry. 2005;42:491–504. https://doi.org/10.1177/1363461505055629.

103. Riddick S. Improving access for limited English-speaking consumers: a review of strategies in health care settings. J Health Care Poor Underserved. 1998;9(Supplemental):S40–61.
104. Institute of Medicine committee on understanding and eliminating racial and ethnic disparities in health care. Unequal treatment: confronting racial and ethnic disparities in health care. Washington, DC: National Academy Press; 2002.
105. Loue S, Wilson-Defosse A, Limbach K. Identifying gaps in the cultural competence/sensitivity components of an undergraduate medical school curriculum: a needs assessment. J Immigr Min Health. 2015;17(5):1412–9.
106. Liaison Committee on Medical Education Competencies Revision, 2015. At: https://www.lcme.org/publications/2015-16-functions-and-structure-with-appendix.pdf.
107. Brown M. An introduction to the discourse on competency-based training (CBT). In: Deakin University Course Development Centre, editor. A collection of readings related to competency-based training. Victoria, Australia: Victorian Education Foundation, Deakin University; 1994. http://files.eric.ed.gov/fulltext/ED384695.pdf. Accessed 30 July 2020.
108. Kaslow NJ, Rubin NJ, Bebeau M, et al. Guiding principles and recommendations for the assessment of competence. Pro Psychol Resear Pract. 2007;38(5):441–51. https://doi.org/10.1037/0735-7028.38.5.441.
109. Rubin NJ, Bebeau MJ, Leigh IW, et al. The competency movement within psychology: an historical perspective. Pro Psychol Resear Pract. 2007;38(5):452–62. https://doi.org/10.1037/0735-7028.38.5.452.

Suggested Reading

American Association of Medical Colleges. Core Entrustable Professional Activities for Entering Residency; 2014. Retrieved from https://www.aamc.org/download/427456/data/spring2015updatepptpdf.pdf.

APA Cultural Formulation Interview. Patient Version; 2013. Retrieved from http://www.dsm5.org/Pages/Feedback-Form.aspx, and Informant Version, at: http://www.multiculturalmentalhealth.ca/wp-content/uploads/2013/10/2013_DSM5_CFI_InformantVersion.pdf. Accessed 30 July 2020.

American Psychiatric Association. Practice Guidelines for the Psychiatric Evaluation of Adults. Washington, DC: American Psychiatric Publishing; 1995.

Baranyi A, Meinitzer A, Stepan A, et al. A biopsychosocial model of interferon-alpha-induced depression in patients with chronic hepatitis C infection. Psychother Psychosom. 2013;82(5):332–40. https://doi.org/10.1159/000348587.

Barker V, Gumley A, Schwannauer M, et al. An integrated biopsychosocial model of childhood maltreatment and psychosis. Br J Psychiatry. 2015;206(3):177–80. https://doi.org/10.1192/bjp.bp.113.143578.

California Department of Mental Health. DMH Information Notice No: 02–03. Addendum for Implementation Plan for Phase II Consolidation of Medi-Cal Specialty Mental Health Services—Cultural Competence Plan Requirements; 2003, superseding (California) DMH Information Notice No: 97–14. Addendum for implementation plan for phase II consolidation of Medi-Cal specialty mental health services—cultural competence plan requirements; 1997. Retrieved from http://www.dmh.cahwnet.gov/DMHDocs/docs/notices02/02–03_Enclosure.pdf. Accessed 30 July 2020.

Cené CW, Johnson BH, Wells N, et al. A narrative review of patient and family engagement: the "foundation" of the medical "home". Med Care. 2016;54(7):697–705. https://doi.org/10.1097/MLR.0000000000000548.

Federal Interagency Working Group on Limited English Proficiency, 2003. Overview of Executive Order 13166. Retrieved from http://www.lep.gov/

Group for the Advancement of Psychiatry. Cultural Assessment in Clinical Psychiatry. Washington, DC: American Psychiatric Publishing; 2002.

Internet World Stats. Internet users in the world-Distribution by world regions; 2011. http://www.internetworldstats.com/stats.htm. Accessed 30 July 2020.

Lim RF. Clinical manual of cultural psychiatry. Arlington, VA: American Psychiatric Publishing; 2006.
Lim RF, Lu FG, Hilty DM. Impact of socio-cultural factors on health care disparities. In: Behavior and medicine. 5th ed. Wedding, Stuber. New York, New York; 2010. p. 289–304.
Lu FG. Annotated bibliography on cultural psychiatry and related topics. February 2005. Retrieved from http://www.nami.org/Template.cfm?Section_Fact_Sheets1&Template_/ContentManagement/ContentDisplay.cfm&ContentID_22156. Accessed 30 July 2020.
National Standards on Culturally and Linguistically Appropriate Services; 2001. Available at http://www.omhrc.gov/templates/browse.aspx?lvl_2&lvlID_15. Accessed 30 July 2020.
New Freedom Commission on Mental Health. Achieving the Promise: Transforming Mental Health Care in America. Final Report. DHHS Publication SMA-03–3832. Rockville, MD, DHHS, 2003.
PEW Research Center, Internet Survey; 2013. Retrieved from http://www.pewinternet.org/~/media//Files/Reports/PIP_HealthOnline.pdf. Accessed 30 July 2020.
Rosenthal TC. The medical home: growing evidence to support a new approach to primary care. J Am Board Fam Med. 2008;21(5):427–40. https://doi.org/10.3122/jabfm.2008.05.070287.
Shore JH. Telepsychiatry: videoconferencing in the delivery of psychiatric care. Am J Psychiat. 2013;170(3):256–62. https://doi.org/10.1176/appi.ajp.2012.12081064.
Smedley BD, Stith SY, Nelson AR, editors. Unequal treatment: confronting racial and ethnic disparities in health care. Washington, DC: The National Academies Presses; 2002.
Tseng WS, Strelzer J. Culture and psychotherapy. Washington, DC: American Psychiatric Publishing; 2001.
United States Census Bureau. An older and more diverse nation by midcentury; 2008. Retrieved from http://www.census.gov/newsroom/releases/archives/population/cb08-123.html. Accessed 30 July 2020.
United States Census Bureau. Rural Assistance Cen, crit rural sites (2005) Rural Health Information Hub, Grand Forks; 2001. Retrieved from https://www.ruralhealthinfo.org. Accessed 30 July 2020.
Weissman JS, Betancourt J, Campbell EJ, et al. Resident physicians' preparedness to provide cross-cultural care. JAMA. 2005;294(9):1058–67. https://doi.org/10.1001/jama.294.9.1058.
World Health Organization. Telemedicine opportunities and developments in member states. Results of the second global survey on eHealth. Geneva; 2011.
Yellowlees PM, Hilty DM, Mucic D. Global/World wide telehealth: international perspectives of telepsychiatry and the future. In: Mucic D, Hilty DM, editors. Key issues in e-mental health. New York: Springer; 2016. p. 233–50.
Zalpuri I, Liu H, Stubbe D, et al. A competency-based framework for social media for trainees, faculty and others. Acad Psychiatry. 2018;42(6):808–17.

Religion, Spirituality, and Mental Health

7

Hannah Cherian Sweet and Rachel Ann Paul

Introduction

The relationship between religion and mental health varies by class, gender, religious denomination, and other factors. The most accurate predictor of religiosity is geography. While religious identification is declining in Western Europe and North America, it is growing in other regions. In Pew Research Center telephone surveys conducted in 2018 and 2019, 65% of American adults described their religious affiliation as Christian, which illustrated a 12% decrease over the past decade [1]. Meanwhile, the religiously unaffiliated share of the population, including those who selected atheist, agnostic or "nothing in particular," increased to 26% from 17% in 2009 [1]. It is important to recognize that those who identify as atheist or agnostic might still consider themselves to be spiritual. In addition, those that consider themselves to be religious might be "culturally religious," where they participate in the traditions of their religion (e.g., Shabbat dinner on Friday), but may not be traditional "true" believers. In contrast to Western Europe and North America, 84% of the world's population identifies with a religious group [2]. Members of this demographic are generally younger and produce more children; thus religious identification continues growing worldwide.

Until the early nineteenth century, psychiatric disorders were managed and treated by religious leaders. A major change occurred when Charcot and Freud associated religion with hysteria and neurosis. This created a divide between religion and psychiatry, which has only started to change in the past few decades. One

H. C. Sweet (✉)
UCSD Division of Child & Adolescent Psychiatry, Rady Children's Hospital,
San Diego, CA, USA
e-mail: hcsweet@health.ucsd.edu

R. A. Paul
Department of Psychiatry, Rady Children's Hospital, San Diego, CA, USA
e-mail: rpaul@rchsd.org

S. H. Koh et al. (eds.), *Diversity in Action*,
https://doi.org/10.1007/978-3-030-85401-0_7

sign of change was in 1994 when the Diagnostic and Statistical Manual of Mental Disorders, fourth edition (DSM-IV) included the V-code of "religious or spiritual problems" with the purpose of helping professionals better understand their patient's beliefs and rituals. The current DSM-5 recommends this V-code "category can be used when the focus of clinical attention is a religious or spiritual problem. Examples include distressing experiences that involve loss or questioning of faith, problems associated with conversion to a new faith, or questioning of other spiritual values which may not necessarily be related to an organized church or religious institution" [3]. Additionally, religious elements may be a symptom of several diagnoses or affect how symptoms are interpreted (e.g., hallucinations may be culturally normative in some religions).

There is wide acceptance that religiosity plays a role in the presentation and treatment of psychiatric diagnoses, but how much of a role, and to what degree, remains unclear. Religion provides us parameters for what a religious client may need in terms of support. Spirituality is more subjective and has no clear guidelines for what a patient believes in, how they view mental health, medications, and the level of need necessary for support. While these are separate belief domains, they often go hand in hand when understanding support needs. If a patient was not religious before onset of symptoms, do we chalk up the religiosity as a symptom of mental illness or treat the person using religion as a protective factor? When is religiosity determined to negatively impact mental health functioning, and when is it incorporated into treatment planning and positive coping mechanisms? Also, who are mental health experts to decide what is hyper-religiosity or not, and if it is disordering a patient's life? Culture is decided by the people within it; if someone's religion or spiritual beliefs no longer fit, is that a disorder? Like with all things, there is a spectrum that describes the relevance of spirituality and religion in the context of a culture. On this spectrum, the majority of individuals linger close to the median and have some faith basis or spirituality structure in their lives. Those who flank the ends of the spectrum hold religion as a large cornerstone of their daily functioning or do not view religion or spirituality as any part of their life. It is essential to find out for each individual person their need and level of support.

Even though religious belief is the majority worldwide, physicians in psychiatry are much less likely to believe in God or be affiliated with a specific religious organization [4]. Compared with other physicians, psychiatrists are more likely to be without religious affiliation (17% *v.* 10%), less likely to believe in God (65% *v.* 77%), less likely to attend religious services at least twice monthly (29% *v.* 47%), and less likely to rely on God for strength and support (36% *v.* 49%) [4]. However, it would be a gross mistake for mental health providers, including psychiatrists, to disregard religion and spirituality when considering treatment because of their personal biases in this area, given the prominence within patient populations.

Religious beliefs can be associated with both positive and negative psychological effects. A negative psychological effect of religious involvement manifests with excessive devotion to religious practice that may result in family discord, particularly in areas of sexuality. Speaking broadly, religion places an emphasis on guilt, sin, and a disregard for personal individuality and autonomy. Positive psychological effects of religiosity increase with being active in one's religious organization. Positive outcomes include a greater sense of optimism and hope, self-esteem, meaning and purpose in life, increased social support, a decrease in suicidality, and higher marital satisfaction [5].

Background

Religious affiliation creates a shared culture affecting one's beliefs, practices, routines, responsibilities, and attitudes. Paul Tillich, one of the most influential theologians of the twentieth century, stated:

> Religion as ultimate concern is the meaning-giving substance of culture, and culture is the totality of forms in which the basic concern of religion expresses itself. In abbreviation: religion is the substance of culture; culture is the form of religion. Such a consideration prevents the establishment of a dualism of religion and culture. Every religious act, not only in organized religion, but also in the most intimate movement of the soul, is culturally formed [6].

Religion is specific to different geographical cultures, and it does not easily translate between cultures. Even when missionaries convert different regions of the world to a different religion, there is variation in the religious practices between the converts and the original.

Throughout human history, many cultures have viewed mental illness as a form of religious punishment or demonic possession. During the Neolithic Era, primitive humans would chip a hole into the skulls of mentally ill individuals to release the evil spirits. Ancient Hindu and Punjabi scriptures attribute anxiety and depression, in part, to disrespecting the gods. In ancient Mesopotamia, priest-doctors treated mentally ill individuals with rituals to drive out evil spirits. In ancient Egyptian, Indian, Greek, and Roman writings, mental illness was characterized as a personal or religious dilemma. In ancient China, the mentally ill were concealed by their families for fear that the community would believe that the affliction was the result of immoral behavior by the individual and/or their relatives.

Hippocrates, a Greek physician who is considered the "father of medicine," was the first to attribute the cause of mental illness to natural occurrences in the human body, particularly pathology in the brain, rather than supernatural forces. During the Middle Ages, mentally ill individuals were believed to be possessed by a demon. Conceptions of madness in the Middle Ages in Europe were a mixture of the divine, diabolical, magical, and transcendental. Madness was thought to be a punishment for sin or a test of faith and character. Hebrews believed that all illness was inflicted upon humans by God as punishment for committing sin, and since Hebrew physicians were also the religious leaders, the treatment did not proceed further. Arab historic texts contain discussions of mental disorders, where some thought they were caused by possession by a djinn (genie), which could be either good or demon-like. Christian theology endorsed various therapies, including fasting and prayer for those estranged from God and exorcism for those possessed by the devil.

Throughout history and modern times, religion has been profoundly intertwined with mental health. Religious preoccupations in obsessive-compulsive disorder (OCD), hyper-religiosity in mania, and delusions of omnipotence are all known psychiatric symptoms. The very nature of these religious experiences is considered pathological. At the same time, religious beliefs and being part of a religious organization are considered protective when assessing suicide risk factors. Belief in God has shown to be comforting to those struggling with anxiety and depression. This complicates things, because it is up to mental health providers to decide when the client's religion is pathological, protective, neither, or both. To address this, clinicians are encouraged to do the following:

1. Obtain information about patients' religious and cultural values.
2. Liaison with one or more well-informed members from the same cultural-religious background.
3. Consider whether religious functioning is problematic.
4. Consider whether religious functioning has been affected by psychopathology.
5. Consider how religion is being used in coping, attending to contextual factors.

Vignette 1

George is a 22-year-old Filipino American male with no previous psychiatric history who was referred to an outpatient clinic after initially presenting to the emergency room for missing several weeks of class. George, along with his family, had always been very active in the Catholic Church. Religion is a large part of his Filipino culture, so he regularly attended youth group and Sunday Mass and served as an acolyte. His family participated in daily devotional prayer, and he was encouraged to attend confession. George was baptized as an infant and attended confirmation preparatory classes. When George entered his teenage years, he would occasionally express desire to skip church with his family Sunday mornings, stating he would rather relax or study. During George's third year in college, he started reading the Bible nightly. This progressed from a devotional in the evening to several hours every day. His family often noticed him in the backyard using his rosary. Eventually, his mother heard from their priest – George attended confessional at the cathedral so often that he was missing classes. By then, his grades started dropping and his parents insisted that he seek assessment. When he finally presented to clinic, a semi-structured interview with George and his parents, as well as the Yale-Brown Obsessive Compulsive Scale was administered, and he was given a diagnosis of OCD. George was started on sertraline and referred for Exposure and Response Prevention (ERP).

This case highlights several important points – often, nonpathological religious practices can precede pathology. Along the continuum, when should a mental health provider intervene?

Culturally Competent Care

The traditional model of culturally competent care is to ask about religion as a check box item and to be cued into any typical alerts. For example, if a patient identifies as Jehovah's Witness, this alerts the provider to be aware of certain medical restrictions, specifically, in regard to blood transfusions. However, more subtle nuances of religious and spiritual beliefs hold just as much importance to culturally competent care.

When caring for clients, it is important to consider a "person in environment" approach. It would not make sense to treat a person in a silo without considering their family and societal systems. Clinicians must ask themselves – what is the norm for that person's environment and what do they view as important? As a clinician, it is vital to not only speak with the patient but also their family, if possible. Do their religious/spiritual practices look similar or different than their family/friend group? When determining pathology, this is an important factor to consider. While something might seem extreme to one person, viewing it in context provides a clearer picture. An example of this is the Hasidic Orthodox Jewish population. If, without context, you had a patient from this religious group share that they pray multiple times a day, before handwashing, meals, when waking up, and when going to bed; that they cannot have certain foods touch or eaten at the same meal time, that they even have separate sinks, plates, and silverware; and that they must wear their hair in a certain way and cannot go in public if part of their head is not covered, this may sound like the beginnings of an OCD diagnosis. When considering this person's behavior in the context of their community, it does not seem strange or pathological. Instead, they fall within the normal standards set by their religious beliefs and community. If this same person presented in your office and all these behaviors were new onset, they were not part of the Hasidic community; then considering pathology would be indicated, especially if these new behaviors were hindering daily functioning. In the Jewish population, none of these behaviors are an issue with how their community and society function, but if this were one person in a different community, it could cause alarm.

When meeting with a patient for the first time, it is valuable to collect a comprehensive history of not just pathology but their strengths, support systems, coping mechanisms, and their outlets of joy. These are essential to understand how they view their life. Also, this information lays the groundwork for helping that person successfully reenter their life with appropriate supports and tools. Obtaining a comprehensive view of a person's culture lays the foundation for treatment. If they find strength in religion, providers can encourage them to connect with an organization that aligns with their belief system or assist them to incorporate the religious or spiritual components that bring them solace.

Understanding the versatile language used is also important as there are no set parameters for the terms "religion" and "spirituality," or how individuals refer to the practices associated with their beliefs. Important information to collect includes learning what a patient calls their belief system, how they refer to a higher power, if they use prayer/meditation, and what religious rituals they engage in. One client might refer to sitting on the ground in silence with mandala beads as meditation, while another might consider that prayer. In a more literal sense, language can be a huge barrier when explaining psychiatric illness, treatment, and medications. A barrier that becomes extremely difficult when coupled with a religious undercurrent. A simple translation usually will not provide complete care. When explaining a serious mental illness to a patient and their family, it is important to have an in-person interpreter who is able to provide cultural context of the religion and belief system of that culture in relation to psychiatric illness. Understanding the difference between being culturally religious and practicing set religious guidelines is an important concept when treating the patient through a culturally competent lens. While traditions are important to the fabric of societies, people who identify with a religion sometimes only do so in a "culturally religious" way. For instance, they might decorate a Christmas tree and hide Easter eggs for their children, but they do not use religion as a source of support or guidance. Knowing this distinction can help guide treatment, and a clinician, in this instance, would be advised to not place significant emphasis on religion when discussing resources in the community.

Not every clinician is expected to be an expert on every religion, subgroup, and spiritual practice. Therefore, it is important to use one's network and resources. Knowing one's limitations, or practicing cultural humility, is vital to providing culturally competent care. For example, a psychiatric team had difficulty communicating the importance of outpatient treatment for a child to the family. The parents did not speak English and were devout in their religion. It was not until they found a community clinic specific to Southeast Asian families that the parents began to engage more in treatment. This community clinic had clinicians who could speak multiple languages native to Southeast Asia and had a shared cultural-religious foundation. In regard to treating a patient through the cultural lens of religion or spirituality, it is necessary to consider how a patient copes and from where a patient draws their strength and resiliency. Even when treating a patient with hyper-religiosity and grandiose thoughts, it is important to not completely disregard these in the treatment. Sometimes a symptom of illness is part of the cure. For example, if reading scripture provides a person peace but was previously used as an avoidance mechanism or became intrusive in their daily functioning, acknowledging the importance of this behavior may be helpful to structuring a more balanced life. The patient may benefit from incorporating it into their day, after completing a needed task, which can provide the patient assurance that their provider views their values and beliefs as important. Consulting with a trained member of the clergy, such as a hospital chaplain, can help a patient parse out how their belief system fits. Often, after a patient in a manic episode or dealing with OCD receives medical treatment, their obsessions or delusional thoughts become less intense. The care and acknowledgement they receive about their beliefs are important to the lifelong sustainability with treatment of their illness.

Vignette 2

Claire is a 12-year-old girl who presented to the hospital for disorganized behavior, hyper-religiosity, and self-injurious behavior. Her injuries were not life threatening, and they were not done with intent to die. Prior to admission, Claire had a diagnosis of attention-deficit/hyperactivity disorder through her school, but she never received psychiatric treatment or medication. She was a typically developing preteen enrolled in a public school in an upper middle-class neighborhood. Claire had a group of friends at school, performed average academically, and attended a youth group at her church. The most recent and pertinent stressor was that her parents separated and lived in different homes. Claire was splitting time evenly between the two households, but due to proximity to her school, she spent most nights at her father's house. Claire's parent brought her to the hospital due to her lack of interest in sleeping, eating, or caring for basic activities of daily living (ADLs). At home, she would climb onto the roof and shout down to cars and passersby religious statements such as "Jesus loves you. Jesus saves." Her parents shared that while the family attended church weekly, they were not extremely religious and never used the phrases the patient shouted. Claire made signs with similar messages to give to people in the neighborhood and to decorate her room. She would shout from her bedroom window day and night resulting in neighbors filing multiple police reports. This behavior was consistent across both parental households, and she stopped attending school several weeks prior to admission.

While in the hospital psychiatric unit, she continued with her erratic behavior, making signs and laying them out in her room in a pattern that could not be disturbed. If the pattern was not "correct," she claimed "the devil would attack" and everyone "would go to hell." Any disruptions to her drawings, signs, and shouting statements caused her distress and concern that the devil would hurt her family and that Jesus would be mad at her. The hospital chaplain met with her in an effort to provide context and comfort, but she was unable to engage productively. She asked insightful questions, but she did not believe the responses if they contradicted her own beliefs. Claire continued to sleep poorly, poor food intake, and needed assistance in completing ADLs in the hospital. Due to Claire's age, staff not only needed parents' permission to medicate but also wanted Claire to assent. Claire's assent was important because without her willingness the likelihood of medication compliance outside of the hospital would be low. After initial discussions, the patient agreed and was started on fluvoxamine to treat her OCD. With medication, better sleep, and ERP therapy, Claire was able to improve her daily functioning and was discharged after 10 days. She was still religiously occupied, but it became a source of comfort instead of a compulsion causing distress.

This case required family input to obtain background information on religious and spiritual needs. The hospital chaplain added the element that the patient is her own autonomous person and her beliefs are valued by the medical staff. While religiosity was a symptom of her OCD, it was also used as part of her treatment to distinguish between shared beliefs and her own obsessions and compulsions.

Training and Education

The first step in evaluating patients is simply obtaining information. As much as possible, the practitioner should maintain a neutral and accepting viewpoint. Consider starting with questions such as the following:

- Are you a member of a religious community?
  - If yes, follow-up questions include:
    How active are you?
    Do you receive support there?
    How does this community feel about your psychiatric treatment?
  - If no, follow-up question:
    Do you have any spiritual beliefs that have shaped your experience?
- Are there religious or spiritual beliefs in your family (even if this is not your personal belief)?

It is important to demonstrate respect for the patient's religious or spiritual beliefs, avoid abrupt transitions from inquiry to support, and adopt a respectful and but neutral position. Even bizarre or clearly pathological religious beliefs should be handled with respect and providers should attempt to understand them. If beliefs do not appear obviously pathological and appear to facilitate coping, then the clinician should consider supporting them. It may be necessary to gently challenge beliefs that are used defensively to avoid making important life changes or attitudinal shifts. If providers assess that certain beliefs should be challenged, a therapeutic alliance is critical. Providers should consult the patient's clergy, if the patient agrees, before challenging beliefs, and discuss why certain aspects appear to be pathologic. Prayer should only be done if the patient initiates a request for it, the psychiatrist feels comfortable doing so, and the religious backgrounds of patient and psychiatrist are similar.

Problems of religion and mental illness may exist together or separately. There are three different types of religious problems that could involve mental health issues:

1. A religious problem with no other psychopathology – for instance, an individual who is anxious about their ability to tithe or volunteer at their religious organization. In this case, the appropriate intervention would be seeking counsel within their religious organization.
2. Parallel religious and mental health problems – for instance, an individual who struggles to maintain their faith after a trauma but also meets criteria for post-traumatic stress disorder (PTSD). In this case, individuals should work concurrently with a mental health practitioner and a religious leader.
3. Religious problems stemming from psychopathology – for example, an individual who seeks confession hourly due to compulsive behaviors associated with OCD – in these cases, providers should focus predominantly on mental health treatment.

When religious issues originate from a mental illness, providers should use a semi-structured interview along with the DSM-5 to determine the appropriate diagnosis. It is important to assess adaptive functioning (preceding and following the religious experience), determine whether symptoms are acute or chronic, maintain a level of openness to exploring spiritual experiences, compare idiosyncratic behavior and beliefs to normative practices in religious/spiritual community (e.g., speaking in tongues, hearing the voice of God), and recognize that psychopathology is often characterized by greater intensity, terror, and decompensation than genuine spiritual experiences. Questions a clinician can ask themselves to lead to the appropriate differential include:

1. Do current behaviors/practices exceed religious injunctions?
2. Does client overemphasize certain practices or beliefs and neglect others?
3. Do beliefs and practices promote wholeness, relatedness, and full humanness?

Disorder Specific Considerations

There are several disorder specific considerations when examining the relationship between pathology and religious and/or spiritual beliefs. Studying this topic presents with many challenges. First, because religious beliefs cannot be randomly assigned to people, research studies are primarily observational and correlational and cannot assume causality. Additionally, determining the amount of religiosity is subjective and self-reported. There are limited quality assessments to measure these concepts and lack of standardization across the field. Furthermore, an individual often has changes in the strength of their religious beliefs throughout their life and periods of increased or decreased involvement within a religious organization and/or community. Individuals that identify or associate with an organized religion have been studied significantly more than those that identify as being spiritual. Therefore, while several studies demonstrate an association between religious or spiritual beliefs and mental health, there are no causal studies, conclusions may be unreliable, findings are nuanced, and studies must be interpreted with these limitations in mind.

Substance Use Disorders

Given that most religions actively discourage the use of substances, it is unsurprising that studies generally indicate negative associations between substance abuse and religious involvement. In a review of 134 studies that examined the relationships between religious involvement and substance abuse, 90% found less substance abuse among the more religious [7].

The majority (nearly 75%) of substance abuse treatment centers use a 12-step model, which involves a religious component. Alcoholics Anonymous (AA) originated the idea for the 12-step model in 1938, when founder Bill Wilson wrote out the ideas that developed through his experience with alcoholism and other alcoholics. He wrote about the positive effects experienced when people struggling with alcoholism shared their stories with one another. Even though success rates in treating substance abuse disorders are low, 12-step programs are more successful than other models. Within the 12 steps, God or a "power greater than ourselves" is mentioned numerous times [8].

Many outpatient and residential substance use treatment programs may incorporate religious elements, such as required attendance of a 12-step program. It is critical to first ask in a neutral and direct manner what the patient's underlying belief system is. When a provider encounters someone resistant to the concept of God or a higher power (for whatever reason), it is important to underline that "God" is a loose term used to represent anything greater than the alcoholic or addict as an individual. Additionally, patients should be made aware of other evidence-based nonreligious support groups, such as Self-Management and Recovery Training (SMART Recovery). Asking about patient's religious beliefs can help inform treatment, prime patient's for appropriate expectations, and utilize religion as a source of strength, support, and resources.

Psychotic Disorders

In hospital settings, one of the hallmark questions to screen for psychotic symptoms is, "Do you hear or see things that other people don't?" If a patient reports that they hear voices when nobody is present, this may indicate the use of an antipsychotic medication. However, certain religious followers pray in order to hear God's voice talking to them. They believe they can hear God, speak directly to God, and this is shared with other members of their religious belief system.

Numerous studies have tried differentiating between schizophrenic or delusional thoughts and religious beliefs. Studies found that there are specific qualities to the visions, voices, and delusions of the psychiatrically ill, even before the onset of the illness [9]. Even when the content of their hallucinations may be influenced by religious ideas or cultural variability, specific qualities including intensity, lack of controllability, and unpleasantness, are more likely to be the result of a psychotic process rather than a religious one.

When psychosis follows a religious experience, the psychosis is more likely to be associated with a mood disorder (e.g., mania) rather than schizophrenia. Moreover, it is likely that the person was a vulnerable individual, with a past history of either psychosis or a premorbid personality. Studies that evaluated the themes of various religious/spiritual delusions report that the most common themes are of persecution by malevolent spirits, being controlled or influenced by spirits, and delusions of grandiosity where the individual feels they are a prophet [10]. Studies also suggest that religious delusions are held with more conviction and pervasiveness than other delusions [9].

Interestingly, the prevalence of religious delusions and hallucinations in patients with schizophrenia varies from country to country. One study reported a higher incidence of religious delusions among schizophrenic patients in predominantly Christian countries than in other populations [11]. Cross-cultural studies that compared people from different ethnic backgrounds suggest, in case of paranoid delusions, Christian patients more often report persecutors to be supernatural beings, compared to Muslim and Buddhist patients [11]. The authors posited this may be due to Christianity being more focused on guilt and forgiveness of sins [11].

Trauma- and Stress or-Related Disorders

Extant literature related to the interaction of religious/spiritual beliefs and trauma- and stress or-related disorders is minimal and with mixed findings. Although some studies found that religion is positively associated with the ability to cope with trauma and may deepen one's religious experience, other studies found that religion has little or negative effects on symptoms of PTSD [12]. One possible explanation for this is that a traumatic event can affect a person's core beliefs and alter their relationship to religion. Potentially moral injurious events can cause psychological distress and completely restructure a person's moral framework [13]. This would differ from person to person as the criteria of an event qualifying as morally injurious is determined by a person's value structure.

Anxiety Disorders

Some studies have examined the relationships between religiosity and specific anxiety disorders such as OCD and generalized anxiety disorder. Contrary to the views of Freud, who saw Western religion as a form of universal obsessional neurosis, empirical evidence suggests that religion is associated with higher levels of self-reported obsessive-compulsive personality traits, but not with higher levels of OCD symptomatology compared to the nonreligious [14]. Religion may encourage people to be scrupulous, but not to an obsessional extent.

The association between anxiety disorders and religious involvement appears to be complex. In a comprehensive review of the relationship between religion and generalized anxiety in 7 clinical trials and 69 observational studies, Koenig and colleagues found that half of these studies demonstrated lower levels of anxiety among more religious people, 17 studies reported no association, 7 reported mixed results, and 10 suggested increased anxiety among the more religious [7]. This suggests the need for a more individualized approach in assessing the role of religion on a patient's anxiety symptoms.

A number of pathways have been discussed in the literature through which religion/spirituality may buffer against depressive and anxious symptomatology, including decreased substance use/abuse, increased support, and emphasis of positive emotions, such as altruism, gratitude, and forgiveness [15, 16]. In addition, religion generally promotes a positive worldview, answers some of the why questions, promotes meaning, can discourage maladaptive coping, and promotes thinking outside oneself [16]. On the other hand, those who question their beliefs or tend to be more prone to guilt, scrupulosity, and following moral rules might show an increase in anxiety symptoms [17].

Mood Disorders

For individuals that find comfort in their religious belief system, rates of depression are often lower. As meta-analysis by Koening and colleagues showed in 93 observational studies, two-thirds found lower rates of depressive symptomatology and diagnoses in people who identified as more religious [7]. In 34 studies that did not find this inverse relationship, 30 found no association, and 4 reported that being religious was associated with more depression [7]. Additional longitudinal research suggests that greater self-reported religiousness predicts more mild symptoms of depression and faster remission at follow-up [7]. Smith and colleagues conducted a meta-analysis of 31 studies that provided spiritual and religious adaptations to group psychotherapies noting a medium effect size (d = 0.56) [18]. This meta-analysis concluded that spiritually oriented psychotherapy may be beneficial to individuals with primary diagnosis of depression, anxiety, and adjustment disorders [18].

However, religious beliefs and variables are not always related to better mental health outcomes. Some studies have found inverse relationships between depression and religious identification [7]. Factors such as denomination, race, sex, and types of religious coping may affect the relationship between religion or spirituality and depression. Negative religious coping (e.g., being angry with God, feeling let down), endorsing negative support from the religious community, and loss of faith correlate with higher depression scores [19]. In general, people of Jewish descent, Pentecostals, and those with no affiliation report higher rates of depression than other religious groups [20]. Higher rates of depression in people of Jewish descent, particularly those who are not actively religious, have been documented in both cross-sectional and longitudinal studies [20]. A variety of factors may explain why people of Jewish descent at least appear to be at higher risk, including that they may be more likely to report depressive symptoms and seek help from mental health professionals. Depression rates appear highest in Jewish people of Eastern European descent, and there has long been speculation that genetic factors may contribute to depression among Ashkenazi Jews [20]. Higher rates of depression in Pentecostals may be due to people with emotional problems self-selecting themselves into Pentecostal groups because of the latter's strong focus on overcoming emotional problems (e.g., many uplifting hymns, strong emphasis on socialization, and positive content of sermons) [20]. Another reason may be the emphasis placed on evangelism by Pentecostals, leading to drawing of members from lower socioeconomic groups that may be at higher risk for depression and other mental illnesses [21].

Depression is important to treat not just because of the emotional distress but also because of the increased risk of suicide. Since religious involvement is often associated with less depression, less anger and hostility, lower rates of substance abuse, greater social support, and better coping with stress, it should not be surprising that religion is also related to less suicide [22]. Furthermore, most religions of the world condemn suicide. A systematic review of this literature, presented in the 2001 and 2012 editions of *Handbook of Religion and Health*, identified 141 studies that examined the relationship between religiosity and completed suicides, attempted suicides, or attitudes toward suicide [12]. Of those, 106 studies (75%) found an inverse relationship between the 2 factors, and only 4 studies (<3%) found more suicide attempts, completed suicide, or positive attitudes toward suicide among people with more religious or spiritual involvement [12].

Recommendations

The essential components for mental health practitioners considering religious issues in diagnosis and treatment are to:

1. Obtain information about patients' religious and cultural values.
2. Liaison with one or more well-informed people from the same cultural-religious background.
3. Consider whether religious functioning is problematic.
4. Consider whether religious functioning has been affected by other psychopathology.
5. Consider how religion is used in coping, with emphasis placed on contextual factors.
6. Help patients clarify how their religious beliefs and practices influence the course of illness. Refrain from giving religious advice. Whatever one's religious background, the professional's moral stance should be neutral, with no attempt to manipulate the patient's beliefs. Clinicians must be aware of how their own religious beliefs affect the therapy process. Direct religious intervention, such as the use of prayer, remains controversial.
7. Remain alert to the need for religious sensitivity and the need to become educated about specific beliefs and practices. At times, patients' religious views may conflict with medical/psychotherapeutic treatment, and clinicians must endeavor to understand the patient's worldview and, if necessary, consult with clergy or religious leaders. It may be appropriate to involve members of the religious community to provide support and to facilitate rehabilitation.
8. Religion or spirituality may have therapeutic implications for mental health. Randomized-controlled trials indicate that religious interventions (e.g., spiritual meditation, pastoral services) among religious patients enhance recovery from anxiety, substance use, and mood symptoms [23]. Psychoeducational groups that focus on spirituality can lead to greater understanding of problems, feelings, and spiritual aspects of life [24].

Conclusion

In order to treat patients through a culturally competent lens, it is important to examine all aspects of their life, including religious and spiritual beliefs. This is an individualized and personal experience, so asking background questions, gaining insight into belief systems, and appreciating the role it plays in a patient's world are important. Mental illness is heavily influenced by a person's understanding of how they exist in the world and their relationship to the importance of human life. While religion can often provide comfort to those experiencing depression and be a protective factor against suicide, it can also cause internal turmoil to those who are concerned their actions are sinful or become a preoccupation or part of a delusion. Throughout history mental illness and religion were linked, including beliefs that mentally unwell were possessed by demons, displeased a higher power, or not on the virtuous path. Even now, religious problems may present with psychiatric disorders such as psychosis, OCD, and mania or independent of them. Treatment historically focused on religious healing. With the Western medicine movement, we now look to different methods of treatment, including pharmacological approaches. However, within the medical model, it is still crucial to address the religious undercurrent. It is often important for mental health professionals to consult religious leaders to gain further insight into protective or maladaptive aspects of religious beliefs and assess functioning and the context in which it presents. Even when a religious preoccupation presents as a psychiatric symptom, gaining insight into the importance and specific benefits may help with treatment planning and coping. It is important to assess adaptive functioning so that the clinician can understand when a client is using maladaptive coping skills. Obtaining history that determines religious involvement predating psychiatric symptoms can provide diagnostic clarification and provide a path toward treatment. Distinguishing whether religious focus is symptomatic or protective (or neither) is essential, but it is also important to remember that even when religiosity is attributed to psychopathology, it may be incorporated into treatment.

Summary of High-Yield Points

- Throughout human history, many cultures have viewed mental illness as a form of religious punishment or demonic possession.
- Although religious identification is increasing worldwide, it is declining in Western Europe and North America and is lower in psychiatrists than other types of physicians [2, 4].
- It is important to obtain a religious and spiritual history of each patient, including understanding how religion and spirituality fits into their life, if at all, where they gain support and strength, the cultural and community context of their environment, and identified resources and supports in the community.

- Mental health professionals may consider liaising with one or more well-informed people from the same cultural-religious background, or religious leaders, to better understand and support their patient.
- Religious themes are a symptom in many psychiatric disorders. For example, loss of faith is common in depression and PTSD, religious preoccupations or compulsions may be part of an anxiety disorder, and grandiose or delusional religious beliefs may be symptoms of bipolar or psychotic disorders [3].
- Overall, most studies have found religious and spiritual identification to be associated with positive mental health outcomes including lower rates of suicidal behaviors, substance abuse, and depression and greater social support, optimism, and meaning and purpose in life [5, 23].
- When distinguishing between pathological or nonpathological religious experiences consider adaptive functioning preceding and following the religious experience, determine whether symptoms are acute or chronic, maintain a level of openness to exploring spiritual experiences, compare idiosyncratic behavior and beliefs to normative practices in religious/spiritual community (e.g., speaking in tongues, hearing the voice of God), and recognize that psychopathology is often characterized by greater intensity, terror, and decompensation than genuine spiritual experiences.

References

1. Smith G, et al. US decline of Christianity continues at rapid pace. October 2019. https://www.pewforum.org/2019/10/17/in-u-s-decline-of-christianity-continues-at-rapid-pace/.
2. Sherwood H. Religion: why faith is becoming more and more popular. August 2018. https://www.theguardian.com/news/2018/aug/27/religion-why-is-faith-growing-and-what-happens-next.
3. American Psychiatric Association. Diagnostic and statistical manual of mental disorders. 5th ed. American Psychiatric Publishing; 2013.
4. Curlin FA, Odell SV, Lawrence RE, et al. The relationship between psychiatry and religion among US physicians. Psychiatr Serv. 2007;58:1193–8.
5. Appel J. Is religion good or bad for us? The psychology of belief. https://medium.com/thrive-global/.
6. Tillich P. In: Kimball RC, editor. Theology of culture. Oxford University Press; 1959. p. 42.
7. Koenig HG, McCullough ME, Larson DB. Handbook of religion and health. Oxford University Press; 2001. p. 514–54.
8. Connors GJ, Tonigan JS, Miller WR. A longitudinal model of intake symptomatology, AA participation, and outcome: retrospective study of the project MATCH outpatient and aftercare samples. J Stud Alcohol. 2001;62:817–25.
9. Appelbaum P, Robbins P, Roth L. Dimensional approach to delusions: comparison across types of diagnoses. Am J Psychiatry. 1999;156:1938–43.
10. Mohr S, Borras L, Betrisey C, Pierre-Yves B, Gilliéron C, Huguelet P. Delusions with religious content in patients with psychosis: how they interact with spiritual coping. Psychiatry. 2010;73:158–72.
11. Stompe T, Ortwein-Swoboda G, Chaudhry HR, Friedmann A, Wenzel T, Schanda H. Guilt and depression: a cross-cultural comparative study. Psychopathology. 2001;34:289–98.
12. Koenig HG, King DE, Carson VB. Suicide. In: Handbook of religion and health. 2nd ed. New York: Oxford University Press; 2012. p. 174–90.

13. Evans WR, Stanley MA, Barrera TL, et al. Morally injurious events and psychological distress among veterans: examining the mediating role of religious and spiritual struggles. Psychol Trauma. 2018;10:360–7.
14. Abramowitz JS, Jacoby RJ. Scrupulosity: a cognitive–behavioral analysis and implications for treatment. J Obsessive Compuls Relat Disord. 2014;3(2):140–9.
15. National Center on Addiction and Substance Abuse at Columbia University. So help me god: substance abuse, religion and spirituality. November 2001.
16. Pargament KI, Koenig HG, Perez LM. The many methods of religious coping: development and initial validation of the RCOPE. J Clin Psychol. 2000;56:519–43.
17. Harris JI, Schoneman SW, Carrera SR. Approaches to religiosity related to anxiety among college students. Men Health Relig Cult. 2002;5:253–65.
18. Smith TB, Bartz J, Richards PS. Outcomes of religious and spiritual adaptations to psychotherapy: a meta-analytic review. Psychother Res. 2007;17:643–55.
19. Ano GG, Vasconcelles EB. Religious coping and psychological adjustment to stress: a meta-analysis. J Clin Psychol. 2005;61:461–80.
20. Levav I, Kohn R, Golding JM, Weissman MM. Vulnerability of Jews to affective disorders. Am J Psychiatr. 1997;154:941–7.
21. Koenig HG, George LK, Meador KG, Blazer DG, Dyck PB. Religious affiliation and psychiatric disorder among protestant baby boomers. Hosp Community Psychiatry. 1994;45(6):586–96.
22. Rasic DT, Belik SL, Elias B, et al. Swampy Cree Suicide Prevention Team. Spirituality, religion and suicidal behavior in a nationally representative sample. J Affect Disord. 2009;114:32–40.
23. Lucchetti G, Lucchetti ALG, Avezum A. Religiosity, spirituality and cardiovascular diseases. Rev Bras Cardiol. 2011;24:55–7.
24. Hefti R. Integrating religion and spirituality into mental health care, psychiatry and psychotherapy. Religions. 2011;2:611–27.

Biculturalism: The Case of Two North American Neighbors

8

Bernardo Ng and Nancy Catherine Colimon-Ardila

I will build a great wall—and nobody builds walls better than me, believe me—and I'll build them very inexpensively. I will build a great, great wall on our southern border, and I will make Mexico pay for that wall. Mark my words. Donald J. Trump, President of the United States of America, 2016–2020

The closeness between the United States and Mexico is more than just a relationship between two governments. Enrique Peña Nieto, President of the United States of Mexico, 2012–2018

Introduction

According to the Merriam-Webster dictionary, the noun *biculturalism* and the adjective *bicultural* are defined as relating to, or including, two distinct cultures [1]. The cultural aspects of "two neighbors" are presented in this chapter. The neighbors are the United States and the United Mexican States, as per their proper political names; for purposes of this chapter, they are referred to as the United States (US) and Mexico, their more commonly used names.

B. Ng (✉)
Department of Psychiatry, University of California San Diego, San Diego, CA, USA

Sun Valley Behavioral Medical and Research Centers, Imperial, CA, USA

Nuevo Atardecer, Geriatric Center, Mexicali, BC, Mexico

Mexican Psychiatric Association, Mexico City, Mexico
e-mail: bng@sunvalleyb.com

N. C. Colimon-Ardila
Nuevo Atardecer, Geriatric Center, Mexicali, BC, Mexico

Mexican Psychiatric Association, Mexico City, Mexico

Colombian Association of Biological Psychiatry, Bogotá, Colombia

S. H. Koh et al. (eds.), *Diversity in Action*,
https://doi.org/10.1007/978-3-030-85401-0_8

Territories once occupied by Spain, France, and Great Britain turned into a land shared by two countries that have grown next to each other for centuries. Despite their differences in geographical extension, population size, official language, and economic power, they maintain a vibrant interaction in cultural and commercial trade and a bidirectional flow of people and goods. This interaction is so robust that the culture of people growing up in either country is greatly influenced by the culture of the other country. This chapter addresses the concept of biculturalism and how it influences the manifestation and prognosis of mental illness, based on models proposed by Cohen [2] and by Chen and Padilla [3]. Relevant issues such as self-esteem, prosocial behavior, religion, socioeconomic status, and region of the country are covered [2–4]. The chapter starts with a historical review from the fifteenth to the twentieth century focused on events that illustrate the beginning of the relationship between these two countries, with differences and similarities, and the subsequent impact on their cultural foundations. The next part of the chapter recounts specific historical events, where the American and the Mexican cultures have interacted, followed by the migration phenomena, and the neighbors' border region. Then, sociocultural models of biculturalism and illuminating clinical vignettes are presented. The chapter closes with clinical recommendations, a summary of high yield points, and comments regarding how biculturalism is likely to prevail and flourish in the relationship of these two neighboring countries.

Background

Biculturalism in the Context of Culture

Biculturalism embodies the degree to which individuals internalize relationships, attitudes, behaviors, and values from two cultural systems and develop the competence needed to successfully respond to demands from both. It incorporates the ability to simultaneously navigate and integrate inherited and host cultural domains, and it is therefore expected to be beneficial for behavioral adjustment and mental health outcomes [5]. Biculturalism is not only applicable to immigrants and children of immigrants but also may apply to individuals who live in a region shared by two different cultures.

Biculturalism predates the concepts of multiculturalism, which can be defined as ethnic or cultural pluralism. When two or more cultures are prevalent in a region, setting, family, or individual, there is often a combination of contention and balance between the two. The relationship between the majority and minority culture plays a role in identification and adoption of cultural practices. Acculturation refers to assimilation into a dominant or prevailing culture. Differences in acculturation are often seen in first-generation immigrants compared to second-generation immigrants. Additionally, specific behaviors can be classified into three categories: monoculturalism, blended or fused biculturalism, and alternating biculturalism. Fusion, or blended biculturalism, integrates both cultures, while alternating biculturalism describes an individual shifting behaviors between the two cultures depending on context.

Historical Significance Between the Two Countries

This section is a non-comprehensive description highlighting events and historical context that pertains to the relationship between the two countries. The section will give some historical and cross-cultural context in working with patients identifying as bicultural.

Numerous indigenous civilizations that emigrated from Asia once occupied US and Mexico land. These groups were distributed throughout the American continent, with different forms of societal and governmental organization, until they were "discovered" by Christopher Columbus in 1492. Within decades of this news reaching Europe, fierce colonization took place with Spain, Netherlands, France, Denmark, and Great Britain occupying these territories through the sixteenth century. By the early seventeenth century, Spain occupied all of Mexico and most of the western half of the United States, while Great Britain, and France occupied the rest of the US territory [6, 7].

I. *The United States*

In 1776 the United States declared its independence from Great Britain, engaging in military combat until the Treaty of Paris was signed in 1783. The new nation gained quick recognition of its emancipation throughout the western world. At the time, the United States occupied most of the eastern seaboard, up to the Mississippi River. The United States had an established economic system that rapidly adapted to its new life as a free nation and went through a phase of military strengthening and territorial expansionism during the first half of the nineteenth century. Under the Monroe doctrine, aiming to avoid additional interventions from Europe, the United States expanded in all directions until modern borders with Canada and Mexico were defined.

From 1861 to 1865, under the presidency of Abraham Lincoln, the United States engaged in the Civil War. During these years, the United States was at risk of separating into two nations. Yet, the war kept the Union together and slavery was abolished. During the rest of the nineteenth century, the United States became a key player in the Industrial Revolution. The country's economic strength was represented by iconic figures such as financier John P. Morgan, oil magnate John D. Rockefeller, and steelmaker Andrew Carnegie. The beginning of the twentieth century was one of economic growth until the stock market crashed in 1929. The first decades of the century are considered "progressive" movements: women were allowed to vote, labor unions grew stronger, the Federal Reserve was created, and the Panama Canal was built.

After the recovery from the 1929 economic crash, the United States successfully went through the First and Second World Wars and in 1946 was one of the protagonists of the Cold War era. The dominant themes at the time were preventing communism throughout the American continent, enhancing civil rights, and the technological arms race. By the end of this century, the New York Stock Exchange prevailed as the financial leader in the world, and free trade became the name of the game [6, 8].

II. *Mexico*

In 1810, Mexico declared its independence from Spain and engaged in military combat until the Treaty of Cordoba was signed in 1821. Various factors prevented Mexico from entering a path of societal and economic growth. Civil unrest continued with persistent conflict and armed outbreaks between conservatives and liberals. Economic progress was hindered by persistent financial demands from the Vatican and other European countries. Two foreign interventions occurred during this century, one from the United States and one from France. The former came with the loss of half its territory, and the latter with the imposition of an Emperor, who was defeated in 1867 by Mexican army general Porfirio Diaz.

Diaz was elected president in 1876, and while he allegedly worked to have Mexico join the Industrial Revolution, the country started the twentieth century in a serious state of poverty and inequality, unable to transition to democracy. Under those circumstances, an insurgent military action, known as the Mexican Revolution, emerged in 1910 causing Diaz's resignation and ending in 1922. Despite the newly instituted postrevolutionary government, it took decades to transition from a military government to a civil government. The dominant themes during this time focused on attaining a military loyal to its president, a fair distribution of agricultural land, public education, and the diplomatic relationship with the United States and the Vatican. The relationship with the Vatican was so delicate that a war broke from 1926 through 1929, known as the "Mexican Crusade" [7].

By 1935 labor unions propagated. In 1938 came the expropriation of power and oil and aggressive distribution of farming land, including the distribution of land owned by Americans in Mexico. The rest of the twentieth century was controlled by political figures of one political party, whose dominance ended in 1994 after the assassination of their presidential candidate. Also, in 1994, Mexico joined the North American Free Trade Agreement (NAFTA), which is further explained below. While the nation's economic growth varied throughout the years, poverty and socioeconomic inequality persisted [6, 7].

III. *Shared Historical Events*

(a) *Guadalupe-Hidalgo treaty (1848)*

Mexico's economic and political instability during the nineteenth century prevented its government from properly controlling its borders. In 1836, the state of Texas separated from Mexico, gained recognition by Great Britain in 1841, and soon after joined the United States. In 1845, the United States declared war on Mexico under the presidency of James Polk. As a result of this war, the Treaty of Guadalupe-Hidalgo was signed in 1848, and the territory from Texas to California, up to the Canadian border, became part of the United States [6, 7].

(b) *California Gold Rush (1849)*

In 1848, there were slightly over 157,000 people in California (31st state of the Union), of which 150,000 were Native Americans, 6500 of Spanish and/or

Mexican descent known as "Californios," and fewer than 800 were non-Native Americans. By the mid-1850s, there were over 300,000 arrivals due to the Gold Rush, including Americans, Mexicans, Chinese, and other Latin Americans. Violence against "foreign miners," including Mexicans, erupted. Beatings, rapes, and murders became common, even against Mexican-Americans, due to their phenotype [9, 10].

(c) *French invasion to Mexico (1861–1865)*

In 1861, due to Mexico's persistent political uncertainty, Spain, France, and Great Britain sent troops to secure their existing financial interests. Negotiations were successful with Spain and Great Britain followed by the removal of their troops, but not with France. In 1862, Napoleon III invaded Mexico, and in 1864 declared the Austrian Archduke Maximiliano of Hesburgh as the new Emperor of Mexico. A year later, US President Andrew Johnson revived the Monroe doctrine, and France ceased its military support to continue occupying Mexico. Nonetheless, Emperor Maximiliano remained in Mexico to defend his position until he was captured, judged, and executed in 1867 [6–8].

(d) *The 18th Amendment of the US Constitution prohibiting the production, transportation, and sale of intoxicating beverages (1919–1933)*

While the 1920s marked a violent and dry period in many regions of the United States, it was an era of prosperity in various Mexican cities near the US border. The industries of food, beverages, and entertainment flourished, with US celebrities and wealthy citizens traveling to spend days to weeks at a time in a country where alcohol and gambling were legal [11]. A cultural residue of that bloodstained era in the US persists now with the so-called spring breakers, when American college students spend their spring break in Mexico, frequently at a beach destination (e.g., Cancún, Puerto Vallarta, Los Cabos), where music, alcohol, and drugs are readily available. Spring break currently marks the beginning of the high tourist season at many of these destinations. In 2018, 39% of all Americans traveling internationally went to Mexico [12]. In the border cities, this activity occurs nearly all weekends or holidays throughout the year. High school graduates can drink at the age of 18 in Mexico, which is three years earlier than the legal drinking age in the United States [13].

(e) *Mexican Repatriation (1929–1936)*

Mass deportation of Mexicans and Mexican-Americans from the United States to Mexico, known as the era of Mexican Repatriation, started after the 1929 financial crash. It has been suggested that an anti-Mexican sentiment began before 1929. The sense of despair plaguing the United States during the financial crisis created a desire for a convenient scapegoat, and they found it in the Mexican community. It is estimated that nearly two million children and adults were deported, of which 60% were birthright US citizens. Given that the identification of those to be reported was by their phenotype, some scholars consider this historical event a process of ethnic cleansing [14, 15].

(f) *Inter-American Conference on Problems of War and Peace (1945)*

Soon after WWII, Mexico was the host of an international meeting with 20 nations, including the United States and most of the Latin American countries. The original goal was to develop a unified front toward the upcoming international order. It was one of the first manifestations of the United States and Mexico working together toward the same goals within the continent. Mexico would take advantage of its natural geopolitical position, as a bridge between the Anglo and the Hispanic sides of the continent [7].

(g) *North American Free Trade Agreement (1994)*

The North American Free Trade Agreement (NAFTA) has been in effect since 1994. It was signed by President George H. W. Bush in 1992, approved by Congress in 1993, and implemented into law by President William J. Clinton on December 8, 1993. While the United States and Canada had a free trade agreement since 1989, the uniqueness of this trilateral agreement was that it involved the participation of two developed countries and one developing country. Mexican President Carlos Salinas de Gortari illustrated this novelty during a conference at Stanford University, stating:

> We want trade, not aid, to generate more employment-- free trade… We do not want to see the century come to an end and find that new (international) arrangements have been made without us. [16]

Nationalists with protectionist views on both sides of the border predicted risks of each countries' sovereignty. Nonetheless, US trade with its NAFTA partners has more than tripled since the agreement took effect. It has increased more rapidly than trade with the rest of the world. Since 1993, US trade with Mexico grew faster than trade with Canada or with non-NAFTA countries. In 2011, trilateral trade among NAFTA partners reached the $1.0 trillion threshold. In 2016, Canada was the leading market for US exports, while Mexico ranked second. The two countries accounted for 34% of total US exports in 2016. In imports, Canada and Mexico ranked second and third, respectively, as suppliers of US imports in 2016. The two countries accounted for 26% of US imports. American businesses such as Walmart and Ford set shop in Mexico. At the same time, Mexican entrepreneurs acquired or started new businesses in the United States and created nearly 3,000,000 US jobs (e.g., Bimbo Bakery) by 2018 [17, 18]. NAFTA critics have highlighted that neither working conditions in Mexico have improved, nor has the economic gap between the United States and Mexico decreased as expected. While the debate continues regarding the met and unmet goals of this agreement, NAFTA has promoted biculturalism [18].

(h) *War on drugs (1970–2019)*

The war on drugs has been lengthy and bloody; it has both allowed the countries to work together, as well as exhibit their corruptible potential. At one point, Mexico was identified as the biggest producer, and the United States the biggest consumer, of illegal drugs [19]. The turn of the twenty-first century marked one of the bloodiest periods in Mexico. A long list of drug cartels fought for the hegemonic control of the market that was eventually seized by the Sinaloa Cartel, led by the famous "El Chapo Guzman" [19]. During the most violent phase of this era, the US Department of State started to "certify" or "decertify" Mexico as a warning for Americans when considering travel to Mexico. As reasonable as this measure was for the regular citizen, it was also controversial as most of the cartels illegally purchased their guns from the United States. The most painful part of this era has been the number of civilian casualties [20–22]. In the last decade, two events brought this war to an apparent pause. First, the decriminalization of the recreational use of marijuana in California and ten other states decreased the demand for marijuana from Mexico [23]. Second is the ultimate incarceration of "El Chapo," who escaped two out of the three times he was captured and held in maximum-security prisons in Mexico. On his third apprehension, he was extradited to the United States where he has been judged and sentenced to life in prison, plus 30 years at the nation's most secure supermax prison [19]. The latest news of this war is the detention of the former Mexican Secretary of Public Security in 2019 for accepting millions of dollars in bribes from the Sinaloa Cartel [24].

(i) *The United States-Mexico-Canada Agreement (2018)*

The United States-Mexico-Canada Agreement (USMCA), an updated and modernized NAFTA agreement, was signed by presidents Donald Trump from the United States, Enrique Peña Nieto from Mexico, and Prime Minister Justin Trudeau from Canada between 2018 and 2019 and is expected to be implemented in 2020. We have yet to see the agreement's effects on the economies of the three partners and the impact on the biculturalism between Mexicans and Americans [25].

IV. *Migration between the United States and Mexico (twentieth to twenty-first century)*

From 1942 to 1964, a series of bilateral agreements between Mexico and the United States, known as the "Bracero Program," allowed millions of Mexican men to travel to and work in 24 of the US states under primarily agricultural labor contracts. Around 4.6 million contracts were signed, with many individuals signing multiple contracts, making it the largest US contract labor program in history. Outside of this program, Americans and Mexicans have migrated in both directions, both legally and illegally, through the rest of the twentieth and the beginning of the twenty-first century [26].

Beyond the Bracero Program, economics continued to be the main driver for migrations. Young Mexicans, usually men, migrated to the United States looking for better wages and in an effort to avoid the poor working conditions in Mexico. This is mostly represented by unskilled workers in farming and hard labor. These migrants typically settled in western US states such as California, Arizona, Nevada, Oregon, and New Mexico. Yet, migrants have located as far from the border as Ohio, New Jersey, and Illinois. It has been reported that in the last two decades, a shift to more skilled workers has occurred [18]. There are also very affluent Mexicans who own a "second home" in the United States so their children can attend world-renowned schools and enjoy a safer environment. The main destinations of these migrants include cities like Houston, Los Angeles, and Miami [27, 28]. In contrast, most Americans that migrate to Mexico are retirees who are on a fixed income and cannot find the appropriate conditions to live comfortably in the United States anymore. Those that migrate to Mexico find better economic opportunities while enjoying privileged weather. Others experience favorable circumstances to start new business enterprises in a safe environment. The main settlements are by the Pacific Ocean, in the states of Baja California (Ensenada) and Baja California Sur (Los Cabos). Other areas chosen by those with better economic conditions are in the states of Jalisco (Puerto Vallarta), Nayarit (Nuevo Vallarta), and Guanajuato (San Miguel Allende) [29–31]. Migration flow, in both directions, includes documented and undocumented residents. According to the 2018 US Census, Mexican-Americans defined as being of full or partial Mexican ancestry, made up 37.0 million or 11.3% of the entire US population. It is estimated that 4.9 million are undocumented, which represents 13.2% of all those of Mexican descent in the United States. In contrast, Mexico's INEGI (Instituto Nacional de Estadística Geografía e Informática), equivalent to the US Census, reported that in 2015 the population in Mexico was made up of 739,168 or 0.6% Anglo-Americans. The report also presented that 673,866 were undocumented, which represents 91.2% of all Anglo-Americans in Mexico [32–34]. These numbers are summarized below in Table 8.1.

Table 8.1 Total and percentages of Mexican migrants in the United States and Anglo-American migrants in Mexico

	United States	Mexico
Total population	327,167,439	119,938,473
Total immigrant population from the neighbor country	36,986,661	739,168
% of the host country total population	11.3%	0.6%
Undocumented immigrants from the neighbor country	4,900,000	673,866
% of the total immigrant population from the neighbor country	13.2%	91.2%

Sources: INEGI, US Census

V. *The US-Mexico border region*

In 1983, the two neighbors signed The La Paz Agreement to protect, improve, and conserve the environment of the border region. The US-Mexico border region (USMBR) was then defined as the area of land 100 kilometers (62.5 miles) north and south of the international boundary. It stretches approximately 2000 miles from the southern tip of Texas to California, defining it as the longest border in the world. It has 35 ports of entry for legal transit and large sections with no wall at all. The population living on this stretch of land was estimated to be approximately 15.0 million people in 2010 and is expected to double by 2020 [35]. The USMBR includes 2 sovereign nations, 4 states in the United States, and 6 states in Mexico, encompassing 44 counties and 80 municipalities, respectively, with a total of 15 pairs of sister cities and 25 Native American Nations. The combined population of the four American border states is 70.9 million, and the combined population of the six Mexican border states is 19.9 million [35].

The USMBR is a dynamic region with unique public health, infrastructure, educational, and economic challenges. Its interdependence makes it a natural process to work together with an efficient and faster border, rather than an impenetrable wall. One of the most interesting demonstrations of regional economic development is the CaliBaja Bi-National Mega-Region that concentrates on five strategic areas, advanced manufacturing, agriculture, applied biotechnology, clean technologies, and logistics, with goods and services moving to both sides of the border daily [36]. Another important reason for keeping an open, yet efficient, border is the commercial interdependence at the local level. It is not only the longest but the most frequently crossed border in the world, and hundreds of thousands of workers, students, tourists, and shoppers go to either country on a daily basis. Mexican shoppers represent over a third of retail sales, and Mexican students represent almost half of the school's population of US border cities, such as McAllen, Laredo, and San Ysidro. By the same token, American shoppers represent high drugstore and optometrists' sales in Mexican border cities [37, 38]. The authors of this chapter live and practice in a pair of USMBR sister communities of Imperial County in California and the Municipality of Mexicali, in Baja California. In this community, the most represented ethnicity is formed by people of Mexican descent, who have interacted, for over a century, with an economically dominant community of Anglo-European American descendants. The population of Hispanic origin in Imperial County (80.6%) is more than double the average of Hispanics in the entire state (38.1%) [32].

The debate over the security and efficiency of the current wall has long existed, even before the inflammatory statements made by President Donald J. Trump during his electoral campaign:

> When Mexico sends its people, they're not sending the best. They're not sending you, they're sending people that have lots of problems and they're bringing those problems.

> They're bringing drugs, they're bringing crime. They're rapists and some, I assume, are good people, but I speak to border guards and they're telling us what we're getting.

However, the areas without a wall are often inhabitable deserts or mountainous terrain, which are impossible to cross. This is why a "smart wall" has been suggested as a better solution [39].

Biculturalism in the Context of Art, Business, Science, and Entertainment

The twenty-first century has been marked by unprecedented migration. This has increased the interaction of people with different cultural backgrounds in schools, places of work, entertainment centers, churches, and banks, among other settings and scenarios. Consequently, biculturalism and multiculturalism are likely to become the rule, rather than the exception, in our society [40]. This has not come passively, especially between the United States and Mexico. As reviewed, history shows the presence of Mexicans and Americans on both sides of the border for centuries. Some have resulted in such close interaction that bicultural and binational families have originated. In contrast to interracial or interethnic relationships, the descriptor "bicultural families" is used to describe the product of bicultural relationships that foster and promote cultural appreciation of both identities. In addition to shared political and historical events, there are many notable figures and celebrities that encompass the growing pool of biculturals in the United States and Mexico:

(a) Vikki Carr

This singer has music hits in English and in Spanish. Born in El Paso, Texas, to parents with Mexican ancestry. She has earned three Grammy Awards and a Latin Grammy Lifetime Achievement Award.

(b) Alfonso Cuarón

Mexican-born film director who earned 13 Academy Awards, 15 BAFTA Awards, and three Golden Globe Awards. His films include Children of Men, Gravity, and Roma.

(c) Lila Downs

Singer and songwriter. Daughter of Anita Sanchez, singer from Oaxaca, Mexico, and Allen Downs, a professor of art and cinematography from Minnesota. She has earned one Grammy and five Latin Grammys.

(d) Tony Garza.

A lawyer who was the US Ambassador to Mexico from 2002 to 2009. Son of Antonio Garza Sr., from Reynosa, Tamaulipas, and Isabel Garza from Wilson, Texas. Mexico bestowed on him the Águila Azteca award in 2009, which is the highest granted to nonnationals. He was married to Mexican millionaire María Asunción Aramburuzabala Larregui from 2005 to 2010.

(e) Ha*Ash

Pop music duo formed by Ashley Grace and Hanna Nicole Perez. Born in Lake Charles, Louisiana, their music has been a success in Mexico. Their parents are American-born Antonio Perez and Mexican-born Mathilda Mosa. They have earned the Gaviota de Oro at the Viña del Mar International Song Festival.

(f) Jeff Luhnow

General manager and president of baseball operations for the Major League Baseball Houston Astros. He was born in Mexico City and is a graduate of the University of Pennsylvania, Kellogg School of Management.

(g) Mario Molina

Mexican-born chemist who won a Nobel Prize in 1995 and was a professor at the Massachusetts Institute of Technology and the University of California, San Diego.

(h) Selena Quintanilla-Perez

Tex-Mex diva and Queen of Tejano music. Born to Marcella Ofelia Samora of Cherokee ancestry and Mexican-American Abraham Quintanilla Jr. in Freeport, Texas. She earned 1 Grammy, 14 Billboard Latin Music Awards, and 5 BMI Music Awards.

(i) Alfredo Quiñones-Hinojosa

Mexican-born physician who leads the department of Neurological Surgery at Mayo Clinic in Jacksonville, Florida. Born in Mexicali, Baja California to Mexican parents. He was once a migrant farm worker in California.

(j) Bill Richardson

30th governor of New Mexico and the ninth US Secretary of Energy, born in Pasadena, California. Son of William Blaine Richardson Jr., an American bank executive of Mexican descent from Boston, Massachusetts, and María Luisa López-Collada, originally from Mexico City, Mexico.

Culturally Competent Care and Biculturalism

Interaction Between Psychiatry and Biculturalism

Culture refers to the values, traditions, beliefs, language, and interactions that identify a society or a group of persons. These cultural factors include art (e.g., music, literature), religion, gastronomy, economy, education, and impact the way one interacts with their significant other, family, peers, coworkers, and society in general [41]. It has been described extensively that the predominant culture in the United States is individualistic and the one in Mexico is collectivistic (i.e., *familism*), and both factors impact behaviors regarding health and illness [42, 43]. As a first approach, we compare and contrast the following "dimensions of cultural variability" in the United States and Mexico as recommended by Cohen [2].

I. *Religion*

The dominant religion since the inception of both countries is Christian, predominantly Catholicism in Mexico, resulting in a notable difference in the relationship between church, government, and society. Even before its constitution as a free nation, the United States insisted on the freedom of religion. It was the engine that brought together the first immigrants to this land who became the founders of the Union. For centuries, societal and economic growth in the United States has been attained regardless of religious differences or surrounding conflicts. On the other hand, Mexico has struggled with a domineering Roman Catholic Church and its fervent followers which thwarted economic and political growth (e.g., the Vatican challenging commerce with Europe after the Independence War), opposed reformation laws (i.e., conservative vs. liberals), supported the establishment of an Empire (i.e., Emperor Maximiliano), sparked an armed conflict (i.e., Mexican Crusade), instigated the assassination of a president (i.e., Alvaro Obregon), and discouraged the Bracero Program, because it promoted the separation of families [7].

II. *Socioeconomic status*

There has been a clear economic superiority of the United States over Mexico and practically the rest of the world. As highlighted above, both historical and cultural factors delayed economic growth in Mexico. The disparity between the neighbors' economies has been present since the independence from Europe. Mexicans have migrated to the United States looking for better work opportunities, legally or illegally. This has had an inevitable impact on how neighbors relate with each other: as mere neighbors (i.e., early nineteenth century), as one neighbor being weaker and therefore vulnerable to invasions or in need of protection (i.e., Mexican-American

War, Franco-Mexican War), one neighbor being the provider of unskilled workers for the other (i.e., Bracero Program), one being the consumer of illegal drugs produced by the other (i.e., war on drugs), one depending on the shoppers coming across the border from the other country, and the rich neighbor and the poor neighbor or the trade partners (i.e., NAFTA). Socioeconomic status is a dynamic aspect that will not cease to evolve. In the International Monetary Fund's 2020 report, the United States remains as world economy number one and Mexico as number 15 [44].

III. *Region within a country*

For purposes of this chapter, following the Cohen model, this section focuses on specific regions of the two countries. This region is the USMBR, where the biculturalism between these two neighbors originates and thrives. These are two countries with different languages, different flags, and different economies that have converged in a region that has gradually become economically productive and culturally vibrant. While the people share a common indigenous background, their histories and societal evolution strayed considerably for centuries. Not until the last few decades has trade, culture, technology, and migration brought them closer again. One of the most iconic representations of the relationship between these two neighbors is the Cross Border Xpress bridge, which connects the cities of Tijuana in Mexico and San Diego in the United States. This pedestrian tunnel starts at a custom-built station in East San Diego and connects directly into the Tijuana International Airport. It is staffed by migration and custom inspectors of both countries, with the corresponding security filters, allowing transit from one country to the other in a matter of minutes [18].

IV. *Psychiatry and biculturalism*

Biculturalism has become a subject of study in psychiatry and mental health for at least three decades. This stems from studies of cultural identity, acculturation and migration, and its impact on mental health, behavior, cognition, substance use, and personality development [43–46]. A study on cognitive functioning measured by a battery of tests that included the six-item screener (SIS), the Brief-Spanish English Verbal Learning Test (B-SEVLT), the Controlled Oral Word Association, and the Digit Symbol Substitution Test in Mexican-Americans in California showed an association of bicultural engagements (i.e., engaging in activities in both English and Spanish languages) and higher cognitive scores [47]. This was a cross-sectional study of a subsample of the Hispanic Community Health Study/Study of Latinos, limited to adults 45 years of age and older. Other studies have shown that adolescents with higher levels of familism and biculturalism are less likely to internalize conflict and develop low self-esteem [48]. A longitudinal study on adolescent Hispanic immigrants showed that self-esteem, optimism, prosocial behavior, and family relationships were higher in those with greater scores of bicultural identity integration [49]. A study on a sample of Mexican-American adults with nicotine addiction receiving cessation treatment discovered longer periods of abstinence by those with strong American cultural identity and a strong heritage cultural identity [33].

In general, these studies suggest that those that identify as bicultural, or fused with both cultures, have better mental health than those that subscribe to only one culture within the Latin minority. Theorists argue that borrowing values from both cultures and applying them judiciously (e.g., alternating) are more conducive to mental health than indiscriminately subscribing to either culture alone [50]. Furthermore, it demonstrates cognitive and psychological flexibility, an important factor in mental health.

The phenomenon of biculturalism naturally plays an important role in the lives of mental health providers as well. Providers practicing in the United States, who were either born or raised in a different culture, are expected to understand the host culture(s) to properly meet the needs of their patients, without unsubscribing to their original culture [51].

Patient's culture and cultural context, in which their symptoms might develop, are essential considerations in the clinical setting. Biculturalism, however, has not been studied enough to thoroughly understand its impact on patient's state of health, other than the likelihood that it may be associated with better outcomes, better self-esteem, and prosocial behavior. Regardless of how much is currently understood about it, it is undeniable that a segment of the population is bicultural, and research suggests it is a favorable feature.

Vignette 1: Bill

Bill is a 46-year-old medically retired, married, Anglo-American male, who was born in rural Oklahoma and relocated to Imperial County, California, right before puberty. His father was a farm worker and his mother a full-time homemaker. He had difficulties in school likely related to an undiagnosed speech and learning disorder. Bill's parents did not comply with his teachers' suggestion to have him evaluated, even after he dropped out of high school during his sophomore year.

Bill started working in the fields, as his father did, but realized that he needed a better source of income. Eventually, he successfully attained his GED which helped him secure a job at the local power company. This was recognized as a great achievement in his family and neighborhood. In fact, he ended up marrying "the cutest and most desired girl" in his social circle. His job included paid vacation, health insurance, and a retirement plan. He worked as a heavy machine operator and was involved in setting up new electric lines around the county. Bill worked uninterruptedly for 17 years until he injured his back and became disabled.

He filed a workman's compensation claim, and while he was getting his injury addressed, he was accommodated at a desk job. His issues with reading, focusing, and learning new material resurfaced, which generated frustration and fear of getting fired. During the ensuing 3 years, he watched his ability to work diminish, his finances deteriorate, and personally worst of all, his marriage disrupted. Bill discovered his wife was cheating on him, which marked the start of the depressive episode that led him to seek treatment. This event damaged his self-esteem and ultimately resulted in him ending the marriage.

As he engaged in services at the outpatient clinic, he was diagnosed with major depressive disorder, attention-deficit/hyperactivity disorder, specific learning disorder, and a speech disorder. He was offered psychoeducation, psychotherapy, and pharmacotherapy. After various medication trials, he responded to a combination of bupropion, gabapentin, and trazodone. He also underwent a spinal surgery that consisted of an L1, L2, and L3 level laminectomy and fusion. Additional medical issues included hyperlipidemia and class I obesity.

Once Bill's income was restored, he decided to get married again, but this time, he "made sure" to partner with a Mexican woman, as he knew she would "never be unfaithful." He learned this through his cultural exchanges with Mexican classmates and coworkers. In fact, he had learned his way around both sides of the border, and crossing the border was familiar to him. Bill met a single mother with three children, one of them with school problems and substance use. It appears as if he identified with her son and decided to help him. He improved his Spanish language skills, converted to Catholicism, and remarried. Bill adopted all of her children and immigrated them to the United States.

Discussion

Growing up in Imperial County, a primarily Hispanic region, allowed Bill to become familiar with some aspects of the Mexican culture. These included exposure to language, religion, and marriage values. It became his understanding that a Mexican woman, once married, will stay married and will not be unfaithful to her husband, whether happy or not. He considered this characteristic extremely significant to him, so he decided to pursue only women of Mexican descent. It would be reasonable to argue that this marriage was the start of him becoming bicultural, but it is unlikely since his growing up in this community allowed him to learn about Mexican culture since he was a grade school student.

Vignette 2: Sebastian

Sebastian is a 20-year-old male, part-time community college student and employed part-time, who was born in southern California but grew up in Baja California, Mexico. His family includes his Mexican-born father, his Anglo-American-born mother, and two younger siblings.

During childhood, Sebastian crossed the border every day to attend school. He was a top student in his high school and was accepted to a college near San Francisco. He joined a fraternity and focused his attention on socializing over academic performance. Toward the end of his first year, he began using recreational cannabis almost daily. Sebastian was fixated on moving through the ranks among his "brothers." As a result, he skipped classes, failed to turn in assignments, and flunked exams. His breaking point occurred when a girl he liked turned him down, and he subsequently became increasingly paranoid and disorganized. Soon after, he was expelled from his fraternity for erratic behavior.

Sebastian was concerned with a delusional belief that everybody in school suddenly "discovered" he was Mexican. Since he carried his father's surname of Mexican origin, his ancestry was no secret. However, he spoke English with hardly any Mexican accent, and his phenotype was that of a White Anglo-American male; he, therefore, explained that no one had initially suspected he was actually Mexican. Additionally, he was convinced that he would become a millionaire with a brand new "dot.com" venture.

He was hospitalized, and his psychotic symptoms completely resolved only to re-emerge within 6 months when he used cannabis and was hospitalized again. After his second hospitalization, he returned to living with his parents, and after 1 year he was able to return to the local community college and work part-time. His outpatient treatment plan included a combination of quetiapine and divalproex, an outpatient substance abuse program, and a work training program.

Discussion

Sebastian has lived in a bicultural environment since birth. He divided his days, partly in Mexico and partly in the United States. He managed very well across cultures; he was bilingual, enjoyed the cuisine of both countries, and would watch Mexican and American television shows and movies. However, the context where he became ill was different than the one where he grew up. This new social setting and eagerness to fit in may have contributed to his desire to hide his Mexican heritage. Furthermore, this case raises the discussion about the effects, consequences, and availability of cannabis, in particular, social factors determining a greater availability to minorities and potential genetic factors determining a greater biological proclivity of Mexicans and Latinos to become addicted [52, 53].

The clinical vignettes presented here underscore how the encounter of two cultures impacts the manifestation of disease, help-seeking behavior, and treatment response. There are different degrees to which people identify as bicultural, and this usually changes over time (as illustrated in case one) and across contexts (as illustrated in case two). In the clinical field, the phenomenology of disease is an intricate and personal experience where psychological and sociological research findings have to be carefully considered.

Training and Education in Biculturalism

The seminal paper on biculturalism by LaFromboise and colleagues in 1993 defined biculturalism within various sociological models [54]. The models included acculturation, alternation, fusion, and multiculturalism, which gave the basis to understand bicultural competence and adjustment to biculturalism without suffering negative psychological outcomes. This was certainly a breakthrough as earlier sociological theorists proposed that being bicultural, or being of "mixed race," would lead individuals to suffer psychological conflict and identity confusion. This novel perspective proposed that an individual could demonstrate a high level of cultural competence in a second culture while keeping ties with the culture of origin. This required six skills:

1. Knowledge of cultural believes and values in each culture.
2. Positive attitudes toward both cultural groups.
3. Bicultural efficacy.
4. Communication ability.
5. Role repertoire.
6. Sense of being grounded in both cultures [54].

These skills are associated with better psychological and sociological outcomes when compared to individuals that choose to maintain competence in only one culture. Chen and Padilla propose the GEAR model, a theoretical framework to understand and see future development of biculturalism and bilingualism [3]. This model consists of:

1. Psychological *G*rowth: a complex, multilayered, multidimensional network of interrelated self-beliefs.
2. Cognitive *E*xploration: flexibility and creativity related to language and higher order processing.
3. Linguistic *A*wareness: bilingual speakers demonstrate greater sensitivity to different linguistic and cultural contexts.
4. Social *R*einforcement: improved social awareness and appreciation within and between cultural groups.

The GEAR model attempts to provide the basis to study and understand the assets of biculturalism and bilingualism and the common and differential effects of the two features on human behavior. In particular, the model allows for a framework to understand the complex psychological phenomenon of biculturalism, which has evolved from a past negative perspective to a more recent focus on its individual social and psychological advantages.

Researchers have expanded the study of bicultural competence to evaluate its prospective associations with mental health, including internalizing (e.g., depression) and externalizing (e.g., conduct disorder) symptoms. Two components of bicultural competence have been proposed: *comfort* (or affective bicultural competence, such as comfort with language switching) and *facility* (or behavioral bicultural competence, such as ability to switch languages), which span multiple cultural domains (e.g., affiliations, attitudes, behaviors, knowledge, values) [55, 56]. While findings are mixed, studies have suggested that individuals with greater bicultural competence may achieve higher levels of life satisfaction, self-efficacy, prosocial tendencies, and self-esteem and present lower levels of anxiety and depressive symptoms [56, 57, 58].

Consideration of a patient's comfort and facility with biculturalism, as well as their identity integration and flexibility, will likely be relevant to case conceptualization and treatment. A mental health clinician may benefit from improving their ability to identify, address, and utilize aspects of biculturalism to improve health outcomes [3, 59]. Training clinicians in cultural competence has shown to improve care and health outcomes. The question at this point is if biculturalism trainings will be categorized separately or will be an extension of existing cultural competency trainings [60].

Recommendations

The evolution of the understanding of biculturalism from the last three decades suggests that bicultural competence in individuals has a positive impact on the ability to enjoy life and draw social support. It is likely to have an impact on an individual's resilience and the manifestation of mental illness. The impact on treatment outcomes and the clinician's competency to diagnose and treat bicultural individuals is less known. As an initial approach in clinical settings, it is recommended to adopt the use of the Mexican American Biculturalism Scale (MABS) [55], which consists of three domains with nine items each:

1. Comfort, explores the individual's degree of comfort in each culture.
2. Facility, explores the individual's perception as to his/her ability to navigate the demands of each culture.
3. Advantages, explores the advantages and disadvantages the individual finds in each culture in specific situations, such as traditions, group work, and problem-solving.

Additional recommendations for mental health clinicians are to obtain an understanding of the historical context in both countries, seek exposure and experience working with diverse populations, and increase cultural competence broadly. Furthermore, clinicians who provide care for minority and/or bicultural patients should not rush through establishing if the patient belongs to one culture or another but, instead, observe how patients navigate through both cultures and realize that American and Mexican biculturalism is common in both countries.

Conclusion

It is foreseeable that sooner than later, the economic gap between these neighbors will shrink. The International Monetary Fund's 2020 report places the three members of the USMCA trade agreement as follows: the United States as the first economy of the world with a GDP of $20.5 trillion, Canada in tenth place with a GDP of $1.7 trillion, and Mexico as the 15th economy in the world with a GDP of $1.2 trillion [44]. The gap between Canada and Mexico is much smaller than the one between either one of the countries and the United States. Once economic differences are less of an issue, it is conceivable that the bicultural exchanges will be rather scientific, artistic, social, and technological; and traveling between countries will be easier.

It is also expected that the border will be more efficient in stopping drug and human traffickers entering the United States and illegal weapons entering Mexico. Hopefully, the border will become a symbol of two good neighbors, with bicultural members in both societies. In regard to the healthcare field, it is feasible that providers in both countries will continue to enhance their understanding of the "other" culture. In fact, during the writing of this chapter, an agreement was established for the exchange of psychiatry residents from a training program in California, United States, and one in Guadalajara, Mexico, to rotate in the other country as part of their training.

In the meantime, the Day of the Dead will continue to be celebrated in Los Angeles, while Halloween will be celebrated in Mexico City. Mexican cinematographers may win the Academy award again, as they did for three consecutive years. American athletes will be the stars in the Liga Mexicana del Pacífico baseball teams like Águilas de Mexicali, while Mexican athletes will be the stars of Major League Soccer teams like LA Galaxy. National Football League and Major League Baseball teams will continue to play in Mexico City and Monterrey, respectively, during their regular seasons.

Furthermore, bicultural exchanges will continue on the individual, daily, and small scale. Thousands of Mexicans will continue shopping at one of the many Walmart branches in Mexican territory, while thousands of Americans will continue working for Bimbo Bakery in American territories. The Mexican company Alsea will continue to run Starbucks in Mexico, Latin America, and Europe; and Americans will continue dining at El Pollo Loco. Chips and guacamole will continue to be the most popular snack during the Super Bowl, margaritas will the most popular mixed drink, hotdogs will be served with jalapenos, quesadillas will be served with root beer, hamburgers will be served with horchata, and breakfast burritos will help us start the day. As we prepare to host the 2026 FIFA World Cup that will take place in

16 cities of Canada, United States, and Mexico, we continue witnessing a fusion of both cultures sprinkled in daily choices.

Clinicians practicing in the United States should be aware that moving forward there will be more bicultural patients requiring care. With that in mind, clinicians should be prepared to conduct a thorough assessment to improve diagnosis, treatment, and compliance. It is also important to be cognizant that research in bicultural competence is ongoing and assessment tools are already available. Experience with theoretical models, assessment scales, and associated psychological sequelae with bicultural patients can enhance clinical practice.

Summary of High-Yield Points

- The United States and Mexico have been neighbors for centuries. In spite of the commonalities in their origins, the United States and Mexico have departed in language, economy, population, and culture.
- There is an incessant social, economic, commercial, scientific, and cultural interaction between the two countries. Individuals growing up in either country are likely to be exposed to the culture of the other country.
- The US-Mexico border region (USMBR) is the longest border in the world and is a dynamic region with unique public health, infrastructure, educational, and economic challenges.
- Biculturalism is defined as the ability to demonstrate a high level of cultural competence in a second culture while keeping ties with the culture of origin.
- Biculturalism is often associated with better psychological and sociological outcomes for individuals, particularly when an individual develops (1) knowledge of cultural believes and values in each culture, (2) positive attitudes toward both cultural groups, (3) bicultural efficacy, (4) communication ability, (5) role repertoire, and (6) a sense of being grounded in both cultures [54].
- The Mexican American Biculturalism Scale [55] is a self-administered scale that can assist in measuring the level of biculturalism of Mexican-American adolescents and adults by examining the primary domains of bicultural comfort, facility, and advantages.
- The cultural exchange between the United States and Mexico is expected to continue growing.

References

1. Merriam-Webster. Biculturalism. 2020. Available from https://www.merriam-webster.com/dictionary/biculturalism
2. Cohen AB. Many forms of culture. Am Psychol. 2009;64(3):194–204.
3. Chen X, Padilla AM. Role of Bilingualism and biculturalism as assets in positive psychology: conceptual dynamic GEAR model. Front. Psychol. 2019. doi: https://doi.org/10.3389/fpsyg.2019.02122. Available from https://www.ncbi.nlm.nih.gov/pubmed/?term=chen+x+culture+2019+gear
4. Juckett G. Caring for Latino Patients. Am Fam Physician. 2013;87(1):48–54.

5. Safa MD, White RMB, Mahrer NE, Knight GP, Gonzales NA, Pasco MC. U.S. Mexican-origin adolescents' bicultural competence and mental health in context. Cultur Divers Ethnic Minor Psychol. 2019;25(2):299–310.
6. Odegard A. American History in 90 Minutes. The clear, concise, and commonsense guide to American History. 2018.
7. Velásquez-García E. Nueva Historia General de México. México, DF: El Colegio de México; 2010.
8. Schweikart L, Allen MA. Patriot's. History of the United States: from Columbus's great discovery to America's age of entitlement. Revised edition. New York, NY: Penguin group LLC; 2014.
9. Carrigan WD. Forgotten dead: mob violence against Mexicans in the United States, 1848–1928. New York, NY: Oxford University Press; 2013.
10. Carrigan WD, Webb C. When Americans lynched Mexicans.New York Times. 2015. Available from https://www.nytimes.com/2015/02/20/opinion/when-americans-lynched-mexicans.html
11. Castillo-Udiarte R, Pérez-Cruz E, Hidalgo-Vivas G, Tarifeño L, Calvillo AL, Cruz-Piñeiro R. Nadie me sabe dar razón. Tijuana: migración y memoria. México: Ed. Instituto Nacional de Bellas Artes; 2016.
12. Waldrop T. Headed to Mexico for spring break? Travelers warned of risks. CNN. 2019. Available from https://edition.cnn.com/2019/03/09/americas/mexico-travel-alert/index.html
13. World population review. Drinking age by state. USA. 2020. Available from http://worldpopulationreview.com/states/drinking-age-by-state/.
14. Balderrama FE, Rodriguez R. Decade of betrayal: Mexican repatriation in the 1930s. University of New Mexico Press; 2006.
15. Hoffman A. Unwanted Mexican Americans in the great depression: repatriation pressures, 1929–1939. Tucson, AZ: University of Arizona Press; 1974.
16. Wilkinson T. Mexico wants trade, not aid, Salinas says. Los Angeles Times. 1991. Available from https://www.latimes.com/archives/la-xpm-1991-10-01-mn-3515-story.html
17. Villarreal MA, Fergusson IF. The North American Free Trade Agreement (NAFTA). Congressional Research Service. 2017. Report No.: www.crs.gov R42965.
18. Seele A. Vanishing frontiers: the forces driving Mexico and the United States together. New York, NY: Public Affairs; 2018.
19. Mexico Drug War fast facts. CNN. 2013. Available from https://edition.cnn.com/2013/09/02/world/americas/mexico-drug-war-fast-facts/index.html.
20. Emmot R. Timeline: key events in US war on drugs in Latin America. Reuters. 2010. Available from https://www.reuters.com/article/us-drugs-mexico/timeline-key-events-in-u-s-war-on-drugs-in-latin-america-idUKTRE60D4YF20100114.
21. Partlow J, Miroff N. Huge manhunt in Mexico as drug lord Chapo Guzmán tunnels out of prison. Washington Post.2015. Available from https://www.washingtonpost.com/world/drug-lord-chapo-guzman-tunnels-out-of-maximum-security-prison/2015/07/12/90279efe-666a-49fb-aba4-4177bb36f0a0_story.html.
22. Lemon J. Nearly all of Mexico's gun violence is committed with illegal firearms coming from US, officials say. Newsweek. 2019. Available from https://www.newsweek.com/nearly-all-mexico-violence-fueled-illegal-us-guns-1453694.
23. Ballotpedia. California Proposition 64, Marijuana Legalization (2016). Lucy Burns Institute. 2016. Available from https://ballotpedia.org/California_Proposition_64,_Marijuana_Legalization_(2016).
24. Semple K, Villegas P. Arrest of top crime fighter stuns Mexico, where corruption Is all too routine. New York Times. 2019. Available from https://www.nytimes.com/2019/12/11/world/americas/mexico-garcia-luna-indictment.html.
25. Executive office of the president. Office of the United States Trade Representative. Agreement between the United States of America, the United Mexican States, and Canada Text. 2019. Available from https://ustr.gov/trade-agreements/free-trade-agreements/united-states-mexico-canada-agreement/agreement-between.
26. Bracero History Archive. Available from http://braceroarchive.org.
27. Nickell JK. The new and rich immigrants from Mexico: how their money is changing Texas. Nation Time. 2013. Available from http://nation.time.com/2013/01/14/the-new-and-rich-immigrants-from-mexico-how-their-money-is-changing-texas/

28. Meyer EL. For rich Mexicans, parallel lives in U.S. *New York Times*. 2007. Available from https://www.nytimes.com/2007/09/16/realestate/16nati.html.
29. Bolotin C. Why some Americans are not crazy to move to Mexico. *Forbes*. 2018. Available from https://www.forbes.com/sites/chuckbolotin/2018/12/25/why-some-americans-are-not-crazy-to-move-to-mexico/#2f4dc3e94d7f.
30. Kester J. Is it safe to travel to Los Cabos? Forbes. 2018. Available from https://www.forbes.com/sites/forbestravelguide/2018/08/31/is-it-safe-to-travel-to-los-cabos/#d8c0639206af.
31. InternationalLiving. DiscoverthePleasuresofStrollingColonialSanMigueldeAllende. Available from https://internationalliving.com/countries/mexico/san-miguel-de-allende-mexico/
32. US Census Bureau. Hispanic or Latino origin by specific origin. 2018.
33. Castro J. Estadunidenses ilegales en México aumentan 37.8%. Excelsior. 2017. Available from www.excelsior.com.mx/nacional/2017/02/28/1149157#view-1
34. INEGI. Encuesta nacional de la dinámica demográfica. 2018. Available from https://www.inegi.org.mx/contenidos/programas/enadid/2018/doc/resultados_enadid18.pdf
35. US Department of Health & Human Services. The U.S.-Mexico Border Region. 2017. Available from https://www.hhs.gov/about/agencies/oga/about-oga/what-we-do/international-relations-division/americas/border-health-commission/us-mexico-border-region/index.html#
36. Cluster Mapping. Cali Baja Bi-National Mega-Region. Harvard Business School. 2019. Available from https://www.clustermapping.us/content/cali-baja-bi-national-mega-region.
37. Murphy JG. How closing the southern border would slam the U.S. economy. US Chamber of Commerce. 2019. Available from https://www.uschamber.com/series/above-the-fold/how-closing-the-southern-border-would-slam-the-us-economy.
38. Sable-Smith B. American travelers seek cheaper prescription drugs in Mexico and beyond. National Public Radio. 2019. Available from https://www.npr.org/sections/health-shots/2019/02/11/691467587/americans-seek-cheaper-meds-in-mexico.
39. Luck S. Privacy impact assessment update for the Border Surveillance Systems (BSS). Department of Human Services. 2018. Available from https://www.dhs.gov/sites/default/files/publications/privacy-pia-cbp022-bss-september2018.pdf.
40. Hossin MZ. International migration and health: it is time to go beyond conventional theoretical frameworks. BMJ Glob Health. 2020;5(2)
41. Morales A. Valores culturales. Significados. 2019. Available from https://www.significados.com/valores-culturales/.
42. McLaughlin EA, Campos-Melady M, Smith JE, Serier KN, Belon KE, Simmons JD, et al. The role of familism in weight loss treatment for Mexican American women. J Health Psychol. 2017;22(12):1510–23.
43. Rogers AT. Exploring health beliefs and care-seeking behaviors of older USA-dwelling Mexicans and Mexican-Americans. Ethn Health. 2010;15(6):581–99.
44. Silver C. Top 20 economies in the world. Investopedia. 2020. Available from https://www.investopedia.com/insights/worlds-top-economies/.
45. Bhugra D. Migration, distress and cultural identity. Br Med Bull. 2004;69:129–41.
46. Cortés DE, Deren S, Andía J, Colón H, Robles R, Kang SY. The use of the Puerto Rican Biculturality Scale with Puerto Rican drug users in New York and Puerto Rico. J Psychoactive Drugs. 2003;35(2):197–207.
47. Vásquez PM, Tarraf W, Doza A, Marquine MK, Perreira KM, Schneiderman N. The cross-sectional association of cognitive stimulation factors and cognitive function among Latino adults in Hispanic Community Health Study/Study of Latinos (HCHS/SOL). Alzheimers Dement (NY). 2019;5:533–41.
48. Smokowski PR, Bacallao ML. Acculturation, internalizing mental health symptoms, and self-esteem: cultural experiences of Latino adolescents in North Carolina. Child Psychiatry Hum Dev. 2007;37(3):273–92.
49. Schwartz SJ, Unger JB, Baezconde-Garbanati L, Benet-Martínez V, Meca A, Zamboanga BL, et al. Longitudinal trajectories of bicultural identity integration in recently immigrated Hispanic adolescents: links with mental health and family functioning. Int J Psychol. 2015;50(6):440–50.

50. de Figueiredo JM. Explaining the 'immigration advantage' and the 'biculturalism paradox': an application of the theory of demoralization. Int J Soc Psychiatry. 2014;60(2):175–7.
51. Goldner-Vukov M. A psychiatrist in cultural transition: personal and professional dilemmas. Transcult Psychiatry. 2004;41(3):386–405.
52. Melroy-Greif WE, Wilhelmsen KC, Ehlers CL. Genetic variation in FAAH is associated with cannabis use disorders in a young adult sample of Mexican Americans. Drug Alcohol Depend. 2016;166:249–53.
53. Wu LT, Swartz MS, Brady KT, Hoyle RH, NIDA AAPI Workgroup. Perceived cannabis use norms and cannabis use among adolescents in the United States. J Psychiatr Res. 2015;64:79–87.
54. LaFromboise T, Coleman HL, Gerton J. Psychological impact of biculturalism: evidence and theory. Psychol Bull. 1993;114:395–412. https://doi.org/10.1037/0033-2909.114.3.395.
55. Basilio CD, Knight GP, O'Donnell M, Roosa MW, Gonzales NA, Umana-Taylor AJ. The Mexican American biculturalism scale: bicultural comfort, facility, and advantages for adolescents and adults. Psychol Assess. 2014;26(2):539–54.
56. Safa MD, White RMB, Mahrer NE, Knight GP, Gonzales NA, Pasco MC. U.S. Mexican-origin adolescent's bicultural competence and mental health content. Cutlur Divers Ecthinc Minor Pyschol. 2019;25(2):299–310.
57. Wei M, Liao KY, Chao RC, Mallinckrodt B, Tsai PC, Botello-Zamarron R. Minority stress, perceived bicultural competence, and depressive symptoms among ethnic minority college students. Journal of Counseling Psychology. 2010;57(4):411.
58. Carlo G, Basilio CD, Knight GP. The associations of biculturalism to prosocial tendencies and positive self evaluations. Journal of Latina/o psychology. 2016;4(4):189.
59. Marín G, Gamba RJ. Acculturation and changes in cultural values. In: Chun KM, Organista PB, Marín G, editors. Acculturation: Advances in theory, measurement, and applied research. American Psychological Association. 2003;83–93.
60. Govere L, Govere EM. How effective is cultural competence training of healthcare providers on improving patient satisfaction of minority groups? A systematic review of literature. Worldviews Evid-Based Nurs. 2016;13(6):402–10.

Part III

Systems and Settings

Correctional Psychiatry

9

Sanaz Kumar and Philip J. Candilis

Vignette

Mr. A, a 28-year-old single Black male, with a history of depression with psychotic features and posttraumatic stress disorder, was sentenced to 6 months in jail for a misdemeanor drug conviction. Upon admission, Mr. A was evaluated by a staff psychiatrist. Mr. A reported persistent low mood and irritability that was previously partially controlled with SSRI treatment and intermittent therapy. Mr. A did not endorse current symptoms of psychosis, suicidality, or homicidality. He reported that he recreationally uses fentanyl a few times per year and that his last use was 2 weeks ago, at the time of his arrest. The evaluating psychiatrist found that his drug screen was positive for opiates. Given persistent depressive symptoms, she increased Mr. A's SSRI dose and scheduled follow-up in 1 month.

Due to speculation that Mr. A is the target of a local gang, custodial staff housed him in a single-occupant cell in solitary confinement, also referred to as protective custody or segregation. One week later, Mr. A began to experience panic attacks several times per day. At night, these were accompanied by nightmares and waking up in a cold sweat. Mr. A asked the correctional officer on his block to move him back to the general population because he "can't take it anymore." Suspecting that Mr. A was overstating his symptoms, the correctional officer walked away with the time-honored phrase, "If you can't do the time, don't do the crime." Feeling helpless

S. Kumar (✉)
Department of Psychiatry and Behavioral Sciences, George Washington University School of Medicine and Health Sciences, Washington, DC, USA
e-mail: sanazk@gwu.edu

P. J. Candilis
Department of Psychiatry and Behavioral Sciences, George Washington University School of Medicine and Health Sciences, Washington, DC, USA

Saint Elizabeths Hospital, Washington, DC, USA
e-mail: philip.candilis@dc.gov

S. H. Koh et al. (eds.), *Diversity in Action*,
https://doi.org/10.1007/978-3-030-85401-0_9

and frustrated, Mr. A threw his food tray against the wall. Another officer approached the cell and encouraged Mr. A to talk to him. Mr. A shouted back, "You can't help me! Just leave me alone!"

During the next several days, Mr. A refused most of his food trays and communication with staff tapered off. Officers observed him quietly sitting on the end of his bed for hours at a time. One evening during unit rounds, an officer observed blood smeared on Mr. A's cell's floor. She asked Mr. A to tell her what happened, but he remained quiet. After calling for assistance, the officers opened the cell door and realized that Mr. A had been cutting his arm with a plastic fork. Staff immediately transported him to the infirmary for evaluation by medical and mental health providers.

Mass Incarceration and Cultural Implications

Introduction

In US correctional facilities, nondominant populations are disproportionately represented. These groups can include people of color, persons diagnosed with mental illness, and those from backgrounds of social and economic disadvantage [1]. Social inequities from the community are amplified in jails and prisons where resources are limited, autonomy is restricted, and security is the primary objective. These factors coalesce into a unique cultural context within correctional settings. Psychiatrists working there may consequently find themselves navigating an environment that runs counter to their usual clinical expectations.

The Problem of Mass Incarceration

US incarceration rates are the highest in the world. Although the USA accounts for less than 5% of the world's population, it houses almost 25% of the world's prisoners [1]. According to the US Department of Justice's Bureau of Justice Statistics (BJS), about 2.2 million people were incarcerated in state prisons, federal prisons, and local jails on a given day in 2018 [2, 3]. To put this in perspective, this would be equivalent to incarcerating every resident of North Dakota, Alaska, and Wyoming [4].

Of these 2.2 million people, 1.47 million were confined in state and federal correctional facilities, where sentences are longer [2]. State and federal prisons incarcerate individuals who have been convicted of felony charges and are serving sentences of more than 1 year. Around the same time, 738,400 individuals were housed in county and city jails [3]. Jails house individuals who are awaiting trial or have already been convicted of misdemeanor charges. Because the incarceration data only represent snapshots in time, they grossly underestimate the total number of individuals incarcerated, particularly those in local jails where stays are briefer. During 2018, local jails admitted 10.7 million individuals total – nearly 15 times their average daily population [3].

These high incarceration rates raise the question of whether mass incarceration is an American cultural phenomenon. The US rate, at about 700 per 100,000 people, is seven times the average incarceration rate of Western European countries [1]. What accounts for this incongruence among democratic nations?

One hypothesis is that American values, which drive public policy decisions, contribute to this pronounced disparity. In their examination of German and Dutch prison practices, the Vera Institute of Justice, a US nonprofit research and policy organization, concluded that while German and Dutch criminal justice systems emphasize "resocialization and rehabilitation," the US system emphasizes "incapacitation and retribution" [5]. Because the German and Dutch systems focus on offenders' reintegration into society, they use prison sparingly and, instead, address crime through noncustodial sanctions and diversion [5]. Meanwhile, the US cultural emphasis on punishment and accountability favors a more extensive use of confinement [5].

Despite falling crime rates, US incarceration rates continue to rise: there has been a 500% increase in the number of incarcerated individuals in the last 40 years [6]. Experts attribute these changes to several factors. Crime rates may be falling because of demographic changes (e.g., an aging population), economic improvements (e.g., rising income and falling unemployment), and changes in policing tactics (e.g., the advent of community policing) [7]. It is not the case that crime rates are falling because more criminals are behind bars [8]. Rather, experts believe that social policy, such as regulations favoring lengthier sentences, stricter enforcement of laws, and changes in arresting patterns are driving the rise in incarceration [7]. These politically popular practices have led to the creation of what some experts have called a "carceral state" [9].

Cost of Mass Incarceration

The human cost of mass incarceration cannot be overstated. The economic, social, and personal costs of this approach can be seen in government and household budgets, in community and family relationships, and in the actual conditions of confinement. Understanding how this system serves as a stressor on prisoners, families, and communities may assist correctional psychiatrists in appreciating the powerful context of their patients' experiences.

The USA spends more than $80 billion annually incarcerating people [7]. Housing inmates in state prisons costs anywhere from $14,780 to $69,355 annually per person [10]. Consider that in New York, where incarceration costs are high, the cost to house an inmate could cover an annual salary for a teacher or firefighter [11]. Communities pick up the tab for mass incarceration in other ways too. Individuals who are incarcerated are unable to provide financial support for their families, and when fathers are incarcerated, families are 40% more likely to live in poverty [7]. Costs accrue even after one's release from confinement: individuals with criminal histories have more trouble finding employment and earn 10–40% less than those without criminal histories [7]. Prisoners themselves are effectively removed from the work force and are unavailable to pay taxes in their communities.

Social costs of mass incarceration are found in communities across the country. Incarceration affects family relationships: most American prisoners are parents to minor children [12], and these children inevitably pay the price. The President's Executive Office report *Economic Perspectives on Incarceration and the Criminal Justice System* indicates that "Parental incarceration is a strong risk factor for a number of adverse outcomes, including antisocial and violent behavior, mental health problems, school dropout, and unemployment" [7]. Individuals who have been incarcerated are less likely to be engaged in civic and political matters [1]. This holds for their families as well.

Finally, mass incarceration imposes real health and human costs upon individuals within the walls of correctional facilities. As correctional institutions have swelled with inmates, overcrowding has led to unsafe practices in some jurisdictions. In 2011, the US Supreme Court ruled that California's prisons fell short in providing inmates' basic health needs: at a time when these prisons were operating at 200% capacity, overcrowding had strained the capacity of medical and mental health services [13]. Under those circumstances, an inmate died every 6–7 days because of inadequate medical care [13]. Suicidal inmates were confined to telephone-booth-sized cages without toilets, and wait times to see mental health providers were as long as 1 year [13]. As a remedy, the Supreme Court ordered California to immediately reduce the number of incarcerated individuals [13].

Psychiatrists may consequently come to believe that mass incarceration is a dysfunctional social approach that deserves closer scrutiny. Mass incarceration is costly for everyone. Indeed, because they are overrepresented in correctional settings, mentally ill individuals and people of color pay more than their share. Psychiatrists working in corrections must come to appreciate the entire range of cultural and institutional influences on those in US correctional systems and the irreparable costs of these systems.

Overrepresentation of People of Color

People of color comprise a large segment of the incarcerated population. Black and Latinx persons make up more than half of those incarcerated in state and federal prisons, even though they represent less than one-third of the US population [7]. A report by the Sentencing Project, a US advocacy group, found that in state prisons people who are Black are incarcerated at 5.1 times the rate of people who are White [14]. The National Research Council report on the growth of incarceration concluded that Black people were incarcerated at six times the rate for White people, with Latinx people incarcerated at three times the rate for non-Latinx White people in 2010 [1]. These findings highlight a grim reality: nondominant cultural groups are more vulnerable to the idiosyncrasies of the judicial system.

Multiple factors, including arresting and sentencing practices, drive racial disparities in correctional settings. Implicit racial biases in law enforcement have been identified in a number of federal oversight reports [15, 16]. These biases influence who police stop, search, arrest, and detain. The Bureau of Justice Statistics report on contacts between the police and public found that although Black, Latinx, and White drivers were stopped by police at similar rates, Black drivers were about three times as likely as White drivers and two times as likely as Latinx drivers to be searched during a traffic stop [17]. Although evidence indicates that people who are Black and people who are White use street drugs at similar rates [14], drug arrests since the 1970s have been higher for Black people [1]. Similarly, despite equivalent rates of cannabis use among Black and White people, Black individuals are 3.73 times more likely to be arrested for possession [18]. Even after arrest and conviction, harsher sentences for drug crimes disproportionately affect people who are Black [19]. Psychiatrists should be aware of these problematic influences that create racial disparities within the US criminal justice system.

Increasingly, courts are acknowledging that structural racism affects the legal system as it does every other facet of American society, contributing to inequality of opportunity and race disparities in mass incarceration. In June 2020, in the wake of George Floyd's death and subsequent mass protests, Washington Supreme Court Justices acknowledged the judicial system's role in "devaluing Black lives" and enabling "racist court decisions" [20]. In an open letter to the legal community, the Justices wrote, "The devaluation and degradation of Black lives is not a recent event. It is a persistent and systemic injustice that predates this nation's founding. But recent events have brought to the forefront of our collective consciousness a painful fact that is, for too many of our citizens, common knowledge: the injustices faced by Black Americans are not relics of the past. We continue to see racialized policing and the overrepresentation of Black Americans in every stage of our criminal and juvenile justice systems" [20].

Also in June 2020, Bernette Joshua Johnson, Chief Justice of the Louisiana Supreme Court, remarked on the injustices she observes in the criminal legal system. She reflected, "We need only look at the glaring disparities between the rate of arrests, severity of prosecutions and lengths of sentences for drug offenses in poor and African American communities in comparison to those in wealthier White communities, to see how we are part of the problem" [20]. Similarly, the California Supreme Court acknowledged "that the legacy of past injustices inflicted on African Americans persists powerfully and tragically to this day." This court added, "We must acknowledge that, in addition to overt bigotry, inattention and complacency have allowed tacit toleration of the intolerable. These are burdens particularly borne by African Americans as well as Indigenous Peoples singled out for disparate treatment in the United States Constitution when it was ratified [20]."

These sobering remarks echo sentiments sweeping across the nation as many Americans come to terms with an uncomfortable reality: despite progress following the 1960s civil rights movement, the legacy of slavery endures and racism against Black Americans persists – interpersonally, in institutions, and systemically. Psychiatrists working in correctional settings invariably hold these unpleasant truths in mind when assessing and treating patients.

Overrepresentation of People with Mental Illness

Psychiatrists new to the field of correctional mental health may be surprised to learn how many inmates entering correctional facilities are afflicted with mental illness. Such individuals comprise another group that is disproportionately represented in correctional facilities.

For many experts, correctional facilities have become de facto psychiatric hospitals. According to the Treatment Advocacy Center, in 2012, about 356,268 prisoners with serious mental illness (SMI) – defined as illness that results in serious functional impairment – were incarcerated [21]. During that same time, less than 10% as many people with SMI, or approximately 35,000 individuals, were in state hospitals [21]. Three jails, the Los Angeles County Jail (CA), Rikers Island (NY), and the Cook County Jail (IL), are consequently the three largest inpatient psychiatric facilities in the country [22]. Although correctional facilities are not designed to care for individuals with SMI, the reality is that correctional facilities have become a common repository for them.

Some experts fault the deinstitutionalization of the state mental health systems for the relocation of individuals with SMI to correctional facilities [23]. When patients diagnosed with mental illness were released from psychiatric hospitals, many relocated to communities that lacked adequate mental health infrastructure. Limited psychiatric resources in the community – inpatient, outpatient, and residential treatment services – contributed to the large number of incarcerated individuals [24].

The Bureau of Justice Statistics (BJS) report *Mental Health Problems of Prison and Jail Inmates* underscores the pervasive nature of mental illness behind bars. This study found that 50% of inmates had a mental health problem as defined by current mental health symptoms or symptoms within the past 12 months [25]. By contrast, the National Institute of Mental Health reports that 18.9% of individuals in the USA suffered from any mental illness in 2017 [26]. Further review of BJS data revealed that 15% of state prisoners and 24% of jail inmates reported symptoms consistent with psychosis, 23% of state prisoners and 30% of jail inmates reported symptoms of major depression, and 43% of state prisoners and 54% of jail inmates reported symptoms consistent with mania [25]. Moreover, about three-fourths of individuals incarcerated in jails met criteria for substance use disorders [25]. Inmates with mental illness constitute a significant portion of correctional populations, and their presence clearly affects the culture of these institutions.

Right to Treatment in Correctional Institutions

Prisoners are the only group in the USA with a constitutional right to medical treatment. Because of the inability of prisoners to obtain their own medical care in a total institution (an institution that controls all of their behavior), the Supreme Court in 1976 held that "deliberate indifference to serious medical needs of prisoners" violated the Constitution's Eighth Amendment, the prohibition against cruel and unusual punishment [27]. Through this ruling, inmates who are post-conviction have a protected constitutional right to medical treatment, albeit at a standard below general malpractice (i.e., "deliberate indifference" falls below the negligence required of a malpractice case). The Constitution also guarantees pre-trial detainees medical treatment through the 14th Amendment's due process clause – the Constitutional passage that assures citizens in the individual states substantive and procedural rights. Prisoners' right to mental health treatment was supported in a subsequent federal ruling. In 1977, in the landmark case of *Bowring v. Godwin*, the federal court ruled that there was "no underlying distinction between the right to medical care for physical ills and its psychological or psychiatric counterpart" [28]. Together, these cases provide the foundation for incarcerated individuals' protected right to medical and mental health care.

Currently, the American Psychiatric Association (APA) expects that clinicians provide "the same quality of mental health services to each patient in the criminal justice system that *should be available* in the community [emphasis in original]" [29]. The APA intentionally sets a higher standard for prisoner mental health treatment than community mental health treatment because adequate services are not always available in open society [29]. This means that psychiatrists working in correctional settings are expected to provide optimal care despite sub-optimal settings and resource limitations [30]. When resource limitations interfere with appropriate service delivery, providers have, at a minimum, the responsibility to voice their concerns to administrative staff.

Challenges of Practicing in Correctional Settings

Although there are many parallels between correctional and community psychiatry, the unique nature of correctional systems creates specific challenges. The culture clash of healthcare and security, the restriction of formularies and other resources, and the implicit social bias that creates this unique population all contribute to an environment that may be unfamiliar to many clinicians.

Typical Responsibilities

Most psychiatrists working in correctional settings provide direct psychiatric care. In this context, common responsibilities include the routine diagnosis of mental illness, medication management, and performance of risk assessments.

Some facilities offer psychiatrists administrative positions or other leadership roles; for example, psychiatrists may serve as directors of mental health services for facilities or groups of facilities within a system. The APA encourages psychiatrists to undertake these positions because they provide opportunities to advocate for patients, improve the quality of mental health service delivery, and prepare patients for community transition [29]. In leadership roles, psychiatrists will have a voice at the table with custodial leadership. In those cases, psychiatrists may communicate resource needs more effectively, improve psychiatric care within agencies, and facilitate productive relationships between providers and correctional staff. Providers and patients all benefit when psychiatrists assume leadership positions in correctional settings.

Cultural Differences: Penal System Versus Mental Health System

The mental health paradigm is inherently at odds with the penal system. A 2015 Human Rights Watch report detailing the use of force on inmates with mental illness asserts that "The institutional culture within many corrections facilities is antithetical to—indeed hostile to—accommodating the needs of prisoners with mental disabilities" [31]. Whereas the US criminal justice system may be seen primarily as punitive rather than rehabilitative, psychiatrists are fundamentally healers who treat patients with compassion, regardless of their offenses. The disparate roles of correctional staff and clinical staff may consequently give rise to disparate professional cultures and attitudes.

In understanding the correctional paradigm, consider that correctional facilities exist first and foremost to house individuals who violate the law. Custodial staff is responsible for maintaining security and order, enforcing institutional regulations, and facilitating daily operations. Correctional officers are front line staff; they interact directly and consistently with inmates. Their jobs are challenging, particularly given common staffing shortages and problems with prison crowding. If correctional officers fail to detect security threats, the costs could be high – incarcerated individuals or other staff members could be seriously harmed. For this reason, correctional officers are trained to be vigilant in observing and attending to suspicious behavior. Keeping a security-first mindset helps them maintain safety as they perform professional duties.

Psychiatrists, as medical professionals, are trained to treat illness and alleviate suffering. Although psychiatrists, like correctional officers, also observe behavior closely, they are not usually looking for evidence of rule-breaking. Typically, psychiatrists seek behavioral clues that reflect their patients' emotional distress, irrational thinking, or cognitive impairment. Psychiatrists and correctional officers therefore observe individuals for different reasons, and their observations may lead them to different conclusions.

Such differences in institutional culture may pave the way for misunderstandings, frustrations, and tensions between custodial staff and mental health providers. Correctional officers, for example, may think that clinicians are coddling prisoners when they carefully draw out mental health symptoms and develop multifaceted treatment plans. Psychiatrists' emphasis on treatment to affect behavioral change may seem naive and misguided to custodial staff who suspect prisoners are manipulating the system. At the same time, psychiatrists may believe that correctional staff are impatient or unduly suspicious. These differences in perspective can lead to miscommunications that themselves undermine security and healthcare.

When possible, mental health providers can partner with custodial staff to promote mutual interests. The psychiatrist's job to communicate with patients, collect collateral information, and make psychiatrically sound judgments can successfully intersect the mission of custodial staff. Listening to reports from correctional officers, who spend considerable time with inmates, may be helpful in clarifying diagnoses or assessing treatment interventions. In weighing this data, clinicians may appropriately err on the side of patient health and safety. When mental health needs are effectively addressed, individuals are more likely to demonstrate adaptive, prosocial behavior. This is in the interest of all parties involved.

Ethical Considerations of Professional Practice

Given the security-first mindset that predominates prison culture, custodial staff may occasionally pressure clinicians to depart from their traditional role as medical providers. Physicians may find that requests to breach confidentiality, search patients, or clear inmates for segregation compromise professional medical ethics. Although uncommon, facilities may even ask physicians to collect urine for security evaluations or force-feed patients [32]. Participating in tasks like these that are designed to advance penological interests corrupts the role of treaters, who are primarily responsible for promoting physical and mental health. National and international organizations recognize that although psychiatrists work within correctional settings, their role is not to enforce or advance institutional interests. The APA cautions, "Treating psychiatrists must not participate in making decisions about discipline, because this crosses ethical boundaries" [29]. At the same time, some respected commentators believe that psychiatrists can at least contribute to discussions of whether inmates understand the disciplinary proceedings themselves or whether their mental illness is a mitigating factor [33]. Nonetheless, the 2015 *United Nations Standard Minimum Rules for the Treatment of Prisoners* states, "Health-care personnel shall not have any role in the imposition of disciplinary sanctions or other restrictive measures" [34]. Professional medical ethics governing physician behavior in the community also apply behind bars.

There are other instances where psychiatrists in correctional organizations may be asked to practice outside a direct clinical role. For example, psychiatrists may be called upon to perform court-ordered forensic assessments (e.g., competency to stand trial, criminal responsibility). The APA recommends that psychiatrists avoid performing these types of evaluations on patients they treat or have treated because of the inevitable conflicts between the obligations to the patient and the court [29]. This is the problem of dual, or multiple agency, in which professionals are torn by various allegiances: the patient, the employer, public safety, and the profession itself. Moral philosophers and forensic psychiatrists alike wonder whether any individual can withstand the balancing of their rights against the daunting counterweight of institutional obligations [35].

Professional organizations, including the APA and the National Commission on Correctional Health Care (NCCHC), offer guidance to providers who practice in correctional institutions. NCCHC, for example, prioritizes the health and wellness of individual patients, leaving solitary confinement to the administrative process [36]. Reviewing such standards may help psychiatrists clarify their professional obligations and effectively respond to ethical dilemmas.

Boundary Challenges

In correctional settings, prisoners, custodial staff, and clinical providers are all vulnerable to adopting an "us vs. them" mentality. When psychiatrists take sides, their neutrality is compromised, and they risk falling short in delivering the standard of care. Custodial and clinical staff can express strong emotional reactions or personal judgments about prisoners who have committed violent crimes, particularly those who have committed sex crimes or harmed children. Participating in derogatory conversations, however, biases providers against their patients and clouds clinical judgment. Further, therapeutic alliances can be jeopardized if prisoners detect providers' and officers' negative feelings.

Conversely, there are risks when psychiatrists overidentify with patients. Some clinicians view prisoners as victims of an unjust judicial system and may wish to rescue them from unfortunate circumstances [37]. Individuals who are incarcerated in turn may perceive these qualities in their providers and exploit them for personal gain. These prisoners may make inappropriate requests (e.g., permission for personal calls, assistance with legal defense, requests for outside items) that providers or other custodial staff members feel compelled to honor. In one famous case, a prison tailor in New York brought tools to two inmates, who then used them to escape. The tailor poignantly described how she became involved in the prisoner's scheme stating, "I believe I helped … [them] escape because I was caught up in the fantasy. I enjoyed the attention, the feeling both of them gave me, and the thought of a different life" [38]. Psychiatrists should be cautious if they feel inclined to depart from traditional clinical responsibilities. In these cases, immediate self-reflection and consultation with colleagues is critical in clarifying appropriate boundaries. Otherwise, repercussions for staff and patients can be serious.

Resource Limitations

Mental health resources, including providers and psychotropic medications, may be more limited in correctional facilities than in community settings. Some jails and prisons do not meet professional mental health staffing recommendations [24]. For example, in 2016, The Boston Globe reported that 7 of 15 prisons in Massachusetts were classified as federally designated health professional shortage areas in mental health. These facilities employed less than 1 psychiatrist per 2000 inmates [39]. A 2018 study from the University of Michigan School of Public Health surveyed 20 correctional facilities from 6 states and found that 80% of the reporting facilities lacked adequate behavioral health staff to meet inmate needs [40]. Eighty-five percent of facilities reported difficulty filling open behavioral health positions, and 70% reported difficulty retaining competent behavioral health staff [40].

For staffing in prisons, the APA recommends one full-time equivalent psychiatrist for every 150–200 patients with serious mental illness (SMI) on psychotropic medications [29]. In jails, where the turnaround is shorter and the acuity greater, the recommendation is 1 full-time psychiatrist for every 75–100 patients [29]. When facilities are clinically understaffed, psychiatrists experience pressure to accept large caseloads and compress treatment sessions. But resource limitations do not justify inadequate mental health treatment. Consequently, clinicians have a responsibility to communicate staffing needs to supervisors, facility administrators, and even legislators.

In addition to feeling the crunch of clinical understaffing, providers may feel constrained by prison pharmaceutical formularies. In correctional facilities, cost may limit the availability of psychotropic medication. Pharmaceuticals are expensive; in some states, they average 14% of prison healthcare spending [41]. A large portion of pharmaceutical spending may fund antipsychotic medications: in 2012, California spent 20% of its $144.5 million pharmaceutical budget on antipsychotic medications [42]. To cut these costs, correctional facilities may strictly limit medication choices. In some facilities, they do so by limiting the psychiatric formulary to a few first-generation antipsychotic medications and other older agents [43]. This practice, which dramatically restricts treatment options, may be why some experts have concluded that psychiatric treatments in correctional standards deviate from the accepted standard of care [30]. Because requesting non-formulary medications is a tedious process by design, providers may be reluctant to make such requests. Advocating to administrators about appropriate medication access, like concerns about understaffing, remains important.

Security Restrictions

Correctional treatment settings differ from community treatment settings in their security protocols, which can interfere with the reliable delivery of mental health services. Escorting patients to providers' offices can be time and labor intensive, particularly when prisoners are in restrictive housing units and require handcuffs and shackles prior to transport. Facilities may limit the number of individuals in a patient waiting area, and waiting for patients may interrupt clinical workflow. Further, providers may be unable to make scheduled appointments for stretches of time secondary to movement restrictions, especially unit head counts. Given the importance of institutional security, providers have limited work-arounds to improve service delivery and consistency.

Security limitations extend to practitioner relationships with the prisoners themselves. There are occasions when providers may learn about potentially dangerous behavior (e.g., plans to riot, escape, assault others) and must legitimately report to the authorities. This is best done in the context of clear communication with patients about the limits of confidentiality and a robust informed consent process prior to starting treatment.

Concerns about security and drug diversion may also drive clinicians' prescribing practices. In correctional facilities, medications are a form of currency. Medications can be sold for money, bartered for items of interest, or traded for sexual favors. Given elevated rates of substance misuse among inmates, medications with mind-altering properties like benzodiazepines, stimulants, opiates, and even antipsychotics have great diversion potential. As a result, some clinicians may be reluctant to prescribe these medications even when they are clinically indicated.

Threats to Confidentiality

Psychiatrists appreciate that patient expectations of confidentiality are essential to the development of strong therapeutic alliances. Because security constraints in correctional settings can compromise privacy (i.e., officers within earshot of doctor-patient conversations), psychiatrists may find themselves making extra efforts to maintain confidential communication with patients. They may avoid "cell-side" or "cell-door" encounters, insisting that patients be evaluated in private examination rooms whenever possible. When examination room doors must be open for security purposes, providers may speak softly to limit others overhearing confidential communications. As in the community, confidentiality limits do include obligations to report suicidality and homicidality. However, psychiatrists working in correctional settings may indeed break confidentiality in cases of security threats like plans to riot or escape.

Mental Health Stigma

Social stigma associated with mental health treatment may be more prevalent in correctional settings than in all of community mental health. As the Boston Globe's Spotlight team describes, "The prison environment itself is a major obstacle to treatment: In a culture ruled by aggression and fear, the trust and openness required for therapy are exponentially harder to achieve" [39]. Prisoners with mental illness may therefore be less likely to seek treatment because other prisoners may view them as weak or vulnerable. They may be intimidated, robbed, or sexually assaulted because of their status. Liberal psychiatric screening practices, specialized mental health units, mental health rounds, and public education about mental illness are all strategies that may facilitate access to treatment for those who are reluctant to seek it themselves.

Implicit Racial Bias

Psychiatrists working in correctional settings must also be mindful of how implicit racial biases within the profession may affect provision of mental health services. In 2020, American Psychiatric Association (APA) President Jeffrey Geller acknowledged the impact of these biases within psychiatry's largest and most prominent organization, the APA [44]. Dr. Geller asserted, "The history of the APA, going back to its very roots in the 1700s, is scarred with structural racism and racist ideas. While efforts have occurred over the years to rectify this problem, particularly by Black psychiatrists, as a field and organization we still have a very long way to go" [44]. To bring awareness to systemic racism within the profession, Dr. Geller formed the APA Presidential Task Force to Address Structural Racism Throughout Psychiatry. This task force was charged with the mission to study the profession's history of structural racism, communicate its impact on mental health, and develop actionable recommendations for change [44].

Implicit clinician bias is not benign and can have serious consequences for patients of color. Studies have found that Black patients are more likely to be diagnosed with schizophrenia than affective disorders when compared to White patients [45]. One recent study of more than 1600 patients in an outpatient mental health center found that clinicians underemphasize the relevance of mood symptoms among Black individuals compared with other racial-ethnic groups [46]. These findings are concerning given that schizophrenia carries a poorer prognosis than affective disorders. Further, treatment of psychotic illnesses may not address affective symptoms, and antipsychotic medications are associated with potentially irreversible metabolic and movement side effects.

Psychiatrists may take some well-established steps to reduce the effects of implicit bias. They should practice self-awareness and challenge internalized assumptions about people of color. Slowing down during clinical evaluations and consciously taking the time to assess each patient as an individual – rather than a member of a stereotyped group – are essential. Maintaining a reflective mindset, as opposed to a reactive one, should be the goal. In addition, psychiatrists may take implicit association tests, attend race equity trainings, and consult frequently with colleagues.

Special Considerations When Working with Patients in Correctional Settings

Individuals with mental illness, a population that is disproportionately represented in correctional institutions, face unique challenges in confinement. Compared to individuals without mental illness, individuals with mental illness are more likely to commit suicide, experience victimization, and be confined to solitary. Consequently, psychiatrists often find that trauma-informed approaches and emphasis on individual safety are essential when working with these patients.

Suicide Risk

As a population, incarcerated individuals are at increased risk for suicide. In jails, suicide has been the leading cause of death since 2006: suicide accounted for roughly one-third of all jail deaths in 2016 [47]. In prisons, suicide accounted for 6.8% of all deaths in 2016 [48]. By contrast, national suicide rates in the population at large are considerably less; in 2016, suicide accounted for 1.6% of all deaths [49]. Correctional organizations are increasingly recognizing that suicide in prisons and jails is a public health crisis and that suicide prevention programs are integral components of their mental health delivery systems.

Individuals who are incarcerated encounter many stressors that contribute to suicidality. They may be particularly vulnerable to feelings of hopelessness, helplessness, and anxiety as their cases make their way through court. The APA cautions that individuals who are incarcerated are at higher risk for suicidality at certain times: upon admission, when facing new legal problems, after receiving bad news, following trauma, after experiencing rejection, as mental illness is exacerbated, and when housed in administrative segregation [29]. Given the dynamic and unpredictable experience of incarceration, mental health clinicians should screen for suicidality and associated risk factors at every clinical encounter. Researchers have identified associated risk factors including mental illness, substance use disorders, psychosocial stressors associated with incarceration, problems with support networks, and conditions of confinement [50].

Trauma and Victimization

Not only are individuals with mental illness more likely to harm themselves when incarcerated, but they also are more likely to be harmed. According to BJS data, prisoners with mental health problems are already more than twice as likely to report a history of past physical or sexual abuse [25]. About 6.3% of individuals identified with serious psychological distress in prisons reported sexual abuse by another inmate; by contrast, this rate is only 0.7% among those without mental illness [51]. The well-known National Prison Rape Elimination Commission Report confirmed that mental illness increased inmates' risk for sexual abuse by other prisoners [52]. Authors of a 6-month survey that examined 13 prisons in a mid-Atlantic state prison system concluded that 1 in 12 male prisoners with mental illness reported sexual victimization, compared to 1 in 33 male prisoners without mental illness [53]. Given these findings, screening for trauma and victimization is a necessary component of mental health evaluations and, like suicide screening, should occur at every clinical encounter.

In recent years, there has been compelling data suggesting that LGBTQIA prisoners are particularly vulnerable to sexual victimization. BJS data found that 39.9% of transgender adult individuals in prisons and 26.8% in jails reported sexual victimization between 2011 and 2012 [51]. By contrast, 4.0% of cisgender individuals in prisons and 3.2% of those in jails reported sexual victimization [51]. Further, among prisoners who identified as nonheterosexual, 12.2% reported sexual victimization by another inmate compared to 1.2% of those who identified as heterosexual [51].

Behavioral Challenges

Incarcerated individuals with mental illness are more likely to be charged with violating prison rules than their nonmentally ill counterparts [25]. They are more likely to engage in certain disruptive behaviors like property destruction, fire setting, and fecal smearing [54]. They are also more likely to be charged with physical or verbal assault on staff members or other inmates [25]. A report by Human Rights Watch (HRW) explains, "Prison is challenging for everyone, but prisoners with mental disabilities may struggle more than others to adjust to the extraordinary stresses of incarceration, to follow the rules governing every aspect of life, and to respond promptly to staff orders" [31]. The implications of this disruptive behavior are profound: they may result in disciplinary solitary confinement or use of force. Advocacy for more mental health resources may counter one particular HRW report that concluded that misuse of force against prisoners with mental health problems is widespread [31].

Solitary Confinement

Background

Solitary confinement, or segregation, is a prison within a prison: individuals' autonomy, physical movement, and opportunities for social contact are even more restricted than in the general population. Social inequities are also more pronounced. BJS data demonstrate that individuals who are younger, without high school diplomas, and members of the LGBTQIA community are more likely to spend time in solitary confinement than their counterparts [55]. Individuals with mental illness are also disproportionately affected by segregation practices [55].

In correctional settings, segregation technically refers to the practice of removing individuals from the general population and confining them to dedicated cells for 22–24 hours a day. Placement may occur for a variety of reasons, including disciplinary and protective purposes. Administrators may wish to discipline prisoners from the general population or protect members of a minority gang or incarcerated former police officers. Individuals in segregation reside in special housing units (SHUs or "shoes") within correctional facilities. The most violent and disruptive offenders may be confined to supermaximum security prisons (supermax), highly secure institutions in which prisoners are "single-celled" for an indefinite period of time with minimal human contact [56]. Other names for segregation include restrictive, segregated, or secure housing; colloquially, segregation may be called "the box" or "the hole."

Segregation may be classified by its intended purpose: protective custody, administrative segregation, and disciplinary segregation. Protective custody is intended to protect individuals who are vulnerable to abuse or harm and often include transgender persons or prisoners who have committed sexual offenses. Administrative segregation is designed to isolate individuals who pose a risk to others or the security of the facility (e.g., gang members). Finally, disciplinary segregation punishes prisoners who violate institution rules by possessing contraband or assaulting correctional officers.

In the Federal Bureau of Prisons, a segregated housing unit cell is typically 60 to 80 square feet and contains a bed platform, toilet, sink, and a narrow window [57]. In other facilities, cells may be as small as 50 square feet, smaller than a standard parking space [58]. Some SHU cells lack windows and are illuminated with artificial light all day and night [54]. In those settings, environmental stimuli are abnormal [59]. Furnishings tend to be sparse, and personal items, such as reading materials and toiletries, are restricted and subject to search.

Even more crucially, meaningful human contact and social activities are limited. In some jurisdictions, inmates are only permitted one phone call or social visit per month [60]. Contact visits and congregate activity (e.g., dining, religious services) are typically prohibited [54]. In fact, in some cases, visits may only occur by closed-circuit television [54]. Direct contact with security staff is minimal and may consist only of the brief conversation when food trays are delivered through slots in the cell door. Contact with other inmates is also restricted but might occur during the 1 hour recreational break each day. Prisoners may develop creative ways to communicate between cells. Using the doors or vents, prisoners may "fly a kite," surreptitiously casting handwritten notes along a string across the cell block. Because opportunities to participate in educational, vocational, and therapeutic programming are uncommon, inmate activity in segregation is uniquely limited.

By the Numbers

Precise numbers of individuals in restrictive housing are hard to come by due to differences in definitions and lack of systematic tracking [57, 61]. Based on data collected from 43 prison systems, the Association of State Correctional Administrators (ASCA)-Liman 2018 nationwide survey on restrictive housing estimated that approximately 61,000 prisoners were in restrictive housing across the USA in the fall of 2017 [62]. These numbers do not account for individuals in jails, juvenile facilities, military, and immigration detention centers. This study also found that among survey respondents, on average 4.6% of prisoners were in restrictive housing. Further, Black prisoners comprised a greater percentage of the population in segregation than they did in the total custodial population [62].

The Government Accountability Office calculated that the Bureau of Prisons confines about 7% of inmates in segregated housing units [63]. BJS data estimates that on an average day in 2011–2012, up to 4.4% of state and federal inmates and 2.7% of jail inmates were held in restrictive housing [55]. This report also concluded that nearly 20% of prison inmates and 18% of jail inmates spent time in restrictive housing in the previous 12 months or since incarceration at their current facility.

The 2018 ASCA-Liman survey also collected data on lengths of stay in segregation: 54.4% were in segregation under 3 months, 26.9% from 3 months to 1 year, and 19.1% for more than 1 year [62]. The Federal Bureau of Prisons, which houses 129,430 inmates in custody, reported that 8.3% of all prisoners were in restricted housing as of July 2020 [64]. Around 30% of this group, or 3413 inmates, were in restricted housing for more than 90 days [64].

Perhaps because of the stresses on inmates and institutions, there has been a trend in recent years to decrease the number of segregated inmates. In 2016, the Federal Bureau of Prisons reported a 25% reduction of restricted housing population since 2012 [57].

Mental Illness and Segregation

It is not uncommon for individuals with mental illness to be confined in segregation. BJS data demonstrate that solitary confinement is closely associated with mental health problems: among those experiencing psychological distress, 29% of individuals in prisons and 22% of those in jails were housed in segregation at some point during the previous 12 months [55]. Further, about a quarter – 26% of prison inmates and 23% of individuals in jails – who had been told they had mental illness also reported a history of time in restrictive housing. By contrast, around 15% of individuals incarcerated in prisons and jails with no symptoms of mental health problems were in restrictive housing units during the same period [55].

These findings have been replicated in other studies. In one study, Cloyes et al. (2006) assessed 87 male supermax security unit prisoners and found that 29% of them showed evidence of mental illness [65]. A significant number met the study's criteria for "serious psychosocial impairment." A Danish study that compared 133 inmates in solitary confinement to 95 non-solitary inmates found that the incidence of psychiatric illness was 28% in those who were segregated as opposed to 15% in those who were not [66].

Individuals with serious mental illness may struggle to follow institutional rules and may be confined to segregation as punishment [67, 68]. As previously described, they may have difficulty managing their emotions, leading to altercations with custodial staff and disruptive behaviors [67, 68]. Providers who work in correctional medicine appreciate how mental health symptoms can prolong segregation stays; in its position statement on solitary confinement, the National Commission on Correctional Health Care (NCCHC) asserts, "Continued misconduct related to [prisoners'] underlying mental health issues, which is often exacerbated by their isolation, can result in their being held in solitary confinement indefinitely" [36].

In facilities where mental health resources are limited, disciplinary segregation may become the default placement for individuals with mental illness who are disruptive and inconvenient [67, 69]. This is part of the incentive for systems to develop specialized mental health units or residential treatment programs which specialize in the treatment and support of mentally ill prisoners who have problems functioning in the general population.

Psychological Impact of Segregation

Conditions of segregated housing may exacerbate mental illness or contribute to the development of new psychopathology. A growing body of literature details potential adverse psychological effects associated with solitary confinement [67, 70]. Although some of these studies and reports have been criticized for their methodologic limitations [61, 71], this literature contributes to the increasing objections to segregation practices, particularly when applied to individuals with serious mental illness. At the same time, one well-known but counterintuitive study with stronger methodology did not substantiate the connection between psychological decline and administrative segregation [72].

Several experts have posited a psychiatric profile for prisoners in solitary confinement. In *A Sourcebook on Solitary Confinement*, criminologist Sharon Shalev hypothesizes that "three main factors are inherent in solitary confinement – social isolation, reduced environmental stimulation, and loss of control over almost all aspects of daily life" [73]. These factors all contribute to the distress associated with segregation. Stuart Grassian, a psychiatrist who studied solitary confinement early on, hypothesizes that limited environmental stimulation and social isolation, two hallmark features of solitary confinement, together exert a synergistic and toxic effect on mental health [74]. Based on his evaluation of hundreds of prisoners, Grassian posits that segregation is associated with a specific psychiatric syndrome – often referred to as "SHU syndrome" – characterized by hyper-responsivity to external stimuli, perceptual distortions, panic attacks, paranoia, poor impulse control, obsessional thinking, and other thinking problems. Craig Haney, a social psychology professor, reached similar conclusions during his study of 100 prisoners at California's notorious Pelican Bay State Prison, a supermax facility [67]. Haney found that almost all prisoners suffered from nervousness/anxiety, chronic lethargy, ruminations or intrusive thoughts, oversensitivity to external stimuli, irrational anger and irritability, confused thought processes, difficulties with attention/memory, and a tendency to withdraw socially. Among this group, 70% felt that they were on the verge of an emotional breakdown [67]. Haney theorized that prisoners with mental illness were particularly vulnerable and "at greater risk of having this suffering deepen into something more permanent and disabling" [67].

Other surveys and studies demonstrate the potential psychological impact of solitary confinement. One multi-site study found that among individuals who were recently released from incarceration, those from solitary confinement were more than two and a half times as likely as those who were not in segregation to report PTSD symptoms [75]. Another study in Denmark found that the incidence of adjustment disorders among prisoners in solitary confinement was double that of other prisoners [66]. In his work, psychiatrist Terry Kupers asserts that almost all individuals in supermax facilities report problems with anxiety, sleep, focus, and memory [68]. Findings like these have led the NCCHC to conclude that even individuals without a history of mental illness may experience a "deterioration of mental health" in solitary confinement [36].

These vulnerabilities can turn out to be life-threatening. Suicide and self-injury occur disproportionately in segregated housing units. In a large study of the New York jail system, Kaba and colleagues found that self-harm was associated significantly with being in solitary confinement at least once [76]. This seminal study examined more than 240,000 incarcerations and 2000 acts of self-harm. The authors calculated that although "7.3% of admissions included solitary confinement, 53.3% of acts of self-harm and 45.9% of acts of potentially fatal self-harm occurred within this group" [76].

Supporting data from a Texas study similarly suggests that individuals in solitary confinement are five times more likely to commit suicide than those in the general population [77]. Further, in 2013, experts concluded that prisoners housed in California's segregation units were 33 times more likely to kill themselves [78]. Raymond Patterson, who served as a psychiatric expert for this case, calculated that 47% of the 15 completed suicides that occurred in the first 6 months of 2012 took place in secured housing units [79].

Youth who are confined and isolated are even more vulnerable. The US Attorney General's Task Force on Children Exposed to Violence concluded that "Confined youth who spend extended periods isolated are among the most likely to attempt or actually commit suicide" [80]. One study, which examined juvenile suicides in confinement (e.g., juvenile detention centers, reception centers, training schools, ranches, camps, and farms), concluded that half the victims were on room confinement at the time of the death [81].

The psychological impact of segregation may persist after release from incarceration. One study that followed 230,000 individuals released from incarceration in North Carolina revealed devastating effects associated with a history of solitary confinement [82]. The authors found that when comparing individuals who spent any time in restrictive housing with those who had not, individuals in the former group were 24% more likely to die in the first year after release, especially from suicide (78% more likely) and homicide (54% more likely) [82]. This solitary confinement group was also 127% more likely to die of an opioid overdose within the first 2 weeks after release [82].

Mental Health Screening and Monitoring in Segregation

Given the prevalence of mental illness, self-harm, and suicide in solitary confinement, correctional systems are developing protocols that provide improved access to mental health services. To facilitate greater access, the APA recommends that institutions conduct mental health screening prior to placing individuals in segregation; this evaluation may include a suicide risk assessment and an assessment of whether an individual's psychiatric illness could worsen in segregation [29]. There is, however, controversy about how involved physicians should be in this process. The NCCHC asserts, "Health staff must not be involved in determining whether adults or juveniles are physically or psychologically able to be placed in isolation" [36]. Similarly, the World Health Organization (WHO) states that "doctors should not collude in moves to segregate or restrict the movement of prisoners except on purely medical grounds, and they should not certify a prisoner as being fit for disciplinary isolation or any other form of punishment" [83]. It is not yet clear how professional roles can avoid the conflict between facilitating the use of segregation and protecting inmates from its effects.

After individuals are moved to solitary confinement, frequent mental health rounds may promote early detection of psychiatric decompensation or the emergence of symptomatology. Individuals at risk, or with early symptoms, may then be referred to psychiatrists for more comprehensive assessments and treatment planning. Inmates without histories of mental illness are also vulnerable to psychological distress. Regular screening in restrictive housing units can be useful for anyone entering that highly controlled environment.

Barriers to Treatment in Restricted Housing Units

Individuals in solitary confinement confront many other kinds of barriers that impede the efficient delivery of mental health services. From a staffing standpoint, transporting inmates from segregation is time and labor intensive. Before inmates can meet with clinical providers, they are often searched and shackled. Escorts are first required to transport individuals to infirmaries and then to supervise them as they await their appointments.

Physical barriers may also impair the quality of a therapeutic relationship between healthcare providers and prisoners in solitary confinement. In some facilities, providers evaluate patients through a glass partition or while inmates are confined to a metal cage. In other facilities, evaluations are conducted "cell-side" via slots on the door or by telephone or speakers. Consequently, prisoners are reluctant to speak openly about mental health symptoms due to their all too reasonable concerns that officers and others may overhear information that can make them a target.

Security regulations and resource limitations also restrict access to therapeutic activities like individual therapy, group therapy, and life skills development [59, 69]. In segregated housing units, it is not uncommon for mental health treatment to consist primarily of psychotropic medication management without therapy [69]. In some facilities, clinicians deliver therapeutic services despite security restrictions. For example, groups may be conducted while individuals are separated in "therapeutic modules" [57], which resemble large phone booths [84]. These are rolled into position and arranged in a semicircle or classroom lineup that does little to facilitate group interaction.

Skepticism of prisoner requests for mental health services may prevent or delay access to treatment. Kristin Cloyes, a researcher who studies correctional health programs, puts it this way, "Doubts about the authenticity of symptoms and concerns of manipulation and malingering are a central focus for SMU [special management units] staff, who may interpret decompensation as a strategic manipulation for softer conditions" [65]. In a culture where corrections officers are the gatekeepers of clinical access, privileges, and contact with the outside world, this can be a significant hurdle for prisoners to overcome.

Movement Away from Segregation

Given the psychological impact of segregation, national and international organizations have been increasingly critical of segregation practices; in some cases, they have called for an end to the practice.

In the USA, psychiatric and correctional health organizations have advocated for limited use of solitary confinement. In 2012, the APA contended that "Prolonged segregation of adult inmates with serious mental illness, with rare exceptions, should be avoided due to the potential harm to such inmates" [85]. Similarly, in 2016, the NCCHC issued a position statement criticizing both prolonged use and application to vulnerable populations [36]. In unequivocal terms, the organization asserted, "Prolonged (greater than 15 consecutive days) solitary confinement is cruel, inhumane, and degrading treatment, and harmful to an individual's health." The NCCHC also recommended that mentally ill individuals, juveniles, and pregnant women "be excluded from solitary confinement of any duration" [36].

Perhaps reacting to such strong sentiments, the US government has steered away from segregation. From 2012 to 2016, the Federal Bureau of Prisons decreased the number of prisoners in restrictive housing by almost one quarter [57]. In 2016, President Obama vowed to adopt the US Department of Justice (DOJ) recommendations to further reduce the use of segregation [86]. He prohibited use of solitary confinement as punishment for prisoners who commit low-level infractions and banned its use for juvenile offenders in the federal prison system. Demonstrating an appreciation for the vulnerabilities of those with serious mental illness (SMI), the DOJ had already recommended that inmates with SMI not be segregated unless they posed an immediate and serious danger and no reasonable alternative existed [57]. Further, the DOJ asserted that suicidality and active psychosis are contraindications to segregation.

Internationally, proposals calling for the near elimination of solitary confinement are ubiquitous. In 2013, Physicians for Human Rights (PHR) recommended that solitary confinement be used "only in very exceptional cases, for as short a time as possible, and only as a last resort" [87]. Barring "exceptional circumstances," United Nations (UN) Special Rapporteur on Torture, Juan Méndez, called for countries to prohibit solitary confinement [88]. He asserted that in some cases solitary confinement may "amount to torture or cruel, inhuman or degrading treatment or punishment" [88]. In the *United Nations Standard Minimum Rules for the Treatment of Prisoners*, the UN prohibits solitary confinement when prisoners have mental or physical disabilities that would worsen if placed in solitary [34]. Further, the organization continues to prohibit use of solitary confinement for women and children. This movement to reduce the use of solitary confinement appears to be gaining momentum.

Vignette Discussion

Taking these themes into consideration, a discussion of Mr. A's case can raise some critical issues. Mr. A presents to the infirmary following self-injurious behavior. Staff may be skeptical of his behavior, but clinicians must not make assumptions and should consider a number of themes. Mr. A has experienced changes in mood and appetite, panic attacks, and nightmares, all of which may have been exacerbated by his stay in solitary. Psychiatric evaluation therefore begins with a thorough suicide risk assessment followed by assessment for symptoms of depression, anxiety, posttraumatic stress disorder, psychosis, and mania. Because the clinician knows that illicit substances are available in jail and that Mr. A has a history of opiate use, she will rule out any ingested substances that could contribute to his presentation. To obtain collateral information, she speaks with the correctional officers who report that Mr. A has appeared more quiet and socially withdrawn during the past few days. He has not been receiving communication through the informal "kite-flying" process on the block.

During the risk assessment, Mr. A reports to the psychiatrist that he does not care if he dies. He says, "What's the point of living? Whether I live a clean life or mess up it feels like the system is against me anyway." He tells the psychiatrist about the many times he has been stopped and searched as a pedestrian because he was "in a high crime area" or because the police thought he "did not belong" in the neighborhood. Acknowledging that Black men are disproportionately targeted by law enforcement, the psychiatrist validates Mr. A's experiences. Using a trauma-informed approach, the psychiatrist listens empathically, while Mr. A describes the frequent violence he witnesses in his neighborhood, his struggles to make ends meet, and his guilt about letting down his kids. He describes vivid nightmares and flashbacks during this incarceration along with feelings of numbness. Mr. A also reports frustration that he was placed in protective custody when he doesn't feel targeted at all.

The psychiatrist and Mr. A collaboratively develop a comprehensive treatment plan. Both agree that his depression, anxiety, and PTSD have been exacerbated in jail. Mr. A agrees to suicide monitoring on the mental health unit. The psychiatrist optimizes Mr. A's antidepressant given his report that it helped in the past. She schedules him for weekly appointments with a cognitive behavioral therapist. Mr. A declines the psychiatrist's recommendation that he also join the men's trauma group but says he will alert the doctor if he changes his mind. Meanwhile, the psychiatrist asks that a housing supervisor meet again with Mr. A to determine whether general population is more appropriate than protective custody.

During the next 48 hours, while Mr. A remains on suicide monitoring, the psychiatrist sees him daily. Mr. A denies suicidal ideation during that period. He is released to the general population. During the next 2 months, Mr. A's visits with the psychiatrist are tapered from weekly to monthly. Meanwhile, he continues to meet with his therapist weekly and improves his understanding of the connection between his thoughts and feelings. Mr. A increases contact with his family via phone and letters and reports that he feels less isolated. During the subsequent 2 months, Mr. A reports improved mood, less anxiety, and fewer panic attacks. As his sentence comes to an end, he and the unit social worker begin discharge planning, including transition to community mental health services.

Conclusion

When setting foot inside prisons and jails, psychiatrists may feel like they have entered uncharted territory. They may be surprised by the amplification of the community's inequities, especially the overrepresentation of individuals with mental illness and nondominant populations. They may be uncomfortable with the seemingly harsh "security-first" mindset of custodial staff. They may be frustrated by resource limitations like staff shortages and restrictive formularies. Moreover, psychiatrists may be uncomfortable with the realization that many of their patients are in segregated housing, a setting where human contact is limited, mental health symptoms may be exacerbated, and facilitating access to treatment is cumbersome.

Cultural competence in correctional psychiatry requires an understanding of all the social forces driving social and racial disparities in the judicial system. Alongside this is the recognition of the distinct roles of officers and clinicians and the appreciation for how resource limitations and security profoundly shape day-to-day experiences for both inmates and providers. Segregation in particular is the setting where all these influences converge to create a unique vulnerability for prisoners.

Despite the many challenges of working in correctional psychiatry (summarized in Table 9.1), providers may rest assured that the psychiatric standard of

Table 9.1 Challenges and interventions of practicing psychiatry in correctional facilities

Challenges of practicing psychiatry in correctional facilities	Interventions
Risk of boundary crossings	Practice self-reflection Avoid rescue fantasies and overidentification with patients Seek supervision from colleagues
Resource limitations (e.g., staffing, restricted formularies)	Apply for positions that provide direct access to custodial leadership, these offer opportunities to advocate for patients' needs
Threats to confidentiality	Inform and remind patients of these risks at each encounter Avoid "cell-side" assessments Use private examination rooms Speak softly, and be mindful of surroundings
Mental health stigma	Implement liberal screening practices Offer public education to improve awareness about mental illness (e.g., informational trainings, groups, posters)
Implicit racial bias	Practice self-awareness and challenge internalized assumptions Slow down when assessing patients from nondominant cultures to avoid risk of reflexive judgments Make an effort to see each patient as an individual, rather than a member of a stereotyped group Take implicit association tests, attend bias, culture, and race equity trainings

care does not change when they enter correctional facilities. Practicing in accordance with professional ethics is an expectation, not a choice. Comprehensive diagnostic evaluations and targeted treatment plans serve patients well. And when providers observe system weaknesses, dangerous practices, or inadequate services, they can practice a well-informed advocacy that supports patients and systems alike.

Summary of High-Yield Points

- Despite falling crime rates, US incarceration rates continue to rise and are among the highest in the world.
- Mass incarceration disproportionately affects people of color and people with mental illness. Its effects cannot be overstated and include significant economic, social, health, and human costs on individual, family, community, and national scales.
- Prisoners have a right to medical treatment including psychiatric care. However, there are challenges to delivery and implementation of treatment, including resource limitations, mental health stigma, and security restrictions.
- Psychiatrists working in jails and prisons are confronted with the challenges of a penal system where punishment and security, rather than treatment and rehabilitation, are primary objectives.
- Segregation, or solitary confinement, may exacerbate mental illness or contribute to the development of new psychopathology. National and international organizations have been increasingly critical of segregation practices; in some cases, they have called for an end to the practice.
- Individuals in correctional organizations, particularly those with mental illness, are at increased risk of victimization including physical and sexual assault, as well as self-harm and suicide.

References

1. Travis J, Western B, Redburn S. The growth of incarceration in the United States: exploring causes and consequences. Washington, DC: The National Academies Press; 2014.
2. Carson E. Prisoners in 2018. Bureau of Justice Statistics: Department of Justice; 2020.
3. Zeng Z. Jail inmates in 2018. Department of Justice, Bureau of Justice Statistics; 2020.
4. The United States Census Bureau. State population totals: 2010–2019. 2020. Available from: https://www.census.gov/data/tables/time-series/demo/popest/2010s-state-total.html#par_textimage_1574439295
5. Subramanian R, Shames A. Sentencing and prison practices in Germany and the Netherlands: implications for the United States. New York: Vera Institute of Justice; 2013.
6. The Sentencing Project. Fact sheet: trends in U.S. incarceration. 2019. Available from: https://sentencingproject.org/wp-content/uploads/2016/01/Trends-in-US-Corrections.pdf
7. Executive Office of the President of the United States. Economic perspectives on incarceration and the criminal justice system. 2016. Available from: https://obamawhitehouse.archives.gov/sites/default/files/page/files/20160423_cea_incarceration_criminal_justice.pdf

8. Gainsborough J, Mauer M. Diminishing returns: crime and incarceration in the 1990s. Washington, DC: The Sentencing Project; 2000.
9. Hernández KL, Muhammad KG, Thompson HA. Introduction: constructing the Carceral State. J Am Hist. 2015;102(1):18–24.
10. Mai C, Subramanian R. Price of prisons 2015: examining state spending trends, 2010–2015. New York: Vera Institute of Justice; 2017.
11. Teichner M. The cost of a nation of incarceration. Cbsnews.com. 2015. Available from: https://www.cbsnews.com/news/the-cost-of-a-nation-of-incarceration/
12. Glaze LE, Maruschak LM. Parents in prison and their minor children. U.S. Department of Justice, Bureau of Justice Statistics; 2008.
13. Brown v. Plata. 563 US 493 (2011).
14. Nellis A. The color of justice: racial and ethnic disparity in state prisons. The Sentencing Project; 2016.
15. United States Department of Justice. Justice Department announces findings of two civil rights investigations in Ferguson, Missouri. 2015. Available from: https://www.justice.gov/opa/pr/justice-department-announces-findings-two-civil-rights-investigations-ferguson-missouri
16. U.S. Department of Justice Civil Rights Division. Investigation of the Baltimore City Police Department. 2016. Available from: https://www.justice.gov/crt/file/883296/download
17. Eith C, Durose M. Contacts between police and the public, 2008. U.S. Department of Justice, Bureau of Justice Statistics; 2011.
18. Edwards E, Bunting W, Garcia L. The war on marijuana in black and white. New York: American Civil Liberties Union; 2013. Available from: https://www.aclu.org/sites/default/files/field_document/1114413-mj-report-rfs-rel1.pdf
19. Kansal T. Racial disparity in sentencing: a review of the literature. Open Society Foundations; 2005. Available from: https://www.opensocietyfoundations.org/uploads/764bf150-13d8-4330-b08b-b04ae313308f/disparity.pdf
20. State court statements on racial justice. Ncsc.org. 2020. Available from: https://www.ncsc.org/newsroom/state-court-statements-on-racial-justice
21. Torrey EF, Zdanowicz MT, Kennard AD, Lamb HR, Eslinger DF, Blasotti MC, et al. The treatment of persons with mental illness in prisons and jails: a state survey. Treatment Advocacy Center. 2014. Available from: https://www.treatmentadvocacycenter.org/storage/documents/treatment-behind-bars/treatment-behind-bars.pdf
22. NPR. NPR. 2011. Available from: http://www.npr.org/2011/09/04/140167676/nations-jails-struggle-with-mentally-ill-prisoners
23. Yohanna D. Deinstitutionalization of people with mental illness: causes and consequences. VM Am Medica Assoc J Ethic. 2013;15(10):886–91.
24. Fellner J. Viewpoint: pain and punishment for persons with mental disabilities behind bars in the USA. Int J Prison Health. 2015;11(3). https://doi.org/10.1108/IJPH-07-2015-0017
25. James DJ, Glaze LE. Mental health problems of prison and jail inmates. U.S. Department of Justice, Bureau of Justice Statistics; 2006.
26. NIMH. Mental illness. Nimh.nih.gov. 2019. Available from: https://www.nimh.nih.gov/health/statistics/mental-illness.shtml#part_154785
27. Estelle v. Gamble, 429 U.S. 97 (1976).
28. Bowring v. Godwin, 551 F.2d 44 (1977).
29. American Psychiatric Association. Work Group to Revise the APA Guidelines on Psychiatric Services in Correctional Facilities. Psychiatric services in correctional facilities. 3rd ed. Arlington: American Psychiatric Association; 2016.
30. Appelbaum KT, Trestman RL, Metzner JL. The future of correctional psychiatry evolving and recommended standards. In: Trestman RL, Appelbaum KL, Metzner JL, editors. Oxford textbook of correctional psychiatry. New York: Oxford University Press; 2015. p. 404–7.
31. Human Rights Watch. Callous and cruel: use of force against inmates with mental disabilities in US jails and prisons. 2015. Available from: https://www.hrw.org/report/2015/05/12/callous-and-cruel/use-force-against-inmates-mental-disabilities-us-jails-and

32. Pont J, Stöver H, Wolff H. Dual loyalty in prison health care. Am J Public Health. 2012;102(3):475–80.
33. Metzner J, Dvoskin J. An overview of correctional psychiatry. Psychiatr Clin N Am. 2006;29(3):761–72.
34. United Nations Office on Drug and Crime. United Nations Standard Minimum Rules for the Treatment of Prisoners (the Nelson Mandela Rules). Vienna. Available from: https://www.unodc.org/documents/justice-and-prison-reform/GA-RESOLUTION/E_ebook.pdf
35. Candilis PJ, Weinstock R, Martinez R. Forensic ethics and the expert witness. New York: Springer; 2007.
36. Statement P. Solitary confinement (isolation). J Correct Health Care. 2016;22(3):257–63.
37. Gage B. Working inside the walls. In: Trestman RL, Appelbaum KL, Metzner JL, editors. Oxford textbook of correctional psychiatry. New York: Oxford University Press; 2014. p. 35–40.
38. Sanchez R, Hanna J, Martinez M. Joyce Mitchell pleads guilty to helping inmates escape–CNN. CNN. 2015. Available from: http://www.cnn.com/2015/07/28/us/new-york-prison-break-mitchell/index.html
39. Russell J, Cramer M. There may be no worse place for mentally ill people to receive treatment than prison. BostonGlobe. 2016. Available from: https://apps.bostonglobe.com/spotlight/the-desperate-and-the-dead/series/prisons/
40. Buche J, Gaiser M, Rittman D, Beck A. Characteristics of the behavioral health workforce in correctional facilities. Behavioral Health Workforce Research Center at the University of Michigan; 2018. Available from: http://www.behavioralhealthworkforce.org/wp-content/uploads/2016/09/Y2FA2P1_BHWRC_Corrections-Full-Report.pdf
41. Pew Charitable Trusts; John D. and Catherine T. MacArthur Foundation. State prison health care spending. 2014. Available from: http://www.pewtrusts.org/~/media/assets/2014/07/stateprisonhealthcarespendingreport.pdf
42. CBS Sacramento. California prison system under federal review for anti-psychotic drug spending. Sacramento.cbslocal.com. 2013. Available from: http://sacramento.cbslocal.com/2013/05/01/california-prison-system-under-federal-review-for-anti-psychotic-drug-spending
43. Daniel AE. Care of the mentally ill in prisons: challenges and solutions. J Am Acad Psychiatry Law. 2007;35(4):406–10.
44. American Psychiatric Association. APA Presidential Task force to address structural racism throughout psychiatry begins its work. Psychiatry.org. 2020. Available from: https://www.psychiatry.org/newsroom/news-releases/apa-presidential-task-force-to-address-structural-racism-throughout-psychiatry-begins-its-work
45. Office of the Surgeon General (US); Center for Mental Health Services (US); National Institute of Mental Health (US). Mental health: culture, race, and ethnicity: a supplement to mental health: a report of the Surgeon General. Rockville: Substance Abuse and Mental Health Services Administration; 2001. p. 67–8.
46. Gara M, Minsky S, Silverstein S, Miskimen T, Strakowski S. A naturalistic study of racial disparities in diagnoses at an outpatient behavioral health clinic. Psychiatr Serv. 2019;70(2):130–4.
47. Carson A, Cowhig M. Mortality in local jails, 2000–2016 – statistical tables. US Department of Justice, Bureau of Justice Statistics, Bureau of Justice Statistics; 2020.
48. Carson A, Cowhig M. Mortality in state and federal prisons, 2001–2016 – statistical tables. US Department of Justice, Bureau of Justice Statistics; 2020.
49. Kochanek K, Murphy S, Xu J, Arias E. Mortality in the United States, 2016. Hyattsville: National Center for Health Statistics; 2017.
50. Hughes KC, Metzner JL. Suicide risk management. In: Trestman RL, Appelbaum KL, Metzner JL, editors. Oxford textbook of correctional psychiatry. New York: Oxford University Press; 2015. p. 237–44.
51. Beck A, Berzofsky M, Caspar R, Krebs C. Sexual victimization in prisons and jails reported by inmates, 2011–12. Bureau of Justice Statistics, U.S. Department of Justice; 2013.
52. National Prison Rape Elimination Commission. National Prison Rape Elimination Commission report. 2009. Available from: https://www.ncjrs.gov/pdffiles1/226680.pdf

53. Wolff N, Blitz CL, Shi J. Rates of sexual victimization in prison for inmates with and without mental disorders. Psychiatr Serv. 2007;58(8):1087–94.
54. Arrigo BA, Bullock JL. The psychological effects of solitary confinement on prisoners in supermax units: reviewing what we know and recommending what should change. Int J Offender Ther Comp Criminol. 2008;52(6):622–40.
55. Beck A. Use of restrictive housing in U.S. prisons and jails, 2011–2012. Bureau of Justice Statistics, U.S. Department of Justice; 2015.
56. Mears DP. Evaluating the effectiveness of supermax. 2006. Available from: https://www.ncjrs.gov/pdffiles1/nij/grants/211971.pdf
57. U.S. Department of Justice. Report and recommendations concerning the use of restrictive housing. 2016. Available from: https://www.justice.gov/archives/dag/file/815551/download
58. Shames A, Wilcox J, Subramanian R. Solitary confinement: common misconceptions and emerging safe alternatives. 2015. Available from: https://storage.googleapis.com/vera-web-assets/downloads/Publications/solitary-confinement-common-misconceptions-and-emerging-safe-alternatives/legacy_downloads/solitary-confinement-misconceptions-safe-alternatives-report_1.pdf
59. Metzner JL, Fellner J. Solitary confinement and mental illness in U.S. prisons: a challenge for medical ethics. J Am Acad Psychiatry Law. 2010;38(1):104–8.
60. Baumgartel S, Guilmette C, Kalb J, Li D, Nuni J, Porter D, et al. Time-in-cell: the ASCA-Liman 2014 national survey of administrative segregation in prison. 2015. Available from: https://papers.ssrn.com/sol3/papers.cfm?abstract_id=2655627
61. Appelbaum KL. American psychiatry should join the call to abolish solitary confinement. J Am Acad Psychiatr Law. 2015;43(4):406–15.
62. The Association of State Correctional Administrators, The Liman Center for Public Interest Law at Yale Law School. Reforming restrictive housing: the 2018 ASCA-Liman nationwide survey of time-in-cell. The Arthur Liman Center Yale Law School; 2018. Available from: https://law.yale.edu/sites/default/files/documents/pdf/Liman/asca_liman_2018_restrictive_housing_revised_sept_25_2018_-_embargoed_unt.pdf
63. U.S. Government Accountability Office. Improvements needed in Bureau of Prisons' monitoring and evaluation of impact of segregated housing. 2013. Available from: http://www.gao.gov/assets/660/654349.pdf
64. Federal Bureau of Prisons. BOP statistics: inmate release numbers. Bop.gov. 2020. Available from: https://www.bop.gov/about/statistics/statistics_inmate_shu.jsp
65. Cloyes KG, Lovell D, Allen DG, Rhodes LA. Assessment of psychosocial impairment in a supermaximum security unit sample. Crim Justice Behav. 2006;33(6):760–81.
66. Andersen HS, Sestoft D, Lillebaek T, Gabrielsen G, Hemmingsen R, Kramp A. A longitudinal study of prisoners on remand: psychiatric prevalence, incidence and psychopathology in solitary vs. non-solitary confinement. Acta Psychiatrica Scandinavica. 2000;102(1):19–25.
67. Haney C. Mental health issues in long-term solitary and "supermax" confinement. Crime Delinq. 2003;49(1):124–56.
68. Kupers T. How to create madness in prisons. In: Jones D, editor. Humane prisons. Oxford: Radcliffe Publishing; 2006. p. 47–58.
69. Abramsky S, Fellner J. Ill-equipped: U.S. prisons and offenders with mental illness. New York: Human Rights Watch; 2003.
70. Grassian S. Psychopathological effects of solitary confinement. Am J Psychiatry. 1983;140(11):1450–4.
71. Smith PS. The effects of solitary confinement on prison inmates: a brief history and review of the literature. Crime Justice. 2006;34(1):441–528.
72. O'Keefe ML, Klebe KJ, Metzner J, Dvoskin J, Fellner J, Stucker A. A longitudinal study of administrative segregation. J Am Acad Psychiatr Law. 2013;41(1):49–60.
73. Shalev S. A sourcebook on solitary confinement. London: London School of Economics and Political Science, Mannheim Centre for Criminology; 2008.
74. Grassian S. Psychiatric effects of solitary confinement. Wash Univ J Law Policy. 2006;22:325–83.

75. Hagan BO, Wang EA, Aminawung JA, Albizu-Garcia CE, Zaller N, Nyamu S, et al. History of solitary confinement is associated with post-traumatic stress disorder symptoms among individuals recently released from prison. J Urban Health. 2018;95(2):141–8.
76. Kaba F, Lewis A, Glowa-Kollisch S, Hadler J, Lee D, Alper H, et al. Solitary confinement and risk of self-harm among jail inmates. Am J Public Health. 2014;104(3):442–7.
77. Butler B, Simpson M. A solitary failure: the waste, cost and harm of solitary confinement in Texas. 2015. Available from: https://texascivilrightsproject.org/wp-content/uploads/2019/08/SolitaryReport_2015.pdf
78. St. John P. Court-appointed expert blasts California effort on prison suicides. lattices.com. 2013. Available from: https://www.latimes.com/politics/la-xpm-2013-mar-13-la-me-ff-court-expert-prison-suicide-rate-20130313-story.html
79. Patterson RF. Report on suicides completed in the California Department of Corrections and Rehabilitation January 1, 2012–June 30, 2012. 2013. Available from: http://solitarywatch.com/wp-content/uploads/2013/04/Report-of-Raymond-Patterson-M.D.-on-Suicides-Completed-in-the-CDCR-1-1-2012-to-6-30-2012.pdf
80. Listenbee RL, Torre J, Boyle G, Cooper SW, Deer S, Durfee DT, et al. Report of the Attorney General's National Task Force on children exposed to violence. 2012. Available from: https://www.justice.gov/defendingchildhood/cev-rpt-full.pdf
81. Hayes L. Juvenile suicide in confinement: a national survey. 2009. Available from: https://www.ncjrs.gov/pdffiles1/ojjdp/213691.pdf
82. Brinkley-Rubinstein L, Sivaraman J, Rosen D, Cloud D, Junker G, Proescholdbell S, et al. Association of restrictive housing during incarceration with mortality after release. JAMA Network Open. 2019;2(10):e1912516.
83. Health in prisons: a WHO guide to the essentials in prison health. Available from: http://www.euro.who.int/__data/assets/pdf_file/0009/99018/E90174.pdf
84. Perrien M, O'Keefe ML. Disciplinary infractions and restricted housing. In: Trestman RL, Appelbaum KL, Metzner JL, editors. Oxford textbook of correctional psychiatry. New York: Oxford University Press; 2015. p. 71–5.
85. American Psychiatric Association. Position statement on the segregation of prisoners with mental illness. American Psychiatric Association; 2012.
86. Obama B. Barack Obama: why we must rethink solitary confinement. washingtonpost.com. 2016. Available from: https://www.washingtonpost.com/opinions/barack-obama-why-we-must-rethink-solitary-confinement/2016/01/25/29a361f2-c384-11e5-8965-0607e0e265ce_story.html
87. Corrandini M, Huskey K, Fujio C. Buried alive: solitary confinement in the US detention system. Physicians for Human Rights; 2013. Available from: https://s3.amazonaws.com/PHR_Reports/Solitary-Confinement-April-2013-full.pdf
88. Solitary confinement should be banned in most cases, UN expert says. UN News. 2011. Available from: https://news.un.org/en/story/2011/10/392012-solitary-confinement-should-be-banned-most-cases-un-expert-says#.WVFiFLGZPX8

Shifting Gears: Cultural Assimilation into Primary Care

10

Teresa Pan, Rahul Lauhan, Jeanne Maglione, and Alan Hsu

The Culture of Primary Care

A discussion about the culture of primary care inherently involves a discussion about the culture of medicine in general, as primary care is the face and foundation of healthcare. The array of factors impacting the culture of primary care mirror the numerous definitions of culture, a "multifaceted, encompassing linguistic, religious, educational, class, and many other dimensions of difference, which intersect in complex ways in the life experience and identity of any one individual" [35]. Sir Liam Donaldson, former Chief Medical Officer for England, defines culture as a "complex set of values, beliefs, and assumptions that define the ways in which a firm goes about its business" [5]. This begs the question, what definition should one choose? A choice that is further complicated by the dynamic nature of culture itself. Despite the challenges in the definition and ever-evolving nature of culture, Janelle Taylor, medical anthropologist, emphasizes that disputing these facts promotes little benefit, and she encourages analyzing the relation between the components themselves [35]. To this end, we limit the discussion of culture in primary care to a few critical aspects: the history of medicine and primary care, the business of primary care, a shift from physician-centric to patient-centered practice, and the organizational structure of practice in primary care. This is by no means an exhaustive list but an initial point to start a discourse. The evolving components of primary care culture and the relationship between interprofessional education, interprofessional practice, models of care delivery, and measurement-based care will be explored and further analyzed using vignettes of patients and provider experience.

T. Pan · R. Lauhan · J. Maglione · A. Hsu (✉)
Department of Psychiatry, VA San Diego Healthcare System/University of California San Diego, San Diego, CA, USA
e-mail: teresa.pan@va.gov; Rahul.lauhan@va.gov; jeanne.maglione@va.gov; Alan.Hsu@va.gov

S. H. Koh et al. (eds.), *Diversity in Action*,
https://doi.org/10.1007/978-3-030-85401-0_10

One does not have to look far to get a sense of the common perceptions of medicine. Physicians in popular culture are often depicted as lone geniuses equipped with powers of detection and knowledge which solve complex patient presentations, as seen in popular television. These pictorials sometimes accurately reflect the history of medicine and the structure of medical education. Traditionally, medical schools focused on the development and education of the medical student in direct competition with their colleagues – often an isolating experience. Student doctors acquire knowledge and develop the ability to distill patient reports into meaningful clinical narratives, something patients do not participate in, with the goal of alleviating suffering. This is an inherently one-sided approach which medical schools have sought to change over the years through advances in curriculum [35]. These changes are reflected in the evolution of patient care models leading to revisions in the business and structure of medical practice and transforming the culture of primary care and medicine.

Historically, it was common for the physician, the focal point of medical service, to be the sole owner of and care provider in their practice. Providers and institutions worked against each other to obtain their shares of the population served. Clinicians took call far more frequently, and their office staff were seen as a necessary tool for the functioning of the business. Naturally, a volume-based reimbursement model was the cornerstone of business, and office visits were scheduled reactively due to patient need or physician request. The success of a practice was typically measured by revenue and net collections [15]. The unintended consequences of this physician-centric model included soaring medical costs, increased wait times, limited access to care, provider burn out, and low patient satisfaction leading to a push for reform and a transition to patient-centric culture.

The Institute of Medicine (IOM) defines patient-centered care as "providing care that is respectful of and responsive to individual patient preferences, needs, and values, ensuring that patient values guide all clinical decisions" [18]. The patient-centered care model posits the primary care provider as the lead in an interdisciplinary care team that encourages cooperation and collaboration between patients and providers. It has been adopted as a standard of how primary care is organized and delivered [15]. The patient-centered medical home was first conceptualized by the American Academy of Pediatrics in 1967 denoting a central location of archiving a patient's medical record. This was then expanded and adapted to the primary care setting in the early 2000s with the following core principles: (1) each patient has an ongoing relationship with their personal primary care provider, who leads an interdisciplinary team that cares for the patient, (2) care is delivered with a "whole person orientation" throughout the stages of a patient's life, (3) care is coordinated and integrated across the healthcare system; and (4) mechanisms are put in place for monitoring of performance as well as continuous quality improvement [14].

An overhaul of primary care practice requires change at all levels within an organization and creates opportunity for conflict. In many settings, these changes were met with initial resistance. Doctors value their autonomy and were previously trained in a long-ingrained culture where they were the center focus. With the patient-centered medical home model, physicians were asked to relinquish some of this independence in favor of a more population and team-based approach to care. This new model emphasized performance evaluation of the system itself [16, 29]. The resulting tension can be explored in the competing values model of culture types for organizations, which was introduced by Cameron and Freeman in 1991. In this model, organizations can be described in terms of two categories with contrasting factors – organizations with an internal vs. external focus and with mechanistic vs. relationship-based processes. Internally focused organizations prioritize internal smoothing and integration, whereas externally focused organizations focus on competition and differentiation. Organizations with relationship-based processes value flexibility, individuality, and spontaneity, whereas mechanistic-type organizations value control, order, and stability [29].

As patient-centered care focuses on collaboration and innovation, there is a need to change to a practice with an external focus with relationship-based processes, known as a "developmental culture." Close coordination between directive management styles, facilitative styles, and staff is imperative to the success of this shift [29]. The push to deliver rapid systemic change may lead managers to adopt an authoritarian style, which is thought to produce fast but short-term change. This style can lead to conflict with physicians and their autonomy, which in turn may impact quality of care, patient satisfaction, and provider job satisfaction. Several studies highlight the positive outcomes associated with the transition in practice, such as those that propose team-based approaches as instrumental to decreased burn out, greater provider and patient satisfaction, and improved health outcomes [38].

As the culture of primary care changes, so does the relationship between primary care and other systems, notably mental health. The culture of primary care encompasses systematic differences that enhance team-based communication and collaboration. For example, primary care emphasizes team-based workflow, panel management, health promotion, and disease prevention for population-based care, which are elements not usually addressed in mental health care practices [30]. Additionally, there has been a push to include more novel psychiatric treatment elements into primary care practices, such as measurement-based care, screening, and treatment algorithms based on essential elements of the collaborative care model: team-driven, population-focused, measurement-guided, and evidence-based [3].

Beyond the cultural shift from "solo practitioner" to team-driven care, the shift toward population-focused and measurement-guided care brings in traditional aspects from the discipline of population health [23, 24]. Population health focuses care on health outcomes and resource distribution within the primary care population by using data to identify determinants of health and thus guides application of system-wide interventions to improve advocacy, as well as policy. In order to apply these elements of population-focused care, effective systems, teams, and clinicians (including psychiatry) need to utilize methods of regular data collection and outcome monitoring. Measurement-based care has been long encouraged in tracking of mental health outcomes but was rarely done in practice [25, 26]. However, in primary care, measuring physical health outcomes has long been the standard, such as tracking for management of hypertension and diabetes. Most standard monitoring methods include tools built into the primary care workflow, including screening measures, symptom measures completed at regular intervals, and chart reviews that assess access and utilization of resources. This type of measurement-based care drives evidence-based care.

Interprofessional Education and Practice

As the culture of healthcare has shifted from individual practitioners caring for their patients toward teams composed of members from various professions working collaboratively with patients, the concept of "interprofessionality" has been introduced into the language of healthcare. D'Amour and Oandasan defined interprofessionality as "the development of a cohesive practice between professionals from different disciplines," involving "continuous interaction and knowledge sharing between professionals, organized to solve or explore a variety of education and care issues all while seeking to optimize the patient's participation. Interprofessionality requires a paradigm shift, since interprofessional practice has unique characteristics in terms of values, codes of conduct, and ways of working" [11]. Although, interprofessional and multidisciplinary approaches share some similarities, there are key differences. The use of the suffix "-professional" over "-disciplinary" clarifies the distinction between the inclusion of different professions (e.g., physicians, nurses, pharmacists, psychologists) with the inclusion of different disciplines (e.g., internal medicine, psychiatry, family medicine), whereas the use of the prefix "inter" over the prefix "multi" emphasizes the importance of collaboration toward a common purpose [31].

In 2011, the Interprofessional Education Collaborative – an organization sponsored by the American Association of Colleges of Nursing, the American Association of Colleges of Osteopathic Medicine, the American Association of Colleges of Pharmacy, the American Dental Education Association, the Association of American Medical Colleges, and the Association of Schools and Programs of Public Health – released its report on the Core Competencies for Interprofessional Collaborative Practice [19]. This report delineates core competencies within four interprofessional collaborative practice domains:

1. Values/Ethics for Interprofessional Practice
2. Roles/Responsibilities
3. Interprofessional Communication
4. Teams and Teamwork

These interprofessional competencies were intended to complement the individual professional competencies and to guide efforts in providing interprofessional education. Since 2011, 15 additional national associations have joined the Academy of Nutrition and Dietetics, the American Association of Colleges of Podiatric Medicine, the American Association for Respiratory Care, the American Council of Academic Physical Therapy, the American Occupational Therapy Association, the American Psychological Association, the American Speech-Language-Hearing Association, the Association of Academic Health Sciences Libraries, the Association of American Veterinary Medical Colleges, the Association of Chiropractic Colleges, the Association of Schools and Colleges of Optometry, the Association of Schools of Allied Health Professions, the Council on Social Work Education, the National League for Nursing, and the Physician Assistant Education Association. Large healthcare systems have implemented these recommendations and provided interprofessional education to healthcare students and trainees [9]. However, knowledge of the benefits of collaborative interprofessional clinical training in psychiatry is sparse [28], despite proven benefits for improving students' readiness for interprofessional collaboration [28], attitudes toward interprofessional collaboration [10], and attitudes toward mental illness stigma [27].

By nature, the care of patients with chronic, complex needs requires a collaborative approach. Wagner emphasized the benefit of including nurse care managers and clinical pharmacists [37]. These professionals, with clinical and behavioral skills, work collaboratively with primary care physicians assisting with population-based care, treatment planning, evidence-based management, group consultations, self-management support, and sustained follow-up. Bodenheimer and Grumbach argued that the traditional system of healthcare was designed to address acute illness and was poorly suited for chronic disease management and lacked "a division of labor that would allow non-physician personnel to take greater responsibility in chronic care management. Too often, caring for chronic illness features an uninformed passive patient interacting with an unprepared practice team, resulting in frustrating, inadequate encounters" [6]. They outlined a new model of care termed the Chronic Care Model with six essential elements: (1) community resources and policies, (2) healthcare organization, (3) self-management support, (4) delivery system design, (5) decision support, and (6) clinical information systems. Through the Chronic Care Model, primary care practices would reorganize their processes to provide care in a collaborative and interprofessional manner.

Primary care has increasingly embraced this model. Joining with the American Academy of Pediatrics, which conceptualized the earliest form of the model, in 2007 the American Academy of Family Physicians, the American College of Physicians, and the American Osteopathic Association announced the patient-centered medical home (PC-MH), "an approach to providing comprehensive primary care for children, youth and adults. The PC-MH is a healthcare setting that facilitates partnerships between individual patients, and their personal physicians, and when appropriate, the patient's family." Characteristics of a PC-MH included a patient-centered, physician-led, team-based approach, providing care throughout the patient's lifetime, including acute, chronic, preventive, and end-of-life care, coordinated and integrated across all elements of the health system [22]. Table 10.1 defines many of the key elements critical to the culture of primary care.

Table 10.1 Key terms in primary care models of care

Key Term	Definition	Example
Patient-centered care model	A model of care that integrates patient preferences, needs, and values into all clinical decisions	Patient-centered medical home
Team-based approaches	The provision of health services to individuals, families, and/or communities by at least two healthcare providers who work collaboratively with patients and their caregivers	Primary care and mental health work collaboratively to ensure that well-rounded care is delivered to patients
Population-focused care	The system established to improve the health outcomes of a group of individuals, including distribution of such outcomes within the group	Use of databases to track outcomes for a specific clinic or provider
Measurement-guided care	Using valid and reliable screening instruments of mental and behavioral health concerns into primary care appointments	Care managers routinely administer measures that are followed over time
Interprofessionality	The development of a cohesive practice between professionals from different disciplines	A healthcare professional seeks advice from a healthcare professional in a different field

The Collaborative Care Model

The collaborative care (CC) model was introduced by Jurgen Unutzer, Wayne Katon, and their collaborators via the IMPACT trial [36]. They demonstrated that their collaborative care model for treatment of late-life depression was feasible and significantly more effective than usual care in a wide range of primary care practices. Since the IMPACT trial, CC interventions have been shown to be effective in a wide range of psychiatric conditions (e.g., major depressive disorder, panic and generalized anxiety disorder, posttraumatic stress disorder, bipolar disorder) in a variety of clinics (e.g., primary care, oncology, HIV/infectious disease), medical settings (e.g., academic, VA, community-based centers), and populations (e.g., underserved, minority, geriatric, adolescent) with an array of comorbid medical conditions (e.g., diabetes, coronary artery disease, cancers, pain/fibromyalgia, HIV) [17]. In some cases, such as Katon's TEAMcare trial, a CC intervention was demonstrated to improve outcomes not only for depression but also for other health outcomes such as blood pressure, cholesterol, and glycemic control [40].

Like the patient-centered medical home, the collaborative care model is based on the Chronic Care Model pioneered by Katon [20]. It emphasizes a team-driven, population-focused approach using a measurement-guided, evidence-based method to stepped care [3]. By utilizing standardized and validated measures such as the Patient Questionnaire-9 (PHQ-9) for depression, a team of professionals can provide treatment-to-target with regular monitoring and stepwise intensification of care. Collaborative care systems acknowledge the underlying premise that most patients receive mental health care from nonmental health providers. A recent analysis of Medical Expenditure Panel Survey demonstrated that while the percentage of US adults receiving outpatient mental health services increased from 19.08% in 2004–2005 to 23% in 2014–2015, over three-quarters received their care from general medical professionals only [32]. Previous research demonstrated that treatment of mental health disorders in primary care is often inadequate, with only 25–50% of patients with depressive disorders accurately diagnosed and only 50% of those diagnosed receiving "minimally adequate pharmacologic treatment" [20]. The CC model provides primary care providers with the knowledge-base, framework, and support necessary to provide effective mental health care to their patients.

The primary medical provider provides the majority of care to patients within the primary care setting. The CC model adds a behavioral health (BH) care manager and a psychiatric consultant, as well as some form of electronic registry to enable tracking and review of standard measures (e.g., PHQ-9 scores) to assist with clinical decision-making. Additionally, the patient's role in their own care is emphasized by placing them at the center of the CC team [1]. Figure 10.1 depicts the team structure in traditional primary care models compared to collaborative care models.

The role of the BH care manager can be performed by a variety of professions, including registered nurses, psychologists, clinical social workers, or master's level counselors, and duties include coordinating treatment, referral management, and supporting medication management through periodic telephone follow-up and use

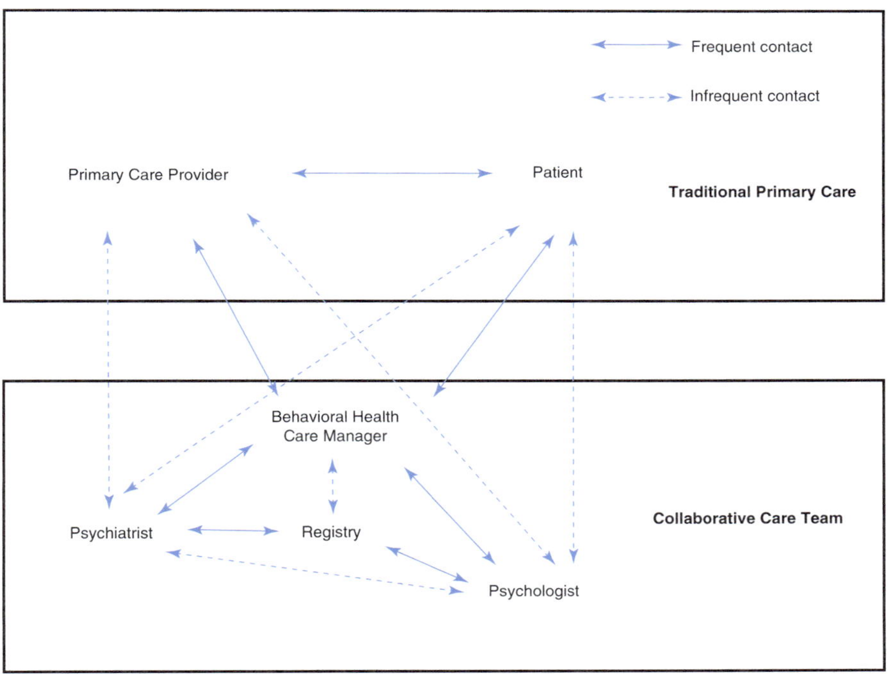

Fig. 10.1 Team structure in traditional primary care compared with collaborative care team

of standard measures. The care manager facilitates communication with the psychiatric consultant and provides brief counseling including motivational interviewing, behavioral activation, and/or problem-solving treatment [2].

The role of the psychiatrist in the CC model includes some responsibilities that differ from traditional psychiatric practice. One of the key distinctions is that direct or formal consultation, in which the psychiatrist assesses a patient face-to-face, is relatively infrequent. In the IMPACT trial, only 5–7% of patients required direct evaluation by the psychiatrist [36], and the overall care of the patient remains with the primary care provider [34]. Psychiatrists practicing in the CC model need to be comfortable providing indirect or curbside consultations and providing recommendations either verbally or via chart note despite not having evaluated the patient. Psychiatrists are also responsible for providing caseload-focused registry review in collaboration with the BH care manager. Together they make decisions based on PHQ-9 or GAD-7 scores and other information to recommend medication adjustments, changes in behavioral approaches, scheduling face-to-face visits, or referral to higher level of specialty mental health care [34]. Psychiatrists also provide education to members of both the primary care and collaborative care team, both formally via presentations or lectures as well as informally. These responsibilities require a psychiatrist to be proficient in interprofessional practice, with a strong understanding of the roles and responsibilities of the other team members and ability to communicate effectively with them.

Measurement-Based Care in Primary Care and Collaborative Care

As primary care has shifted toward integrated, collaborative care that emphasizes the importance of mental and behavioral health, health outcomes such as depression, alcohol use, suicidality, smoking cessation, and other psychosocial risk factors have been included in regular screening measures and outcomes tracking. Screening of behavioral health and substance concerns within primary care promotes early identification of mental health conditions, opportunity to initiate timely interventions, and triage for appropriate referrals [4, 12]. Additionally, measurement-based care enhances clinic outcomes, fosters patient-centered communication and patient involvement in care, as well as increases use of evidence-based treatments [13, 26, 39].

Beyond screening and measurement-based care, practice of psychiatry within the primary care setting may also involve panel management and team-based review of patient outcomes, as noted above. For example, a nurse care manager may employ measurement-based monitoring of patient outcomes within a patient registry to identify lack of symptom improvement or patient concerns that are subsequently relayed to the primary care provider and psychiatrist to inform treatment plan adjustments. Use of panel management for mental health treatment within primary care has demonstrated improvements in patient outcomes, quality of treatment, and evidence-based treatment utilization [7, 8, 33].

Table 10.2 Key differences between a traditional medical model and a collaborative care model

	Traditional medical model	Collaborative care model
Patient's role	Passive	Active participant
Interaction style	More authoritarian	Shared decision-making
Focus of care	Disease centered/ biomedical	Whole health and quality of life/biopsychosocial
Point of contact	MD	Care manager
Outcome measurement	Variable	Measures assessing symptom severity and response to treatment
Relationships	MD to patient	Patient ↔ team, team to population, team to hospital system

Practicing psychiatry in primary care thus requires a shift from traditional psychiatric training to flexibly adapt to the primary care culture of collaborative workflows, infrastructure, shared panel management, and effective use of data through measurement-based care to communicate with patients and other providers. There are many elements to consider in effective implementation of measurement-based care in integrated primary care, such as selection of conditions for screening, population-based screening, selective screening, stepped care screening and assessment, and triage to stepped care interventions [21]. Table 10.2 highlights these key differences between traditional psychiatric models of care and the CC model.

Vignette 1

To illustrate the differences in culture between practicing psychiatry within the traditional medical model and a collaborative care model within primary care, a case contrasting the two approaches is presented.

Mr. S is a married 30-year-old Caucasian male with past medical history significant for obesity, hyperlipidemia, and hypertension. He established care with his primary care physician in 2011. In 2019, he presents for routine follow-up and states that he has been having a difficult time with his emotions as his young daughter had a failing liver transplant. He worries about the loss of another child as he and his wife previously lost a 7-month-old. A chart review also shows history of mood disorder and posttraumatic stress disorder. He denies any substance use with the exception of minimal alcohol intake, which is not above the weekly recommended limits for males. He finds himself suddenly feeling tearful on various occasions and requests to speak with a mental health care provider.

Traditional Model of Care

The primary care physician provides Mr. S with a list of several psychiatrists and psychiatric clinics in the community and recommends he make an appointment to treat his depressive symptoms. The PCP then returns to addressing Mr. S's other comorbid conditions, as he remains obese with uncontrolled hyperlipidemia and hypertension despite being prescribed appropriate doses of medications for these conditions.

Following his visit, Mr. S begins contacting the psychiatrists and psychiatric clinics on the list provided by his PCP. The first two psychiatrists he contacts are not on his insurance panel, and the third is not accepting new patients. He contacts one of the psychiatric clinics and can secure an intake appointment in 2 months. Over the next 2 months, he continues to feel very depressed and begins isolating himself, withdrawing from his wife, engaging in binge eating episodes, oversleeping, and paying less attention to his hygiene. His work performance begins to suffer, and he takes sick days with increasing frequency. He presents to his intake appointment with the psychiatrist at the clinic, where he is diagnosed with major depressive disorder, recurrent, severe without psychotic symptoms, and a rule-out of posttraumatic stress disorder. He reports having tried sertraline in the past, but does not recall the dose or the response. The psychiatrist prescribes sertraline 50 mg daily. He is given a follow-up appointment in 1 month and a referral to a CBT psychotherapist. Mr. S calls to schedule the CBT appointment but is told that there will be a 2-month wait for an appointment, and he declines to schedule.

Mr. S returns to see the psychiatrist in 1 month with unchanged symptoms for a 15-min medication management visit and reveals he had stopped sertraline due to nausea. He is switched to escitalopram 5 mg daily. After about 2 weeks on the new medication, he begins feeling somewhat more energetic and has slightly more motivation, but does not experience any functional improvement. At his next 1 month follow-up, Mr. S's escitalopram dose is further up-titrated to 10 mg, and the psychiatrist counsels him about behavioral activation. He experiences further improvements in energy, mood, and motivation; around this time his daughter's condition has stabilized, and he begins spending more time around his family and engaging in various activities. At his next follow-up, 5 months after initially presenting to his primary care provider, he experiences remission from depressive symptoms. When he next sees his primary care doctor 7 months later, he is still being prescribed escitalopram 10 mg, but his hypertension and hyperlipidemia remain uncontrolled.

Collaborative, Interprofessional Model of Care

The primary care physician sends out an instant message to the primary care mental health integration (PCMHI) team requesting additional services for Mr. S toward the end of his office visit. The patient is seen within 15 min by the behavioral health care manager who screens the patient and gathers more information. The patient reveals that trauma-related symptoms have been getting worse for the past year and he has lost interest in daily activities. The care manager inquires about his treatment preferences; he is interested in both pharmacologic and therapeutic interventions. His depression and anxiety screening scores are elevated: PHQ-9 is 17 and GAD-7 is 14. Noting that the patient has a mental health history and has been on medications in the past, the care manager asks the PCMHI psychiatrist via instant messaging to review the patient's chart and provide medication recommendations. The

PCMHI psychiatrist reviews chart notes and finds that the patient was previously prescribed sertraline by his primary care provider but had discontinued it due to nausea. However, at that time the patient had reported improvement in his symptoms, so no further treatment was pursued. The psychiatrist writes a brief note in the chart summarizing the case as she understands it and recommends – with a caveat that she has not evaluated the patient herself – that a trial of escitalopram 5 mg daily would be appropriate. She knows the patient's primary care physician well, collaborated with him frequently in the past, and is confident that this physician will be willing to order this medication at her recommendation. The care manager also sends a request for the PCMHI psychologist to connect with the patient for brief psychotherapeutic intervention.

Mr. S is seen by the PCMHI psychologist within the next week. Psychotherapeutic interventions initiated include aspects of acceptance and commitment therapy and supportive therapy with an emphasis on behavioral activation. At telephone follow-up with the care manager in 1 month, the patient's PHQ-9 and GAD-7 scores are essentially unchanged, and on the medication adherence questionnaire, Mr. S acknowledges that he is less than 50% adherent to escitalopram. On further questioning, he admits to taking his statin and antihypertensive less than 50% of the time. The care manager provides psychoeducation regarding the importance of daily adherence, and the patient reveals that he does not have a system for ensuring he takes his medications. The care manager arranges for a pill box to be sent to him and assists him with setting up smart phone alarms to remind him to fill his pill box weekly and to take his medications daily. The care manager also alerts both the patient's primary care physician as well as the PCMHI regarding his findings, and they agree on a plan for him to contact the patient again in 1 month for telephone follow-up.

Two weeks later, the PCMHI psychologist meets again with the patient, who reports that he is feeling somewhat more energetic since adhering to escitalopram daily. They work together on a plan for him to take advantage of the increased energy to take part in valued activities with his family and to begin a light exercise program. After another 2 weeks, he is contacted by the care manager. His PHQ-9 rating has dropped to 7 and GAD-7 to 5. He feels satisfied with the effect of escitalopram, does not report any side effects, and has been increasingly active and exercising. He has been able to be present and doting to his daughter, whose condition fortunately stabilizes. Mr. S is also adhering to his statin and antihypertensive on a daily basis. At his next routine follow-up 10 months later with his primary care provider, he has lost 10 pounds, and his cholesterol and blood pressure are within normal limits.

Vignette 2

To further illustrate the differences in culture between practicing psychiatry within the traditional medical model vs. a collaborative care model within primary care, the following case will describe the practice of a psychiatrist in the traditional model and her transition to practice in the collaborative care model.

Traditional Model of Care

Dr. T is an outpatient psychiatrist working full-time in an outpatient clinic. She works 8–4:30 p.m., Mondays through Thursdays, and spends the majority of each day in her private office seeing patients. She has two 60-min intake slots per day: one in the morning at 8 a.m. and one in the afternoon at 1 p.m. The rest of her slots are 30-min follow-ups, but the standard practice in her clinic is that if she has back-to-back 30-min follow-up slots open, they can be used to book an intake. She is expected to maintain 70% of her time seeing patients, with the remaining 30% for administration, note writing, telephone calls, completing patient forms, her own education, and completing required training.

Though she is part of a clinic, in practice Dr. T is solely responsible for the care of her patients. Her schedule is usually booked out for 2–3 months into the future, so if a 1-month follow-up is indicated, she needs to have the schedulers either create a slot during her administrative time or double book the patient. Patients generally call her directly with questions about their medications, requests for forms to be filled out, or the status of their psychotherapy referrals. The psychologists are physically located on the other side of the clinic, and since they are also generally fully booked, they rarely communicate directly about shared patients. When Dr. T needs to communicate with the patient's primary care providers, she has the ability to forward them her note along with her question or comment in a message.

Dr. T is responsible for a patient panel of around 400 patients, though she has not had any contact with some of them in over a year. For several months she had tried keeping track of her patient panel using a password-protected Excel spreadsheet, but this process quickly became too burdensome. Her leadership has been phasing in requirements to use measurement-based care, but Dr. T – along with all of the other psychiatrists and psychologists in the clinic – has been very resistant to the idea, arguing that they obtain the same information in the course of their usual clinical practice and can reference their own notes to get a sense of their patients' trajectories.

Transition to Collaborative, Interprofessional Model of Care

Dr. T, interested in the collaborative model of care, completes the American Psychiatric Association training online. Not long afterward, an opening for a collaborative care psychiatrist is announced for a collaborative care program currently staffed by two care managers and a psychologist. The primary care clinic consists of eight primary care teams, which are comprised of a primary care provider, a registered nurse, a licensed vocational nurse, and a medical assistant. Each primary care team shares one of the two care managers with three other teams and cares for about 1000 patients. After a series of interviews, Dr. T is selected for the position.

Dr. T is excited but nervous about the transition, since she had never practiced in this type of setting before. During her orientation week, she is introduced to a slew of individuals from all different professional backgrounds. Being unfamiliar with the roles of the various team members, she requests and is allowed to shadow a team member from each of the professions in the primary care teams, including primary care mental health, primary care provider, pharmacist, nursing, and administrative staff. Through observing their routines and asking questions about their various tasks, she gains an understanding of how each team member sees their roles and how these roles complement the roles of other team members.

Dr. T learns that there are several staff meetings each month, including an all-staff meeting once per month in primary care, a primary care provider meeting once per month, and a weekly collaborative care team meeting. In her first collaborative care team meeting, she introduces herself describing her training and background, acknowledging that this is her first experience working in collaborative care. Her team describes to her their usual practice; up until now the care managers have been able to do brief targeted assessments of how symptoms affect functioning, brief psychosocial interventions such as problem-solving therapy or behavioral activation, psychoeducation regarding depression/anxiety, and how the primary care providers prescribe medications. The psychologist has typically been seeing patients who need somewhat more involvement such as a brief course of CBT (four to six sessions) for depression, anxiety, or insomnia. The psychologist also provides safety assessments for patients who report suicidal ideation.

Prior to Dr. T's arrival, when a patient needed a medication, the psychologist and care manager offered the primary care provider pharmacologic suggestions, with variable success. They are excited about what Dr. T will be able to bring to the team in terms of being able to provide more specific medication recommendations, education for the primary care providers, as well as both indirect and direct consultations. At her team's suggestion, she coordinates with the primary care clinic leadership to present in both the all-staff and primary care provider meetings to describe her role, highlighting what she will be able to add to the ability of the entire clinic to care for the mental health needs of their patients. She emphasizes that as a single psychiatrist, she cannot possibly see every single patient with a mental health need, but by working as a team, they can meet the needs of the entire clinic population.

At first, Dr. T receives many requests for in-person consultations and encounters some resistance from some of the primary care team members to allow her to provide indirect consultations. She discusses this with the collaborative care team at one of their weekly meetings, and they describe to her the comfort level of each of the primary care providers in the clinic. At their suggestion, she arranges to meet with Dr. C – one of the PCPs, who is most comfortable treating his patient's mental health concerns – and with Dr. L, one of the primary care providers, who is least comfortable. Dr. T learns from Dr. C that his training is in family practice and he had substantial experience working in a rural area with little to no psychiatric care available. He attended several workshops at conferences that increased his familiarity with various psychotropic medications. He has found the collaborative care team a tremendously helpful extension of his ability to provide more detailed assessment and follow-up for his patients. He planned to mostly utilize Dr. T for curbside consultation in a more informal manner and to continue alerting his care manager to follow-up on the treatment plans for his patients. Dr. L, on the other hand, trained in internal medicine at a busy academic center. The center had a prominent department of psychiatry with a sterling reputation but was one in which the traditional psychiatric practice model was emphasized. As a result, Dr. L was taught to refer all his patients with any mental health need to psychiatry and since transitioning to this primary care clinic about a year ago had become increasingly frustrated with the long wait times for the mental health clinics in the system. He had been excited to learn that a psychiatrist was going to be embedded in the clinic and saw this as an opportunity to connect all his patients with a psychiatrist. Dr. T thanked him for his enthusiasm for getting his patients the mental health care they needed and, with his permission, described for him the collaborative care model and the importance of providing stepped care, which meant that in order to meet all of his patients' needs, Dr. L would need to be able to care for the milder presentations. Dr. L expressed a willingness to try but felt a lot of discomfort since his own training included very little psychiatry. Dr. T suggested that they collaborate on creating a brief curriculum that could be delivered at the monthly primary care meeting for the first 5–10 min with the goal of helping Dr. L and his colleagues gain familiarity with psychiatric diagnosis and treatment. Dr. L enthusiastically agreed. Dr. T also reassured Dr. L that she was willing to talk through cases with him, to provide detailed chart review with recommendations whenever he needed, and if she identified a case that was more complex, she would schedule the patient to see her for a consultation.

After about a year adjusting to her new practice, Dr. T has settled into a routine. Each day, she arrives at the clinic and is greeted by chart notifications from the various team members. These typically consist of requests from either the CM or a PCP to review a patient's chart for antidepressant recommendations, notes from the CM reporting on a patient's response to treatment that including measurement-based scales (e.g., PHQ-9 and GAD-7 scores), requests from the PCP or CM to see a patient for consultation, or questions about how to manage a difficult patient. Sometimes, the PCPs contact her directly on instant messaging with their questions, or drop by her office (she usually keeps the door open unless she is seeing a patient). About 50% of Dr. T's time is unscheduled to allow her to be available in real time to her colleagues.

Dr. T does not keep her own panel of patients; rather, she views the entire population of the primary care clinic as the patients her team is responsible for treating. As such, she generally limits the number of times she sees any single patient to two or three visits and most commonly sees a patient only once. Generally, she reserves in-person consultations to patients who are more complex – these can be patients who have had several medication trials in the past, patients who may have more severe forms of mental illness, or patients with multiple comorbidities. Dr. T also takes into account the resources of the greater healthcare system she is part of; when she identifies a patient who can be managed in primary care, she assists the PCPs in treating them and reserves the referrals to the mental health clinic for patients who have more severe or treatment-resistant illnesses.

Dr. T and the collaborative care team continue to meet weekly to discuss how their team functions within primary care and to identify any areas for improvement. She also meets weekly with each of the care managers individually to review their patient panels. Using the care management software, they can search and sort patients by PHQ-9 and GAD-7 scores to identify patients who are not improving, who have severe symptoms, or who would benefit from additional services. She and the team psychologist communicate regularly throughout the week about patients they have both seen to ensure they are on the same page about the treatment plan.

Conclusion

As depicted in the case vignettes, the collaborative model of primary care offers a shifting perspective to allow for more shared decision-making with patients, interprofessional team-based care, and real-time consultation across providers. While there may be some barriers to adopting this model and limitations in practice, these can be overcome through consultation and education. This practice allows for clinic-wide changes to treatment targets and utilizes the entire team to improve the quality and timeliness of care for better patient and population outcomes.

Summary of High-Yield Points

- Practicing psychiatry in the primary care setting requires a shift from a culture of "solo practitioners" to a team-based, collaborative culture.
- The care of patients with complex, chronic care needs requires a collaborative and interprofessional approach.
- Interprofessional practice competencies are specific and can be taught.
- Interprofessional, team-based care models have been created for the care of patients with complex, chronic care needs, including the patient-centered medical home for primary care, and the collaborative care model for the practice of psychiatry within primary care.
- The use of measurement-based care allows for collaborative workflows, infrastructure, shared panel management, and effective use of data enable a team-based approach to treatment and communication between patients and other providers.

References

1. Advancing Integrated Mental Health Solutions (AIMS) Center. Behavioral health care manager. University of Washington; 2020a. Retrieved from https://aims.uw.edu/collaborative-care/team-structure/care-manager
2. Advancing Integrated Mental Health Solutions (AIMS) Center. Team structure. University of Washington; 2020b. Retrieved from https://aims.uw.edu/collaborative-care/team-structure
3. American Psychiatric Association. Dissemination of integrated care within adult primary care settings: the collaborative care model. American Psychiatric Association; 2016.

4. Auxier A, Farley T, Seifert K. Establishing an integrated care practice in a community health center. Prof Psychol Res Pract. 2011;42:391–7.
5. Baker R, Stevenson K. Investigating organisational culture in primary care. Qual Prim Care. 2005;13(4):191–200.
6. Bodenheimer T, Wagner E, Grumbach K. Improving primary care for patients with chronic illness. J Am Med Assoc. 2002;288:1775–9.
7. Bower P, Gilbody S, Richards D, Fletcher J, Sutton A. Collaborative care for depression in primary care. Making sense of a complex intervention: systematic review and meta-regression. Br J Psychiatry. 2006;189:484–93.
8. Chaney E, Bonner L, Vivell S, Cohen AN, Young AS, Rubenstein L. How behavioral healthcare informatics systems interface with medical informatics systems: a work in progress. In: Dewan NA, Luo JS, Lorenzi NM, Dewan NA, Luo JS, Lorenzi NM, editors. Information technology essentials for behavioral health clinicians. New York: Springer; 2011. p. 195–204.
9. Clay M, Garr D, Greer A, Lewis R, Blue A, Evans C. An update on the status of interprofessional education and interprofessional prevention education in U.S. academic health centers. Acad Med. 2018;10:61–6.
10. Curran V, Heath O, Adey T, Callahan T, Craig D, Hearn T, White H, Hollett A. An approach to integrating interprofessional education in collaborative mental health care. Acad Psychiatry. 2012;36:91–5.
11. D'amour D, Oandasan I. Interprofessionality as a field of interprofessional practice and interprofessional education: an emerging concept. J Interprof Care. 2005;19(Suppl 1):8–20.
12. Derogatis LR, Lynn LL. Screening and monitoring psychiatric disorder in primary care populations. In: Maruish M, editor. Handbook of psychological assessment in primary care settings. Mahwah: Erlbaum; 2000. p. 115–52.
13. Dowrick C, Leydon GM, McBride A, Howe A, Burgess H, Clarke P, et al. Patients' and doctors' views on depression severity questionnaires incentivized in UK quality and outcomes framework: qualitative study. BMJ. 2009;338:b663.
14. Erickson SM. The patient centered medical home (PCMH): overview of the model and movement part 1. 2010. Retrieved March 2, 2020, from: https://www.acponline.org/practice-resources/business-resources/payment/delivery-and-payment-models/patient-centered-medical-home/understanding-the-patient-centered-medical-home/what-is-the-patient-centered-medical-home
15. Hauguel JF. Primary care transformation: the changing of a culture. 21 2017. Retrieved March 3, 2020, from https://www.mgma.com/resources/operations-management/primary-care-transformation-the-changing-of-a-cul
16. Hayward R. Why the culture of medicine has to change. BMJ. 2007;335(7623):775.
17. Huffman JC, Niazi SK, Rundel JR, Sharpe M, Katon WJ. Essential articles on collaborative care models for the treatment of psychiatric disorders in medical settings: a publication by the Academy of Psychosomatic Medicine Research and Evidence-Based Practice Committee. Psychosomatics. 2014;55(2):109–22.
18. Institute of Medicine (US) Committee on Quality of Health Care in America. Crossing the quality chasm: a new health system for the 21st century. National Academies Press; 2001.
19. Interprofessional Education Collaborative Expert Panel. Core competencies for interprofessional collaborative practice: report of an expert panel. Washington, DC: Interprofessional Education Collaborative; 2011.
20. Katon W. Collaborative depression care models: from development to dissemination. Am J Prev Med. 2012;42(5):550–2.
21. Kearney LK, Wray LO, Dollar KM, King PR. Establishing measurement-based care in integrated primary care: monitoring clinical outcomes over time. J Clin Psychol Med Settings. 2015;22(4):213–27.
22. Kellerman R, Kirk L. Principles of the patient-centered medical home. Am Fam Physician. 2007;76(6):774–5.
23. Kindig DA. Understanding population health terminology. Milbank Q. 2007;85(1):139–61.
24. Kindig D, Stoddart G. What is population health? Am J Public Health. 2003;93(3):380–3.

25. Lambert MJ, Whipple JL, Hawkins EJ, Vermeersch DA, Nielsen SL, Smart DW. Is it time for clinicians to routinely track patient outcome? A meta-analysis. Clin Psychol Sci Pract. 2003;10:288–301.
26. Lambert MJ, Harmon C, Slade K, Whipple JL, Hawkins EJ. Providing feedback to psychotherapists on their patients' progress: clinical results and practice suggestions. J Clin Psychol. 2005;61:165–74.
27. Maranzan KA. Interprofessional education in mental health: an opportunity to reduce mental health stigma. J Interprof Care. 2016;30(3):370–7.
28. Marcussen M, Nørgaard B, Arnfred S. The effects of Interprofessional education in mental health practice: findings from a systematic review. Acad Psychiatry. 2019;43(2):200–8.
29. Marshall MN, Mannion R, Nelson E, Davies HTO. Managing change in the culture of general practice: qualitative case studies in primary care trusts. BMJ. 2003;327(7415):599–602.
30. Mitchell P, Golden R. Core principles & values of effective team-based health care. National Academy of Sciences; 2012.
31. Oandasan I, Reeves S. Key elements for interprofessional education. Part 1: the learner, the educator and the learning context. J Interprof Care. 2005;19(Suppl 1):21–38.
32. Olfson M, Wang S, Wall M, Marcus SC, Blanco C. Trends in serious psychological distress and outpatient mental health care of US adults. JAMA Psychiat. 2019;76(2):152–61.
33. Oslin DW, Ross J, Sayers S, Murphy J, Kane V, Katz I. Screening, assessment, and management of depression in VA primary care clinics: the behavioral health laboratory. J Gen Intern Med. 2006;21:46–50.
34. Raney LE. Integrating primary care and behavioral health: the role of the psychiatrist in the collaborative care model. Am J Psychiatr. 2015;172(8):721–8.
35. Taylor JS. Confronting "culture" in medicine's "culture of no culture". Acad Med. 2003;78(6):555–9.
36. Unützer J, Katon W, Callahan CM, Williams JW Jr, Hunkeler E, Harpole L, et al. Collaborative care management of late-life depression in the primary care setting: a randomized controlled trial. JAMA. 2002;288(22):2836–45.
37. Wagner EH. The role of patient care teams in chronic disease management. BMJ. 2000;320(7234):569–72.
38. Willard-Grace R, Hessler D, Rogers E, Dubé K, Bodenheimer T, Grumbach K. Team structure and culture are associated with lower burnout in primary care. JABFM. 2014;27(2):229–38.
39. Yeung AS, Jing Y, Brenneman SK, Chang TE, Baer L, Hebden T, et al. Clinical outcomes in measurement-based treatment (COMET): a trial of depression monitoring and feedback to primary care physicians. Depress Anxiety. 2012;29(10):865–73.
40. Katon W, Lin EH, Von Korff M, Ciechanowski P, Ludman E, Young B, Rutter C, Oliver M, McGregor M. Integrating depression and chronic disease care among patients with diabetes and/or coronary heart disease: the design of the TEAMcare study. Contemporary clinical trials. 2010;31(4):312–22.

Psychiatric Care in Residential Care Environments

11

Omar Ghosn, Steven Huege, and Daniel D. Sewell

Introduction

In the USA, 4.2% of individuals 65 years old and older live in nursing homes (NHs) [1]. This estimate does not include older adults living in other proprietary residential environments. Over the past several decades, a spectrum of terms have been coined to describe the various levels of care provided by, and the configurations of, these residential care facilities for older adults including independent living, assisted living, subacute care hospitals, rehabilitative facilities, and retirement communities. In addition to these terms, other terms describing housing options for older adults include senior community, 55 and up community, senior retirement community, senior living community, multilevel senior community, and continuing care retirement community (CCRC). In this manuscript, the term "proprietary residential care environment" is used when referring to all of the above housing options for older adults. If something is unique to a specific housing option, this will be noted. As the older adult population increases, improved understanding of proprietary residential care setting's unique cultural environments will be critical to implementing successful transitions and promoting the health and well-being of older adult patients.

Background

One of the most important distinctions between different proprietary residential care environments is the level of care or support provided. The term retirement community (RT) is an umbrella term which describes a variety of housing options for predominantly independent seniors. An RT is a residential or housing complex that is designed for older adults and is generally age-restricted (e.g., age 55 and older).

O. Ghosn · S. Huege · D. D. Sewell (✉)
Department of Psychiatry, University of California San Diego, San Diego, CA, USA
e-mail: oghosn@health.ucsd.edu; shuege@health.ucsd.edu; dsewell@health.ucsd.edu

S. H. Koh et al. (eds.), *Diversity in Action*,
https://doi.org/10.1007/978-3-030-85401-0_11

Residents are usually partially or fully retired and able to care for themselves without regular nursing or other routine medical assistance; however, assistance from home care agencies is allowed in some communities. RTs offer shared services, amenities, activities, and socialization opportunities [2].

As defined by the American Association of Homes and Services for the Aging (AAHSA), a CCRC is "an organization that offers a full range of housing, residential services, and healthcare in order to serve its older residents as their needs change over time" [3]. CCRCs are communities that attempt to promote a sense of independence in older adults throughout their later years. Another term used to describe a CCRC is multilevel senior community.

Older adults who cannot or choose not to live independently, may reside in an assisted living facility (ALF). It is important to note, however, that there is no standard definition for the term. In some states where assisted living is not licensed or regulated, the term may be used quite loosely. Facilities in these states may not provide the services and care usually associated with assisted living. In other states, the term is used to describe a specific type of housing option that is licensed and regulated by the state government. There are also specialized ALFs that cater to those living with a dementia illness. Synonyms for ALF include board and care home and, if dementia care is provided, special care unit or memory care unit.

The exact number of older adults living in each type of senior housing across the USA is not available due to the heterogeneity of labels and defining features, as well as the lack of central data collection. In 2017, the not-for-profit senior living organization National Senior Campuses reported over 19,000 senior living units across the USA, up from the 15,500 estimate provided in 1998 by the American Senior Housing Association (ASHA) [4]. Currently, it is estimated that one million Americans live in some type of senior living community, and that number is expected to double by the year 2030 [5].

With advancements in life expectancy, all studies predict an increase in both the number of older adults and in the complexity of their needs. In fact, the fastest-growing segment of the US population is the group of individuals older than 85 years. The 85-and-older age group is expected to increase from about three million in 2009 to more than 18 million in 2050 [6]. What's more, projections for the year 2050 predict that approximately 40% of the older population will belong to racial or ethnic minorities [7].

Psychiatric Illness in Residential Care Environments

In the early 1980s, work by the National Citizens' Coalition for Nursing Home Reform, a consumer advocacy group concerned about substandard care in NHs, emphasized residents' rights and the importance of implementing resident assessments. Its Consumer Statement of Principles for the Nursing Home Regulatory System, released in 1983, was endorsed by more than sixty national organizations, presented to the US Department of Health and Human Services, and distributed to all congressional offices [8]. Several of the major issues raised about the quality of NH care were related to its psychiatric aspects; physical and chemical restraints were inappropriately used to control residents' behavior, and psychiatric disorders, primarily depression, were undertreated [6]. In fact, epidemiological studies between 1986 and 1993 uniformly reported high prevalence rates for psychiatric disorders among NH residents [9]. The prevalence of psychiatric disorders among persons newly admitted to a proprietary chain of NHs was found to be 80.2%. In all studies, the most common psychiatric disorder was dementia, with prevalence rates of 50–75% and up to 30% of residents exhibiting behavioral problems [9]. To date, ALFs have not been studied as extensively as NHs, and as described above ALF, licensing or regulation varies by jurisdiction.

Despite the difficulties associated with methods and measurement, evidence to date suggests that quality of life in residential care community environments for older adults is largely determined by the presence of mental health problems and one's subjective sense of well-being [10]. Research also suggests that both the individual's cultural identity, the sensitivity of the treating team toward this identity [11], and the culture of the residential care environment [12] can significantly impact the mental health and perceived quality of life of older adults living in a residential care home. As a result, geriatric psychiatrists play an integral part in the care of older adults residing in NHs and other proprietary residential care environments. The role of geriatric psychiatrists includes advocating for the patient to ensure that they receive optimal care, including appropriate psychiatric treatment. Each resident/patient needs a clinically comprehensive, culturally sensitive, and individualized assessment and treatment plan which addresses medical as well as social and environmental factors as potential contributors to mental health problems. Close monitoring to assess treatment responses and to prevent unwanted side effects is also essential. The 1980's alarm bells warning about NH's low quality of care inspired a series of reforms, public policies, individual initiatives, and innovations which aimed to create and improve the existing practices and standards of care. The movement toward *person-centered care* has been slowly gaining ground in these settings ever since. Still, more needs to be done to improve the health and well-being of older adults living in various residential living environments.

In addition to ensuring comprehensive and individualized care, geriatric psychiatrists and others involved in caring for older adults in proprietary residential living environments are strategically positioned to advocate at various levels of healthcare and community systems. Specifically, advocacy efforts are important within insurance companies, organizations involved in providing housing to older adults, systems of healthcare, government programs, and policy and regulations. Issues include improved architecture which reflects universal design concepts, implementation of new and innovative psychosocial programs, formulation of institutional policies and procedures for assessment, care delivery, training and educating care providers, and monitoring the quality of care being provided in various settings [6, 9]. The education and training that is needed by those who help provide care to older adults living in residential care environments includes knowledge, understanding, humility regarding the cultural identities and characteristics of the individuals for whom they care, awareness of the culture and atmosphere of the residential living environment, and appreciation for the complex intersections of the two. This becomes especially important when addressing situations where conflict arises and may diminish the patient's quality of life.

Some of the cultural aspects and challenges in care are similar across the various housing options for older adults, and some are unique to the specific type of living environment. The case vignette and ensuing discussion are intended to depict the current landscape and challenges a geriatric psychiatrist may face when caring for older adults in proprietary senior living environments.

Vignette

Mr. X is a single 84-year-old Asian male who has been residing in an ALF. He moved to an ALF after careful consideration and with the support of his nephews. He was feeling very lonely at home and struggled to care for himself with limited support and social interactions, other than occasional visits from his nephews. His medical history is notable for hypertension, diabetes, and an old stroke with minimal residual symptoms. He had no past history of psychiatric illness.

Upon arrival to the ALF, Mr. X's mood improved. Staff members described him as socializing well with other residents and, overall, being a positive addition to the community. A few weeks after he moved in, however, Mr. X's nephews contacted the facility director in distress following a visit with their uncle. They requested an urgent psychiatric consultation due to concerns after observing their uncle's unusual disinhibited sexual behaviors and aggression toward other residents. The medical director of the ALF, who was also the patient's primary care provider (PCP), prescribed Mr. X clonazepam to control these problem behaviors while awaiting the psychiatry consultation.

- *A – Is clonazepam a good choice in this case? Are benzodiazepines commonly prescribed for older adults living in a residential care environment? What does the law say about benzodiazepines and antipsychotic prescriptions for older adults?*

Shortly after, Mr. X suffered from a fall overnight and was sent to the emergency department (ED). Imaging revealed no fractures, but his urine analysis indicated a urinary tract infection (UTI). The patient was diagnosed with delirium secondary to his UTI. After Mr. X had spent 12 hours in the ED, he returned to his ALF with an oral antibiotic prescription, and clonazepam was discontinued. Mr. X's nephews could not help asking themselves if this time-consuming and costly visit could have been prevented.

- *B – What personal characteristics make Mr. X more prone to an ED visit?*

Mr. X's nephews were furious about the incident and its subsequent consequences. They blamed the ALF for the delay in diagnosis of the UTI and the associated delay in medical management. Without consulting Mr. X, who was still recovering from delirium, the nephews decided to transfer him to a NH.

- *C – What are the advantages and disadvantages of this decision? What differentiates a NH from an assisted living community?*

Mr. X remained slightly confused and his recovery proceeded slowly in his new environment. He had trouble adapting to his windowless room and smaller bathroom. His mood was low and he did not engage with other residents or staff members. He was often verbally abusive toward staff. At times, he remained disoriented and forgetful of recent events and names. He also developed new-onset urinary incontinence. Staff members accused him of being purposefully incontinent of urine.

- *D – How can we explain Mr. X's behavior? Could his incontinence be an act of protest instead of the symptom of a medical problem like benign prostatic hypertrophy?*

A neuropsychology referral took place and psychometric tests revealed cognitive impairments consistent with the diagnosis of major neurocognitive impairment due to Alzheimer's disease. Donepezil was suggested to slow the progression of his symptoms. Mr. X rejected the diagnosis and showed no insight into his deficits and limitations. His nephews also had trouble coming to terms with the patient's dementia diagnosis, and they did not wish to start medication for what they believed was a normal process of aging.

- *E – Was there a common cultural belief behind Mr. X's and his nephews' reluctance to accept the recommendation for treatment with donepezil?*

Mr. X was uncooperative whenever assistance with activities of daily living was needed. Up to four staff members were required to assist him with personal hygiene and toileting except when J, a nursing assistant, was on duty. Mr. X had slowly begun to trust J and was less distressed and agitated in his presence. J is from Portugal and he enjoyed talking to Mr. X about his travels in Asia. He once brought him traditional Thai food for lunch, and Mr. X was overjoyed.

- *F – What made J different than the other staff members? Could J's approach be adopted by others?*

The NH director noticed J was more successful than other staff members at engaging with different residents in the ALF, including Mr. X. With the director's approval, J tried to provide his co-workers some pointers about how to approach residents with different racial, ethnic, or cultural backgrounds. Initially, J faced a lot of resistance, especially from registered nurses.

- *G – What could be behind the resistance of the RNs, the low attendance at J's presentations, and the limited engagement of some of the staff members during J's workshops?*

One day while assisting Mr. X with personal care, Mr. X made inappropriate sexual comments. He described his desire for intimacy and his yearning for human contact. J set boundaries with Mr. X who apologetically noted he had been lonely and isolated for a long time.

- *H – Do NH residents maintain their libido and interest in intimacy?*

When queried, Mr. X revealed his preference for men and that he identified as homosexual all his life. According to him, no staff member at the different residential placements had bothered to ask him about his sexual orientation. As a result, he did not mention this to others due to his concerns that he would experience homophobia, feel judged, be rejected and not receive the same quality of care as others.

- *I – What made Mr. X so reluctant to share his sexual orientation? How can we address his fear of stigma and discrimination on an institutional level?*

Despite receiving better medical care at the NH, Mr. X insisted on returning to the ALF where he had originally moved and where he was allowed to have his own furniture and personal belongings. At first, his nephews were shocked by this decision. They were concerned about his care and always thought of the ALF as a "progressive crazy house for the elderly," remembering an older woman wandering around barefoot in nightwear, carrying purses and dolls, and talking to herself. Mr. X explained he felt much more at home there, more respected, and more heard. Mr. X's nephews eventually agreed and respected his wishes.

- *J – What makes the person-centered care philosophy and approach so successful?*

Case Discussion and Recommendations for Optimal Treatment

- *A – Pharmacological treatment of behavioral disturbances experienced by older adults living in residential care environments: undertreating or overtreating?*

National concerns about inadequate and inappropriate care for older adults living in residential environments have focused on the overuse of psychotropic drugs in NH residents, especially the misuse of these medications as "chemical restraints" to control patient behaviors [6, 8]. Studies in the 1970s and 1980s reported that approximately 50% of residents had orders for psychotropic medications, with 20–40% being given antipsychotic drugs, 10–40% given anxiolytics or hypnotics, and 5–10% given antidepressants [9]. These prescribing habits were deemed dangerous due to the multiple adverse effects associated with these medications.

In 1987, Congress mandated stricter regulations to reduce unnecessary drug use as part of the Omnibus Budget Reconciliation Act. The first set of regulations, implemented in 1990, focused on antipsychotic drugs, which often were used to control the behavior of NH residents despite concerns about adverse effects (e.g., anticholinergic effects, orthostatic hypotension, extrapyramidal symptoms, and ventricular arrhythmias) and lack of efficacy [13]. The second set of regulations, implemented in 1992, focused on benzodiazepines, which were used routinely despite their association with hip fractures, confusion, and other serious adverse effects [14]. These changes in regulations and policies did inspire some improvements in prescribing practices moderated by medication type and setting. A study evaluating NHs responses to those regulations revealed a marked reduction in antipsychotic drug use but little change in the benzodiazepine prescription trends despite the 1992 regulations. Adoption of the new regulations was found to be significantly greater in facilities with a high score on "resident-centered care philosophy" than in those with a low score. The term "resident-centered care philosophy" describes beliefs and norms that emphasize individualized assessment and psychosocial care, avoidance of restraints, and multidisciplinary collaboration. Reduction in psychotropic drug use was greater in communities that had an organizational culture that was compatible with this philosophy [12, 15, 16].

Despite the federal regulations, unique NH settings and practices played a role in medication prescribing trends. Psychiatric medication overprescribing was not found in all NHs. Some studies found that rural nursing homes were consistently under-prescribing psychotropics, which led to suboptimal treatment of depressive, psychotic, and disruptive behaviors. Under-prescribing was associated with the commonly found limitations encountered in rural long-term care settings, such as reduced availability and accessibility of health professionals and services [17]. Tribal NHs are a commonly referenced example as they are mostly located in rural areas, often have challenges in access and identification, and therefore reduced pharmacotherapy [18, 19].

Over half of residents in senior communities have a diagnosis of dementia, and many have associated behavioral disturbances [9]. There are a number of published sources that outline the proper assessment and treatment of behavioral symptoms in patients living with dementia. Clinicians working with older adults in residential care environments should be very familiar with at least one of these (e.g., the Physician Guidelines for the Screening, Evaluation, and Management of Alzheimer's Disease and Related Dementias; http://championsforhealth.org/alzheimers). Of note, recently the FDA approved the second-generation antipsychotic medication, pimavanserin (Nuplazid), for use with patients living with Parkinson's disease and psychosis. Pimavanserin, is the only antipsychotic to have FDA approval for use in patients with a form of dementia [20]. In general, the important steps when evaluating behavioral symptoms in an older adult living with dementia are:

1. Rule out underlying medical illness as the cause of the behavioral problems.
2. Identify and remove any environmental triggers.
3. Implement behavioral interventions.
4. Use psychiatric medications only when behavioral interventions fail or when the behaviors are so serious that imminent harm is likely to occur.

5. Combine pharmacological, behavioral, and psychological interventions to achieve potentially quicker, safer, and more long-lasting results.

– *B – Are there resident characteristics associated with bad outcomes and more frequent ED transfers from senior residential care environments?*

Residents of senior living communities, and especially NHs, may have complex comorbidities that often challenge the busy ED provider who is trying to differentiate between acute and chronic illness during a time-limited encounter. Likewise, the often chaotic ED environments can be difficult for any patient with a health crisis but are especially challenging for older adults living with a dementia illness. Many transfers from the NH to the ED are believed to be either unnecessary or preventable and may result in more harm than benefit. According to one study, 47 percent of all long-stay NH residents experienced at least one transfer to the ED over the course of a year. At the time of their first ED transfer, 36.4% of the participants were admitted to the hospital, whereas 63.1% of those who visited the ED were not. The median time to first ED visit for the participants with dementia was significantly higher than for the participants with no dementia [21]. Due to the high costs and poor quality of care involved in unnecessary transfers, they have become a target of policymakers and a focus of a Centers for Medicare and Medicaid Services demonstration project [22].

– *C – Nursing homes* versus *assisted living*

NHs have been the primary source of institutional care for older adults since the inception of Medicare and Medicaid in 1987 [23]; however, the combined impact of a growing number of older adults, a shortage of NH beds, the increasing costs of nursing care, the better health of new cohorts of older adults, and dissatisfaction with NH care have increased focus on other care settings [24]. Specifically, awareness has increased regarding the gap in the "continuum" of care between independent senior housing options (that cater to the older adult population with no functional impairments) and nursing facilities (that provide care to the chronically ill and disabled) [24]. As a result, CCRCs and larger NHs have broadened their range of care to bridge this gap, resulting in the stand-alone ALFs, which have increased dramatically since the 2000s. The original ALFs were modeled after Dutch residential settings and aimed to provide an "invisible support system" in a residential setting [25]. ALFs, however, are not subject to the same licensing restrictions and guidelines expressly encouraging aging in place [24]. Furthermore, although the ALF's professional organizations endorse providing a homelike environment, independence, autonomy, and privacy to their residents, facilities that do not subscribe to this philosophy are free to use the same term. In addition, the term ALF is not always used by facilities that do aspire to the type of environment described above [26].

Differences in the culture of the various residential care environment options available to seniors are evident from studies that compared their admissions thresholds. NHs were more likely than ALFs to admit impaired residents, both overall and specific to those with activities of daily living (ADL) impairments. Within ALF facility types, smaller facilities consistently housed the most impaired residents, and traditional facilities consistently housed the least impaired. Adults with ADL, cognitive, and behavioral impairments are most prevalent in younger facilities (less than 5 years old) and those that are for-profit. Facilities with higher rates of resident impairment have more lenient admission policies, provide less privacy, and less resident control—all areas seemingly consistent with the realities of a more impaired population [27]. Given that newer NHs do not differ from traditional and newer model ALFs in the provision of social and recreational services (e.g., exercise, outside entertainment, groups), policy clarity (e.g., holding orientations and staff meetings, distributing newsletters) and resident control (e.g., conducting resident meetings, involving residents in plans regarding activities and room changes) may be indicative of improvements that have been made in the philosophy of NH care. Perhaps because of regulations or an evolution in response to consumer demand and the growth of ALFs, there may be increasingly blurred distinctions between NHs and ALFs [27]. Whether a community is for-profit or not-for-profit also plays a role in the culture and philosophy of the community. For-profit ALFs may face an inherent conflict between optimal resident care and financial constraints/pressures that might be less overt in a not-for-profit facility. In contrast, not-for-profit ALFs sometimes have charitable sources to subsidize residents who cannot afford to pay for their care [28].

The number of choices may make selecting the best option for residential care difficult. There are many guidance sources available for older adults who need help determining what option may be best. In many communities, for-profit businesses that specialize in helping older adults and/or their family members make these decisions now exist. If the decision to move to residential care is made near the end of an inpatient hospitalization, then a hospital social worker may be able to provide guidance. In addition, there are several not-for-profit organizations, such as the local chapter of an Alzheimer's Association, that are also able to help. Lastly, there are a growing number of reliable online sources of information, including information provided by the federal government and by a number of state and local governments, to aid in the decision-making process.

- *D – Impaired residents and nonverbal communication: Can agitation and incontinence be used as communication tools?*

The *need-driven dementia-compromised behavior model* conceptualizes problem behaviors as attempts to communicate unmet needs that, if responded to appropriately, will enhance the individual's overall quality of life [29]. An unmet need can trigger increased levels of frustration, which, in turn, may lead to further dissatisfaction, agitation, and eventually disruptive and dangerous behaviors. In fact, abuse in nursing facilities occurs bidirectionally. It is a "double-edged sword," with staff mistreatment of residents being the most visible edge. However, resident abuse of staff also occurs, but continues basically unnoticed as outsiders primarily focus on the quality of resident care [30].

Furthermore, incontinence is very common in nursing homes and affects approximately 40–75 percent of residents. It is often a major factor in decisions to institutionalize [11]. Incontinence is typically associated with shame and loss of self-esteem. Unfortunately, for restrained or severely debilitated residents, incontinence provides one of the few remaining possibilities for protest. Its most immediate impact is a significant workload increase for staff members which may lead to job dissatisfaction or burnout [31].

- *E – How do different cultural beliefs among various minority groups affect attitudes toward mental health disorders and access to treatments?*

The changing age profile of populations in all western countries means that dementia will become a more significant issue and demands for various supportive services will be greater in the future. A report regarding individuals living with dementia noted less use of services among individuals and their caregivers who belong to certain ethnic minorities when compared to members of other ethnic groups. The authors of this report argued that the needs of this subset of individuals may be unidentified, underrepresented, or unmet [32]. The reasons mentioned in the literature for these observed variations in levels of resource utilization include [33, 34]:

(a) Differences in prevalence rates between the ethnic groups
(b) Cultural deficiencies in the instruments used to assess cognitive function
(c) Differing cultural interpretation of the signs and symptoms of dementia
(d) Different age stratification found in minorities in various countries
(e) The stigma revolving around mental illnesses
(f) A lack of knowledge and understanding of available resources and services
(g) A general reluctance to use health and social resources and services which some members of ethnic minorities may perceive as culturally inappropriate, or even racist
(h) Language barriers, particularly when it comes to first-generation immigrants living with dementia

By 2050, it has been projected that approximately 40% of the older adult population will belong to a racial or ethnic minority [7]. The broad categories used by the US federal government to define ethnic minorities—African Americans, American Indian and Alaska Natives, Asian Americans, Pacific Islanders, and Hispanic Americans—do not capture the broad range of cultural differences that can play a role in defining illness and selecting treatment. Examples of groups in the USA with particular healthcare needs include Ethiopians, Haitians, Holocaust survivors of different nationalities, Hutterites, Laotians, Mexicans, Somalis, Russians, Vietnamese, and people from Eastern Europe and from countries in Central America. Examples of culturally based behaviors in various ethnic and cultural groups include: [1] Russian immigrants may neglect to obtain insurance because they are accustomed to the government's providing healthcare and other necessities by default; Afghans, Bosnians, and Somalis, may be suffering from overlooked posttraumatic stress

Table 11.1 Cultural differences regarding family members serving as caregivers [33, 35]

Ethnic or racial group	Caregiving as a family obligation	Possible reasons for not seeking services
Hispanic Americans	Yes	Stigma about mental illness Illness seen as punishment for past sins
Asian/Pacific Islanders Americans	Yes, mainly oldest son and wife, followed by rest of children if needed	Strong shame and stigma leading to frequent somatic presentations Symptoms seen as natural and untreatable consequence of aging
American Indians	Not typically	Poor services in native regions Symptoms seen as a normal process of aging Little stigma and shame from behavioral problems and confusion in older adults
African Americans	Yes, informal support from extended family, kin, and religious community	Lack of knowledge or awareness of resources Illness caused by various life stressors

disorder (PTSD) resulting from war, torture, or ethnic conflict [36]; and immigrants from Central America and Mexican-Americans may also be at risk for PTSD resulting from violence experienced in their home country, during their journey to the USA, or as a result of experiences associated with attempts to immigrate [37]. San Francisco General Hospital provides a model outlining how to address the range of ethnic minorities represented in their psychiatric inpatients [38]. The department offers different inpatient programs for Hispanic, Asian and Pacific Islander, African-American patients, as well as programs for women, HIV-positive patients, lesbian and gay patients, and forensic patients.

The *Cultural Influences on Mental Health* (CIMH) framework is a useful approach when characterizing cultural factors that develop in a relationship between the patient and the mental healthcare system. This model suggests that various cultural influences contribute to the etiology and development of mental illness and affect how one personally defines symptoms and illness. For example, cultural differences may contribute to the prevalence of mental disorders, influence beliefs about the causes of mental illness, and subsequently impact treatments and interventions [7]. The goal of describing the various cultural influences is not to stereotype groups— as groups are composed of unique individuals— rather, the goal is to sensitize practitioners of various disciplines to ethnocultural issues, values, and needs. Table 11.1 summarizes cultural differences regarding family members serving as caregivers in four different ethnic or cultural groups.

– *F – Do cultural competence trainings work?*

Cultural characteristics represent an integral aspect of all parts of life and play a major role in defining one's self-identity. The degree to which healthcare providers are culturally aware can shape the patient's ability to receive and apply information regarding their own healthcare, which consequently affects their overall health and health outcomes [39]. Educational programs that are sensitive to cultural diversity have the potential to produce culturally responsive healthcare assessments that yield optimal healthcare interventions and practices. For example, the APA practice guideline for treatment of patients with Alzheimer's dementia recently highlighted several cultural characteristics that affect care including symptom presentation, familial acceptance of the behavioral disorder, caregiving style, and size of and support from social networks [7]. Cultural sensitivity trainings for providers have demonstrated increased open-mindedness and cultural awareness, improved understanding of multiculturalism, and enhanced communication quality with members of ethnic and racial minorities. A study on the effectiveness of cultural sensitivity training of foreign-trained medical graduate students found that those who received cultural sensitivity training were more open and resilient, had increased self-confidence and tolerance, were nonjudgmental, were able to deal with ambiguity, and were capable of better understanding others [39]. Those who were trained also exhibited improved skills in assessing verbal and nonverbal cues communicated to them by people who were from different backgrounds than themselves [39].

– *G – Work environment hierarchy in nursing homes: Is a change needed?*

Just as in homes and communities, organizations create their own unique and dynamic cultural environments. It is not uncommon for residential care settings to have tension and conflict between staff members, which may have a significant impact on the residents and the care provided there. For example, in the USA, some NHs struggle with tension between different clinical professions and hierarchies. Nursing aides or certified nursing assistants (CNAs) typically tend to the basic bodily needs of residents, including elimination and incontinence care. Given their frequent contact with blood, feces, sputum, vomit, and urine, aides are very much at risk of becoming ostracized as "polluted people" or "dirty workers," whose sole job is to clean up a mess. Unlike aides, professional nurses in nursing homes are, for the most part, able to evade elimination care, which sometimes creates conflict between CNAs and RNs. Nursing assistants, it seems, are reluctant to accept the postulate that a nursing license exempts its bearer from elimination care or that their lack of license exempts them from being more useful to the residents [38]. Spending consistent time with residents helps CNAs become familiar with residents' patterns of health and behavior and their likes and dislikes. Familiarity with their residents promotes the development of relationships, as well as the CNAs' expertise in making day-to-day care decisions on the residents' behalf. Further, research shows second-career CNAs tend to have altruistic intentions and are more influenced by relationships and the desire to make a difference than by money [40]. More so, they expressed their values and ideals through their work and sought to transform nursing home care. Yet, difficulty retaining these long-term care workers continues to plague nursing homes, as turnover rates approach 100% [41]. Researchers have documented that these CNAs' decisions to leave their jobs were influenced less by hard work and low pay and more by feeling devalued by administration and other staff [40].

The work environment hierarchy may have played a role in the poor response that J received when he was asked to share his approach with other staff members at Mr. X's NH. In a naturalistic survey, one CNA described their experience in the workplace as:

> Transitioning between two worlds: In one world, the institution provides care to numerous frail older adults, while meeting state and federal regulations. In this world, CNAs are replaceable workers. In the other world, the home offers a sense of community and a home-like environment where the residents' individual needs and preferences are attended to. In this world, CNAs are considered valued members of the team and the community. [42]

Successful nursing home communities have demonstrated that they value CNAs by seeking their input in resident care planning, providing mentoring activities, and respecting their work. Important, then, is the adoption of policies and practices that create an atmosphere of valuing and appreciating CNAs' contributions [43]. Whether it is tension between nurses and nursing assistants or conflict between other groups of staff or individuals, these conflicts impact the culture of the residential care environment and need to be identified and resolved to optimize the resident's experience.

– *H – Sexual behaviors in residential care environments. Given the spectrum of possible causes, what is the optimal outcome?*

Sexual expressions remain important for a significant proportion of older people. Despite this, within healthcare systems, the sexual needs of the older adults are often unrecognized and unmet. Frequently, this occurs as a result of negative attitudes and beliefs surrounding sexuality, sex, and sexual desires, especially in older adults [5]. A majority of older adults, even those residing in long-term care environments, maintain some level of sexual interest, albeit at decreased levels. Future cohorts of older adults are expected to have even greater sustained interest in sex, as well as higher frequency of participation in sexual acts, as generational acceptance and perception that sexuality is normal for older individuals increase [44]. Evidence suggests, however, that sexual desire is mediated not only by age but also by psychosocial factors including partner availability, frequency of contact, and generational perceptions of the appropriateness of sexual activity in later life [45], as well as biological factors, including the presence of chronic diseases and the medications used to treat them [46]. For residents living in long-term care settings such as assisted living, these factors are likely to be highly relevant.

Historically, the culture of most residential care environments for older adults has not supported the sexual needs of the residents. Physical aspects of life in a residential care environment are one of the most common and significant barriers to sexual intimacy, such as living in a shared room with only a curtain between the beds for privacy. The cultural beliefs and attitudes of personal and professional caregivers, however, are another common obstacle for sexual expression. Studies have shown that nursing home staff members' attitudes toward sexual behaviors in older adults –which are primarily negative– present another barrier to residents fulfilling their sexual needs [47]. Such attitudes often lead clinical and support staff, including housekeeping and food service team members, and members of the management team to perceive any attempt at sexual expression as inappropriate, even by residents without cognitive impairment. Preferred forms of sexual expression vary widely. Sexuality and intimacy are manifested in various ways, including intercourse, but findings overwhelmingly reveal that intimate touch, hand holding, and other less physically intense expressions are common and valued just as significantly as younger individuals might enjoy more vigorous physical expressions of sexuality [48].

Assisted living policies regarding sexuality were found to be sometimes informal and vague. For example, some assisted living directors instruct their staff to leave quietly when they observe sexual activity in residents' apartments. Facilities' responses to sex and intimacy are context related. Assisted living settings' responses to sex and intimacy are couched in the social context of the situation. Directors and staff rely on the family members' and powers' of attorney wishes and directives. They can be permissive if the family is supportive of relationships but can reinforce limit setting if the family is not accepting the behaviors. If an assisted living setting has a low census of patients, policies may become more flexible. Problematic sexual behavior may be discouraged but impulsive patients will not be banned [48]. Advance directives are generally used to give guidance concerning medical care, not sexual relationships. As directives become more widely used, however, they may also be used to specify other aspects of care the patient wishes to receive when incompetent, including sexual behavior. In fact, "some individuals may feel so strongly about loyalty to a spouse or religious belief that they may include directives concerning future sexual relationships" [49]. Cultural training around the healthy expression of sexual behaviors in older adults may be needed to ensure that older adults who want to remain sexually active receive proper acceptance, education, understanding, and support, even after moving to a residential care community.

- *I – LGBT discrimination exists in residential care environments and nursing homes*

According to the National Gay and Lesbian Task Force, there are currently between 1.4 and 3.8 million lesbian, gay, bisexual, and transgender (LGBT) Americans over the age of 65 [50]. They remain particularly at risk of both homophobia and heterosexism. Homophobia is defined as the unreasonable hatred, prejudice, and fear of LGB people. Transphobia is the term to describe hatred, prejudice, and fear of transgender individuals. Heterosexism and cisgender status function as default assumptions; it is a bias where the heterosexuality and cisgender of most people are presumed. Institutional heterosexism relies on the assumption of heterosexuality as the norm when health services are provided resulting in the needs of LGBT people being neglected [51]. *The LGBT Cultural Competency Project* is an example of a collaborative initiative between multiple partnerships with a primary goal of providing education and awareness of the unique needs and concerns of LGBT older adults who are aging into long-term care communities [51]. Many LGBT older adults are concerned about entering nursing homes due to fears that they will be forced into the closet to avoid being shunned by other nursing home residents for being openly lesbian, gay, bisexual, or transgender. Others fear mistreatment by administrative staff, care staff, and peers [52]. In fact, "invisible" is a recurring description of older LGBT individuals. Although "passing" is used as a survival tactic to protect against discrimination, the trauma for those who have lived their lives openly and honestly but find themselves going back into hiding when "they become ill, vulnerable and dependent on others" should not be minimized [53]. Transgender persons are at particular risk of avoiding institutions and situations where they would be forced to rely on assistance from insensitive and transphobic providers, for example, in vulnerable situations such as bathing [53].

Until June 26, 2015, when the US Supreme Court legalized same-sex marriage in all fifty states, the absence of federal recognition of same-sex unions made same-sex couples ineligible to receive financial and other benefits offered to couples in opposite-sex marriages. As LGBT people age and become more dependent on federal benefits, such as Social Security, Medicare, and Medicaid (none of which were previously extended to same-sex partners), and become more enmeshed in health-care systems that do not grant their partners the same rights as legal spouses, they experience the effects of a lifetime of inequality. These effects can follow a lesbian or gay person into the nursing home setting [54]. Furthermore, for a long time, most retirement communities in the US were faith-based; this meant they could discriminate without bounds because of their exemption from most nondiscrimination statutes. As an alternative to faith-based homes, several retirement communities catering to the LGBT community have now opened around the country. The most well-known of these is called RainbowVision, the first US retirement village designed specifically for gay men and lesbians in Santa Fe, New Mexico [52]. Similar communities now exist in a number of major American cities.

Some nursing homes, including those that do not specifically cater to the LGBT community, have endorsed the *HEALE* curriculum [53]. The *HEALE* curriculum sets a standard for best practices in nursing management and for LGBT cultural competency in geriatric education. The nurses' *HEALE* training has significantly increased knowledge and, as a result, nurses' confidence in providing culturally sensitive care to older LGBT individuals [53]. However, a nationally representative mail-in survey of nursing home social service directors revealed that LGBT cultural trainings are still not the norm. More than 75% of responders reported not receiving any training during the previous 5 years [55]. If the nursing home where Mr. X was living had asked about his sexual orientation and provided him with appropriate options for the expression of his sexuality, it may have reduced the likelihood of inappropriate behavior with J.

– *- J – Person-centered care: What works?*

In the early 1980s, the National Citizens' Coalition for Nursing Home Reform conducted focus groups to learn directly from the nursing home residents their definition of quality. Subsequently, the Institute of Medicine committee on nursing regulation published *Improving the Quality of Care in Nursing Homes*. This was followed by a sweeping set of nursing home reforms, known as the Nursing Home

Table 11.2 The principles of patient-centered care

Patient-centered care principles	Description and examples
1. Resident direction Care and all resident related activities are directed as much as possible by the resident	Residents are offered choices and encouraged to make their own decisions, such as what to wear, when to go to bed, and what time to wake up
2. Homelike atmosphere Practices and structures are designed to be less institutional and more homelike	Small "households" of 10 to 15 residents in the organizational unit. Meals are prepared on the units, and residents have access to refrigerators for snacks
3. Close relationships Relationships between residents, family members, staff, and the community are close	For example, the same group of nurse aides consistently care for a resident (a practice known as *consistent assignment*), in order to increase mutual familiarity and caring
4. Staff empowerment Work is organized to support and empower all staff to respond to residents' needs and desires	Teamwork is encouraged, and additional staff training is provided to enhance efficiency and effectiveness
5. Collaborative decision-making Management enables collaborative and decentralized decision-making	Flattening of the typical nursing home hierarchy and participatory management systems is encouraged. Aides should be given some decision-making authority
6. Quality improvement processes	Systematic quality improvements that are comprehensive and measurement-based should exist

Reform Act, which was incorporated into the Omnibus Budget Reconciliation Act of 1987. The law made nursing homes the only sector of the entire healthcare industry with an explicit statutory requirement for providing what is now called "person-centered care" [8]. This *culture change movement* is a broad-based effort to transform nursing homes from impersonal healthcare institutions into true person-centered environments offering long-term care services. The *culture change movement* represents a fundamental shift in thinking about nursing homes. Facilities are viewed not as healthcare institutions but as person-centered homes offering long-term care services. Table 11.2 summarizes the principles of person-centered care which include not only resident care practices, such as elimination of physical restraints but also organizational and human resource practices and the design of the physical environment.

The culture change to patient-centered care should be recognized as far more than offering amenities or making superficial changes. Rather, it should be treated as an ongoing process affecting overall performance and leading to specific, measurable outcomes. For example, older adults may be well cared for in terms of their healthcare, hygiene, nutritional needs, and housekeeping (quality of care) but still be unhappy. Some of the possible reasons for this unhappiness include consuming unappealing food, being required to bathe in the morning when they prefer an evening shower, awakening to vacuuming in the middle of the night because that is when there is the least amount of foot traffic, and feeling lonely for companionship [56]. Making an effort to keep shower rooms warm can make bathing a more pleasurable experience for residents, reduce staff stress, save time, and avoid agitation [8].

Material objects can be used to help people with dementia maintain connections to past social identities and roles and provide a sense of comfort and security. Handbags, for example, imbued with social and personal meaning, can serve many different functions for women living in care homes. First, the tangibility and accessibility of a handbag can itself provide reassurance, particularly when the owner feels vulnerable. The act of rummaging or sorting through a handbag also provides women in care homes with a "distraction"—a means of looking busy or purposeful when sitting alone in a public space, disguising a sense of discomfort. More so, handbags also provide a "prop" for managing the lack of privacy in care home settings [57]. In the same spirit of using physical materials, a growing body of evidence is showing that dolls provide comfort and companionship for some residents with advanced Alzheimer's disease in their care homes [58]. Felt dolls provide sensory stimulation and seem to promote purposeful activity. Dolls were noted to promote positive changes in behavior, reducing aggression and agitation. They also increase interactions between staff and residents as their interactions expand to discussions and activities relating to the doll, such as folding the doll's clothes together [58]. When integrating the use of a doll into the care of a patient, it is recommended that family members and friends of the patient be educated about the value and purpose of the doll.

Despite widespread recognition of the *culture change movement*, the discovery of deep and enduring cultural change is relatively rare. Several aspects of the nursing home industry, including its workforce, regulation, and reimbursement, have conspired to limit the initiation of culture change practices [8]. The Commonwealth Fund's 2007 National Survey of Nursing Homes found that only 5% of nursing directors said that their facilities completely met the description of a nursing home transformed through *culture change*. Only 10% reported that they had initiated at least seven or more *culture change* practices. Altogether, about one-third reported adoption of some *culture change* practices, and another third said that they were planning to follow suit. But the remaining 40% of the respondents said that they were neither practicing nor planning to commence *culture change* [8].

On the other hand, Green House (GH) NH models, which strive to fully express the tenets of culture change, are gaining in popularity and have elicited great interest among policy, provider, and research stakeholders, in large part because they offer a true alternative to traditional models of nursing home care by focusing on person-centered care and deinstitutionalizing the NH. Between 2011 and 2014, the Robert Wood Johnson Foundation funded an independent evaluation of Green House NHs by four project teams, which were organized under the umbrella of The Research Initiative Valuing Eldercare (THRIVE). The collaborative interrelated research projects of these teams examined GH care processes and outcomes. THRIVE concluded that implementation of the GH model is inconsistent in different homes, sometimes differing from design [59]. Among many recommendations, THRIVE research established the importance of communication and collaboration between and among direct care staff and medical care providers to effect good-quality care [59].

In GH homes, *consistent assignment* of a universal worker who directs care staff, and small homes built around a central living area allow familiarity with residents and provide opportunities for frequent interactions among staff. If used in an optima manner, increased multidisciplinary collaboration might lead to early identification and intervention in response to a resident's change of medical condition, a vital step in quality care. Some GH homes were found to take advantage of these opportunities to improve quality; others did not [59]. Consequently, GH leadership and others promoting *culture change* to improve care should identify and overcome barriers to communication and collaboration. The THRIVE studies suggest that scheduling physician, nurse, and other professional staff visits should be more purposeful, and congregate areas should be used to promote interaction [59].

Conclusion and Recommendations

Be it in traditional NHs, in progressive person-centered nursing homes, or assisted living communities, cultural challenges in care provision are common. An important role of the geriatric psychiatrist on both clinical and institutional levels is to help address these challenges. Practicing cultural competence in long-term facilities requires education about and sensitivity toward different cultural identities including race, gender identity, and sexual orientations. In addition, awareness of the impact of staff hierarchies in residential care environments, implementation of patient-centered approaches, and the removal of common barriers to their adoption are also essential. We conclude with a number of recommendations to help clinicians navigate the potentially challenging yet rewarding task of integrating the cultural identity of an older adult with the culture of the residential care environment:

(a) Be mindful of the location (urban vs rural) and culture, e.g., (traditional vs person-centered) of the residential care environment and the available services and prescribing trends.
(b) Obtain a good history of the nursing home resident and their behavior, which may help avoid costly and unnecessary trips to the ED that are especially difficult for many older adults, especially those living with dementia.
(c) Use your knowledge of the patient and the complexity of their comorbidities to guide the choice of placement in an ALF vs NH. Other factors to be taken into consideration include the size and age of the institutions, their philosophy, and financial sustainability.
(d) Keep an inquisitive mind about interpreting reported disruptive behaviors like agitation or incontinence. Sometimes these behaviors are inspired by unmet needs or unaddressed frustrations.
(e) Be mindful of various religious or cultural beliefs, family traditions and involvement, possible sources of shame or stigma, and culturally influenced interpretations of symptoms— any and all of which can play a major role in explaining the medical diagnoses, prescribed treatments, and recommended supportive services and in establishing reciprocally supportive and rewarding relationships with family members and friends of the resident.
(f) Attend a cultural competency training. These have shown efficacy in increasing humility and tolerance but also reducing judgments and frustrations.

Psychiatrists aiming to ensure a culturally sensitive practice in their facility ought to implement them as part of their pre-employment trainings.

(g) Empower nursing assistants, and recognizing that these team members are a valuable, yet often under-recognized, part of the treatment framework. Ensuring they are heard and given room for creative interventions can play an important role in person-centered care culture.

(h) Remember that sexual behaviors in a nursing home are common and not necessarily a sign of disinhibition, or malintent. A discussion incorporating family preferences, home philosophy, and the residents' values and wishes should guide approaches toward the sexual expression of residents, especially those with a diagnosis of dementia.

(i) Arrange LGBT competency trainings for nursing home staff members to promote culturally sensitive practices and avoid institutional heterosexism and cisgenerism, which have been shown to directly impact the mental health of residents.

(j) Promote a *person-centered* approach in NHs and proprietary residential care environments for older adults. To do this, the psychiatrist must be well-versed in non-pharmacological interventions and take initiative with all parties involved to ensure effective communication and the delivery of holistic care.

Summary of High Yield Points

- In the USA, 4.2% of individuals 65 years old and older live in nursing homes [1], and the need continues to grow as the population of older adults increases.
- There are numerous residential care options for older adults other than nursing homes including independent living, assisted living, subacute care hospitals, rehabilitative facilities, retirement communities, and continuing care retirement communities.
- Psychiatric disorders in older adults living in residential care communities are common. The most common diagnosis is dementia, with prevalence rates of 50–75% [9]. Combining pharmacological, behavioral, and psychological interventions will achieve potentially quicker, safer, and more long-lasting results.
- Many transfers from nursing homes to the emergency departments are believed to be either unnecessary or preventable and may result in more harm than benefit.
- Agitation, incontinence, and aggressive or disruptive behaviors may be forms of communication by impaired and/or nonverbal residents.
- Individuals living with dementia who belong to certain ethnic minorities do not use services to the same degree as members of other ethnic groups. This suggests that the needs of this subset of individuals may be unidentified, underrepresented, or unmet [32].
- Lesbian, gay, bisexual, and transgender individuals have historically avoided proprietary residential care environments due to fears about mistreatment by administrative staff, care staff, and peers [51]. The *HEALE* curriculum is a six-hour LGBTQ cultural competency continuing education training for nurses and heathcare professionals and is provided to nurses and social workers for free care.

- After a series of publications, policies, and laws passed in the 1980s, nursing homes are the only sector of the entire healthcare industry with an explicit statutory requirement for providing what is now called *person-centered care* [8]. However, despite widespread recognition of the *culture change movement*, the transition to deep and enduring cultural change in proprietary residential care environments, including nursing homes, has been relatively rare.
- The geriatric psychiatrist has the important role of ensuring comprehensive and individualized care, addressing clinical and organizational cultural issues, and promoting advocacy and policy recommendations.

References

1. Milne A. The care home experience. Principles and Practice of Geriatric Psychiatry. 3rd ed. Wiley-Blackwell; 2010. p. 78–82.
2. Center for disease control and prevention: considerations for retirement communities and independent living facilities. https://www.cdc.gov/coronavirus/2019-ncov/community/retirement/considerations.html. Accessed 4 Oct 2020.
3. Sanders J. Continuing care retirement communities: a background and summary of current issues. Assistant Secretary for Planning and Evaluation (ASPE), U.S. Department of Health and Human Services; 1997. https://aspe.hhs.gov/basic-report/continuing-care-retirement-communities-background-and-summary-current-issues. Accessed 4 Oct 2020.
4. Gibler KM, Moschis GP, Lee E. Planning to move to retirement housing. Financ Serv Rev. 1998;7(4):291.
5. American senior communities: assisted living statistics – a deeper dive into the demographics. https://www.asccare.com/assisted-living-statistics-a-deeper-dive-into-the-demographics/. Accessed 4 Oct 2020.
6. Sadock, Sadock, Ruiz, editors. Kaplan and Sadock's comprehensive textbook of psychiatry. Geriatric psychiatry. 9th ed. Lippincott: Wolter-Kluwer/Williams and Wilkins; 2009. p. 3932–4258.
7. Daniel J. Cultural beliefs and mental health treatment preferences of ethnically diverse older adult consumers in primary care. Am J Geriatr Psychiatry. 2012;20(6):533–42.
8. Koren MJ. Person-centered care for nursing home residents: the culture-change movement. Health Affairs. 2010;29(2):312–7.
9. American Psychiatric Press. Textbook of geriatric psychiatry. 4th ed. American Psychiatric Press; 2009.
10. Smallbrugge M, Pot AM, Jongenelis L, et al. The impact of depression and anxiety on well being, disability and use of health care services in nursing home patients. Int J Geriatr Psychiatry. 2006;21:325–32.
11. Gabrel C, Jones A. The national nursing home survey vital and health statistics series. Vital Health Stat. 2000;13(146):91.
12. Svarstad B, Mount J, Bigelow W. Variations in the treatment culture of nursing homes and responses to regulations to reduce drug use. Psychiatr Serv. 2001;52(5):666–72.
13. Medicaid State Operations Manual. Provider certification, transmittal, vol. 232. Washington, DC: US Department of Health and Human Services, Health Care Financing Administration; 1989.
14. Medicaid State Operations Manual. Provider certification, transmittal, vol. 250. Washington, DC: US Department of Health and Human Services, Health Care Financing Administration; 1992.
15. Shorr RI, Fought RL, Ray WA. Changes in antipsychotic drug use in nursing homes during implementation of the OBRA-87 regulations. JAMA. 1994;271:358–63.

16. Garrard J, Chen V, Dowd B. The impact of the 1987 federal regulations on the use of psychotropic drugs in Minnesota nursing homes. Am J Public Health. 1995;85:771–6.
17. Coburn AF. Rural long-term care: what do we need to know to improve policy and programs? J Rural Health. 2002;18(Suppl):256–69.
18. Jervis L, Manson S. Suboptimal pharmacotherapy in a tribal nursing home. J Am Med Dir Assoc. 2007;8(1):1–7.
19. Jervis L, Manson S. Cognitive impairment, psychiatric disorders, and problematic behaviours in a tribal nursing home. J Aging Health. 2007;19(2):260–74.
20. Nuplazid: drug information and FAQ. https://www.nuplazid.com/about-nuplazid. Accessed 6 Oct 2020.
21. Lamanthia M. Patterns of emergency department use among long-stay nursing home residents with differing levels of dementia severity. JAMDA. 2016;17:541–6.
22. Unroe KT, Nazir A, Holtz LR, et al. The optimizing patient transfers, impacting medical quality, and improving symptoms: transforming institutional care approach: preliminary data from the implementation of a Centers for Medicare and Medicaid services nursing facility demonstration project. J Am Geriatr Soc. 2015;63:165e169.
23. Korcok M. "Assisted living": developing an alternative to nursing homes. Can Med Assoc J. 1987;137:843–5.
24. Mollica R. The evolution of assisted living: a view from the states. Caring. 2001b;20:24–6.
25. Sullivan JG. Redefining long term care. Contemporary Long Term Care. 1998;21:60–4.
26. Hawes C, Rose M, Phillips CD. A national study of assisted living for the frail elderly. Executive summary: results of a national survey of facilities. Beachwood: Meyers Research Institute; 1999.
27. Zimmerman S. Assisted living and nursing homes: apples and oranges? Gerontologist. 2003;43(Special Issue II):107–17.
28. Dobbs D. The relationship between psychiatric disorders and the ability to age in place in assisted living. Am J Geriatr Psychiatry. 2006;14:7.
29. Algase DBC, Kolanowski A, Whall A, Berent S, Richards K. Need driven dementia-compromised behavior: an alternative view of disruptive behavior. Am J Alzheimers Dis. 1996;11:10–9.
30. Micheal M. Aggressive behaviors among the institutionalised elderly. J Am Geriatr Soc. 1993;41(8):853–6.
31. Lori J. The pollution of incontinence and the dirty work of caregiving in a US nursing home. Med Anthropol Q. 2001;15(1):84–99.
32. Badger F, Cameron E, Evers H. Demented and mentally impaired clients from ethnic minorities. The community care project, no. 10. Birmingham: Health Services Research Centre, University of Birmingham; 1988.
33. Kane M. Ethnoculturally sensitive practice and Alzheimer's disease. Am J Alzheimers Dis. 2000;15(2):80–6.
34. Darker-White G. Minority ethnic groups in dementia care: a review of service needs, service provision and models of good practice. Aging Ment Health. 2002;6(2):101–8.
35. Elliot KS. Working with Chinese families in the context of dementia. In: Yeo G, Gallagher-Thompson D, editors. Ethnicity and the dementias; 1996. p. 89–108.
36. Zucker M. Cultural sensitivity and aging. Psychiatric Serv. 1998;49(6):769–71.
37. Cervantes RC, de Snyder VN, Padilla AM. Posttraumatic stress in immigrants from Central America and Mexico. Psychiatric Serv. 1989;40(6):615–9. https://doi.org/10.1176/ps.40.6.615.
38. Lu FG. Culturally relevant inpatient care for minority and ethnic patients—Ethnic-Minority Psychiatric Inpatient Programs, Department of Psychiatry, San Francisco General Hospital, University of California, San Francisco. Psychiatric Serv. 1987;38(11):1216–7.
39. Majumdar B. Effects of cultural sensitivity training on health care provider attitudes and patient outcomes. J Nurs Scholarsh. 2004;36(2):161–6.
40. Pennington K, Congdon JG, Magilvy JK. Second-career CNAs in nursing homes: tapping an underused resource. J Gerontol Nurs. 2007;33(6):21–8.

41. Scanlon WJ. Nursing workforce: recruitment of nurses and nurse aides is a growing concern (Publication No. GAO-01-750T). 2001.
42. Carpenter J, Thompson SA. CNA's experiences in the nursing home. J Gerontol Nurs. 2008;34(9):25–32.
43. Pennington K, Scott J, Magilvy K. The role of certified nursing assistants in nursing homes. J Nurs Adm. 2003;33:578–84.
44. Hillman J. Sexual issues and aging within the context of work with older adult patients. Prof Psychol Res Pract. 2008;39:290–7.
45. DeLemater J, Sill M. Sexual desire in later life. J Sex Res. 2005;42:138–49.
46. Maurice W. Sexual medicine in primary care. New York: Mosby; 1999.
47. Hajjar RR, Kamel HK. Sexuality in the nursing home, part 1: attitudes and barriers to sexual expression. J Am Med Dir Assoc. 2004;5:S42–7.
48. Frankowski A. Sexuality and intimacy in assisted living: residents' perspectives and experiences. Sex Res Social Policy. 2009;6(4):25–37.
49. Tenebaum E. Sexual expression and intimacy between nursing home residents with dementia: balancing the current interests and prior values of heterosexual and LGBT residents. Temp Pol Civ Rts L Rev. 2011;21:459.
50. Harley DA, Teaster PB. Chapter 2: Sexual minority status. In: Handbook of LGBT elders: an interdisciplinary approach to principles, practices and policies. Springer; 2016. p. 29.
51. Gendron T, Maddux S, Krinsky L, White J, Lockeman K, Metcalfe Y, Aggarwal S. Cultural competence training for healthcare professionals working with LGBT older adults. Educ Gerontol. 2013;39(6):454–63.
52. Hovey J. Nursing wounds: why LGBT elders need protection from discrimination and abuse based on sexual orientation and gender identity. Elder LJ. 2009;17:95.
53. Hardacker C. Adding silver to the rainbow: the development of the nurses' health education about LGBT elders (HEALE) cultural competency curriculum. J Nurs Manag. 2014;22:257–66.
54. Dubois MR. Legal concerns of LGBT elders. In: Kimmel D, Rose T, David S, editors. Lesbian, gay, bisexual, and transgender aging: research and clinical perspectives. New York: Columbia University Press; 2006. p. 195–205.
55. Bell F. Most nursing home social service directors lack training in working with lesbian, gay, and bisexual residents. Soc Work Health Care. 2010;49(9):814–31.
56. Love K, Pinkowitz J. Person-centered care for people with dementia: a theoretical and conceptual framework. Generations. 2013;37(3):23–9.
57. Buse C. Women with dementia and their handbags: negotiating identity, privacy and 'home' through material culture. J Aging Stud. 2014;30:14–22.
58. Higgins P. Using dolls to enhance the wellbeing of people with dementia. Nursing Times. 2010;106(39):18–20.
59. Zimmerman S. New evidence on the green house model of nursing home care: synthesis of findings and implications for policy, practice, and research. Health Serv Res. 2016;51:475–96.

Index

S. H. Koh et al. (eds.), *Diversity in Action*,
https://doi.org/10.1007/978-3-030-85401-0

MIX
Papier aus verantwortungsvollen Quellen
Paper from responsible sources
FSC® C105338

If you have any concerns about our products,
you can contact us on
ProductSafety@springernature.com

In case Publisher is established outside the EU,
the EU authorized representative is:
Springer Nature Customer Service Center GmbH
Europaplatz 3, 69115 Heidelberg, Germany

Printed by Libri Plureos GmbH
in Hamburg, Germany